Clinical Allergy and Asthma Management in Adolescents and Young Adults

T0203800

Clinical Allergy and Asthma Management in Adolescents and Young Adults

Edited by

Ravindran Chetambath and Venugopal Panicker

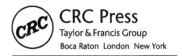

CRC Press
Taylor & Francis Group
Boca Raton London New York

CRC Press is an imprint of the
Taylor & Francis Group, an **Informa** business

First edition published 2022
by CRC Press
6000 Broken Sound Parkway NW, Suite 300, Boca Raton, FL 33487-2742

and by CRC Press
2 Park Square, Milton Park, Abingdon, Oxon, OX14 4RN

© 2022 Taylor & Francis Group, LLC

CRC Press is an imprint of Taylor & Francis Group, LLC

This book contains information obtained from authentic and highly regarded sources. While all reasonable efforts have been made to publish reliable data and information, neither the author[s] nor the publisher can accept any legal responsibility or liability for any errors or omissions that may be made. The publishers wish to make clear that any views or opinions expressed in this book by individual editors, authors or contributors are personal to them and do not necessarily reflect the views/opinions of the publishers. The information or guidance contained in this book is intended for use by medical, scientific or health-care professionals and is provided strictly as a supplement to the medical or other professional's own judgement, their knowledge of the patient's medical history, relevant manufacturer's instructions and the appropriate best practice guidelines. Because of the rapid advances in medical science, any information or advice on dosages, procedures or diagnoses should be independently verified. The reader is strongly urged to consult the relevant national drug formulary and the drug companies' and device or material manufacturers' printed instructions, and their websites, before administering or utilizing any of the drugs, devices or materials mentioned in this book. This book does not indicate whether a particular treatment is appropriate or suitable for a particular individual. Ultimately it is the sole responsibility of the medical professional to make his or her own professional judgements, so as to advise and treat patients appropriately. The authors and publishers have also attempted to trace the copyright holders of all material reproduced in this publication and apologize to copyright holders if permission to publish in this form has not been obtained. If any copyright material has not been acknowledged please write and let us know so we may rectify in any future reprint.

Library of Congress Cataloging-in-Publication Data

Names: Chetambath, Ravindran, editor. | Panicker, Venugopal, editor.
Title: Clinical allergy and asthma management in adolescents and young
    adults / edited by Ravindran Chetambath, Venugopal Panicker.
Description: First edition. | Boca Raton, FL: CRC Press, 2022. | Includes
    bibliographical references and index. | Summary: "This text addresses
    the need for a practical handbook on asthma and allergy in adolescents
    and young adults. This ready reckoner aims to help in understanding
    clinical allergy which is imperative for every physician who is caring
    for patients with asthma given its high prevalence and heterogeneous
    treatment options"—Provided by publisher.
Identifiers: LCCN 2021033270 (print) | LCCN 2021033271 (ebook) | ISBN
    9780367646783 (paperback) | ISBN 9780367646776 (hardback) | ISBN
    9781003125785 (ebook)
Subjects: MESH: Asthma—therapy | Hypersensitivity—therapy | Adolescent |
    Young Adult
Classification: LCC RJ436.A8 (print) | LCC RJ436.A8 (ebook) | NLM QW 900 |
    DDC 618.92/238—dc23
LC record available at https://lccn.loc.gov/2021033270
LC ebook record available at https://lccn.loc.gov/2021033271

ISBN: 9780367646776 (hbk)
ISBN: 9780367646783 (pbk)
ISBN: 9781003125785 (ebk)

DOI: 10.1201/9781003125785

Typeset in Palatino
by KnowledgeWorks Global Ltd.

To my family, friends and students, whose continuous support and encouragement helped me to complete this project.

—R Chetambath

To my wife, Dr Uma, and children, Vaisakh and Vaishnav, for sparing me the time meant for them.

—V Panicker

Contents

Preface

Allergic diseases are complex multifactorial disorders, with interactions of genetic, environmental and socioeconomic factors determining disease expression. Allergic diseases represent one of the most common types of disease globally. They incur a substantial global health burden. The most common allergic diseases are allergic rhinosinusitis and asthma, although one must also note the significant presence of skin allergies, such as urticaria and eczema, and food allergy with gastrointestinal manifestations.

The escalation of allergic diseases over the last few decades has been linked to an increase in environmental pollutants. The prevalence of allergic rhinitis is associated with genetic predisposition, living in urban areas and socioeconomic status, combined with the increased chance of exposure to allergens and automobile exhaust. In asthma, there is also some evidence for geographical variations in its prevalence. Although genetic predisposition is the strongest single risk factor for atopic eczema, air pollutants may aggravate the condition by acting as nonspecific irritants and immunomodulators.

The increased prevalence of all allergic diseases suggests that the prevalence of atopy has increased. Epidemiological information from Switzerland and Japan shows that the prevalence of atopy is increasing in children and young adults. The rising prevalence of allergic disease has resulted in increased use of health services. The prevalence of difficult-to-control asthma and acute severe asthma are also on the rise. The incidence of asthma is higher in children and young adults. Longitudinal surveys suggest that children with mild disease are likely to become asymptomatic as teenagers, whereas those with more severe disease will have symptoms that persist throughout life.

Asthma and other allergic diseases among adolescents and young adults raise some concerns. Loss of school or college days, poor scholastic performance and difficulty in engaging in exercise and recreational activities are bothersome for the individual. Environmental tobacco smoke and peer pressure for vaping and smoking are always factors leading to worsening symptoms in this age group. Children who grow up in large families with exposure to older siblings are likely to experience more childhood infections, and sensitization to common allergens is found to be lower among them. High rates of infection in childhood may protect against the development of atopy and allergic disease.

In this book on *Clinical Allergy and Asthma Management in Adolescents and Young Adults*, we have included chapters on asthma and various other allergic diseases with a focus on real-time issues among adolescents and young adults. We extensively discuss various asthma phenotypes and its management. Other allergic diseases such as urticaria, eczema, angioedema, insect allergy, drug allergy and food allergy are also discussed in detail, as well as allergy testing and allergen immunotherapy. Management of asthma phenotypes using biologics with a view of personalized management is also discussed.

Readers will find this textbook useful to understand the pathogenesis, causes, clinical manifestations, investigations and management of various allergic diseases including asthma among adolescents and young adults. We hope this book will also stimulate students and researchers to study these diseases and develop new diagnostics and treatments for allergic disorders.

We would like to thank all the authors who have contributed chapters to this book and thank the publishers for all their help at every stage of the publication. We would like to particularly thank Himani Dwivedi and Shivangi Pramanik for their tireless efforts, their constant reminders and for putting up with us through the editorial process.

Acknowledgements

We would like to acknowledge our teachers, colleagues, trainees and patients who have been the source of knowledge and inspiration. We would also like to express our immense gratitude to all the authors who, in spite of their busy schedules, especially in the midst of COVID-19, have submitted their work well within the time limit. It was a wonderful experience working with them.

Editors

Ravindran Chetambath, MD, FRCP, MBA, is Professor and Head of Pulmonary Medicine at DM Wayanad Institute of Medical Sciences, Wayanad, Kerala. He was previously Dean of Govt. Medical College, Kozhikode, Kerala. His career has been dedicated to teaching medical students, both undergraduates and postgraduates. His areas of special interests are airway diseases, interstitial lung diseases and sleep disorders. He frequently talks at postgraduate fora, seminars and conferences around the world on various respiratory diseases and has presented research papers at the European Respiratory Science Congress, national conferences on pulmonary medicine and national conferences on tuberculosis. He has 85 research publications to his credit and has contributed chapters to various textbooks. He is the author of (1) *Paediatric Respiratory Illnesses* 2nd Ed., 2014 (Macmillan Medical Communications); (2) *X-Ray Atlas*, 2016 (Macmillan Medical Communications); (3) *Chest X-Ray Illustrated* (Pulmonary Infections, Interstitial Lung Diseases, Pleural Diseases, Lung Tumours), 2016 (Macmillan Medical Communications); (4) *COVID 19 and Lung Lesions*, 2021 (Kothari Publications). He is on the editorial board of *Lung India*, the *Indian Practitioner* and *EC Pulmonology and Respiratory Medicine*. He is a Fellow of the Royal College of Physicians, London, a Fellow of the International Medical Science Academy and a Fellow of the Indian Chest Society. He is currently the Chairman of the Kerala State Chapter of the Indian Chest Society and Editor in Chief of the *Journal of Advanced Lung Health*.

Venugopal Panicker, MD, DNB, DETRD, FCCP, is Professor and Head, Department of Pulmonary Medicine, Govt. TD Medical College, Alappuzha, Kerala. He also holds the post of Principal Investigator, National Occupational Research Centre under the Govt. of Kerala located in Alappuzha. He is a teacher and clinician and is interested in respiratory allergy and asthma. His research interest is mainly on chronic respiratory problems and allergy among coir workers of the Alappuzha District. He has published more than 25 papers in various journals and presented his work in national and international conferences. He is a Fellow of the American College of Chest Physicians (FCCP) and a life member of the European Respiratory Society. He was awarded the "Young Pulmonologist Award" in 2005 by the Academy of Pulmonary and Critical Care Medicine. He is the chief editor of *PULMON*, (the *Journal of Respiratory Sciences*).

Contributors

Saleel Punnilath Abdulsamad
Senior Clinical Fellow
Royal Preston Hospital
Preston, UK

Tisekar Owais Rafique Ahmed
Registrar
Critical Care Medicine
Manipal Hospitals
Bangalore, Karnataka, India

Mahesh P Anand
Professor
Department of Respiratory Medicine
JSS Medical College
JSS Academy of Higher Education & Research
Mysore, Karnataka, India

Paramez Ayyappath
Senior Consultant
Respiratory Medicine and Critical Care
Lisie Hospital
Ernakulam, Kerala, India

Jayaprakash Balakrishnan
Additional Professor of Pulmonary Medicine
Government Medical College
Trivandrum, Kerala, India

Ravindran Chetambath
Professor and Head of Pulmonary Medicine
DM Wayanad Institute of Medical Sciences
Wayanad, Kerala, India

Devasahayam J Christopher
Professor
Department of Pulmonary Medicine
Christian Medical College
Vellore, Tamil Nadu, India

Alpa Dalal
Head
Department of Pulmonary Medicine
Jupiter Hospital
Thane, Maharashtra, India

Jefferson Daniel
Assistant Professor
Department of Pulmonary Medicine
Christian Medical College
Vellore, Tamil Nadu, India

Aratrika Das
Pulmonologist
Narayana Hrudyalaya Group of Hospitals
and
Rabindranath Tagore International Institute of
    Cardiac Sciences
Kolkata, West Bengal, India

George A D'Souza
Professor
Department of Pulmonary Medicine
St John's Medical College
Bangalore, Karnataka, India

Jyothi Edakalavan
Associate Professor of Pulmonary Medicine
Govt. Medical College
Kollam, Kerala, India

Benita Florence
Registrar Trainee
Emergency Medicine
Milton Keynes University Hospital
Thames Valley Oxford Deanery, NHS Trust
Oxford, UK

Bindu Cheriattil Govindan
Associate Professor in Pulmonary Medicine
Government TD Medical College
Alappuzha, Kerala, India

Dodiy Herman
Consultant
Emergency Medicine
Shrewsbury and Telford Hospital, NHS Trust
Shrewsbury, Shropshire, UK

Priyank Jain
Associate Consultant in Pulmonary Medicine
Metro Centre for Respiratory Diseases
Noida, Uttar Pradesh, India

Balachandran J
Professor of Pulmonary Medicine
Travancore Medical College
Kollam, Kerala, India

Aditya Jindal
Consultant and Intervention Pulmonologist
Jindal Clinics
Chandigarh, India

Surinder K Jindal
Medical Director
Jindal Clinics
and
Emeritus-Professor
Postgraduate Institute of Medical Education
    and Research
Chandigarh, India

Tarang Kulkarni
Clinical Associate
Department of Pulmonary Medicine
Jupiter Hospital
Thane, Maharashtra, India

Ajith Kumar
Senior Consultant and Head
Critical Care Medicine
Manipal Hospitals
Bangalore, Karnataka, India

Anitha Kumari
Professor and Head of Pulmonary Medicine
Govt. Medical College
Trivandrum, Kerala, India

Abha Mahashur
Consultant in Pulmonary Medicine
Lilavati Hospital and Research Center
Mumbai, Maharashtra, India

Ashok Mahashur
Senior Consultant in Pulmonary Medicine
PD Hinduja Hospital
Mumbai, Maharashtra, India

Manas Mengar
Consultant
Department of Pulmonary Medicine
Jupiter Hospital
Thane, Maharashtra, India

Mohammed Munavvar
Chest Physician/Interventional Pulmonologist
Lancashire Teaching Hospitals
Preston, UK

Soofia Mohammed
Pulmonologist
Insurance Medical Services
Govt. of Kerala
Kerala, India

Sailal Mohanlal
Consultant and Head
Department of Pulmonary and Critical Care
    Medicine
KVM Hospital
Chertala, Alappuzha, Kerala, India

Saibal Moitra
Pulmonologist
Department of Allergy and Immunology
Apollo Gleneagles Hospital
Kolkata, West Bengal, India

Priti Nair
Senior Consultant Pulmonologist
Ananthapuri Hospital
Thiruvananthapuram, Kerala, India

Sanjeev Nair
Associate Professor of Pulmonary Medicine
Govt. Medical College
Trichur, Kerala, India

Kiran Vishnu Narayan
Assistant Professor
Pulmonary Medicine
Government Medical College
Trivandrum, Kerala, India

Arjun Padmanabhan
Chief Consultant and Head of Department
    of Respiratory Medicine
Kerala Institute of Medical Sciences
Trivandrum, Kerala, India

Lisha Pallivalappil
Assistant Professor of Pulmonary Medicine
Amala Institute of Medical Sciences
Trichur, Kerala, India

Venugopal Panicker
Professor and Head
Department of Pulmonary Medicine
Govt. TD Medical College
Alappuzha, Kerala, India

Sujeet Rajan
Senior Consultant Pulmonologist
Bombay Hospital and Institute of Medical
    Sciences
Mumbai, Maharashtra, India

Vishnu Sharma
Professor and Head of Pulmonary Medicine
AJ Institute of Medical Sciences
Mangalore, Karnataka, India

Nishtha Singh
Consultant
Asthma Bhavan
Jaipur, Rajasthan, India

Virendra Singh
Chief Consultant
Asthma Bhavan
Jaipur, Rajasthan, India

Shajahan P Sulaiman
Additional Professor of Pulmonary
    Medicine
Government TD Medical College
Alappuzha, Kerala, India

Arjun Suresh
Senior Resident
Govt. TD Medical College
Alappuzha, Kerala, India

Rajesh Swarnakar
Director and Chief Consultant Pulmonologist
Department of Respiratory Critical Care,
    Sleep Medicine and Interventional Pulmonology
Getwell Hospital and Research Institute
Nagpur, Maharashtra, India

Deepak Talwar
Director and Chair
Metro Centre for Respiratory Diseases
Noida, Uttar Pradesh, India

Rajesh Venkitakrishnan
Senior Consultant
Department of Pulmonary Medicine
Rajagiri Hospital
Aluva, Kerala, India

PART I
ALLERGY

1 Biology of Allergy

Jayaprakash Balakrishnan

CONTENTS

INTRODUCTION

An allergic condition is a hypersensitivity disorder in which the immune system reacts to substances in the environment that are normally considered harmless. The term allergy encompasses a wide range of conditions. Allergies are the result of an inappropriate reaction to innocuous environmental proteins. It is not a disease in itself. Any substance that is recognized by the body immune system as unsuitable is an allergen. In people with an allergic tendency, the allergens are picked up by certain cells called antigen presenting cells which process them and allow them to be recognised by and to initiate the innate immune system (1). The incidence and prevalence of allergy has increased worldwide in recent decades. The precise cause of this increase is unknown but definitely reflects changes in lifestyle, in particular improvements in housing. Allergic disorders are proposed to result from a complex interplay between genetic and environmental factors. The common risk factors associated with development of allergy includes dust exposure, seasonal changes, number of hours spent outdoors, contact with animals, and so on. Young age, higher socio-economic status, and living in urban area are also factors leading to high prevalence of allergy. Food and medications are other common causes of allergy.

EPIDEMIOLOGY

Allergic disorders are common, and it has been estimated that 15% of the global population has some form of allergic reaction during their lifetime (2). More than 20% of the Indian population suffers from various forms of allergy (3). The prevalence of allergic reactions is increasing globally, and the cause of this is thought to be due to changes in lifestyle, especially improvements in housing. Reduction in breastfeeding has led to a high incidence of atopic eczema. Improvements in public health leading to the elimination of parasitic infections may contribute to allergy through a lack of physiological function for the IgE-mast cell axis. This has been explained by the hygiene hypothesis. Allergy is responsible for approximately 1% of all disability-adjusted life years lost worldwide. People with allergic disorders such as atopic dermatitis, allergic rhinitis, food allergy, and atopic asthma can experience acute signs and symptoms of disease within minutes of exposure to the associated allergens (4). They can also typically develop long-term changes in the affected tissues after repeated exposure to these allergens over a period of weeks to years.

Allergic diseases that have long been associated with lifestyle show an increasing prevalence in Western and Asian countries. Now efforts are made to investigate and find out the sensitization and disease patterns, which are a prerequisite to organizing adequate health care, such as diagnostic and therapeutic options and standards. Current epidemiological data from each country together with recent insights into the pathogenesis of immune reactions provide new strategies for the management of diseases such as allergic rhinitis, asthma, atopic dermatitis, mast cell-driven diseases, and drug allergy.

Understanding the pattern of allergic diseases in immigrants can provide further insight into the role of the environment. The risk of atopy

DOI: 10.1201/9781003125785-1

increases with duration of residence, younger age at migration, or birth after migration as compared to migration after birth (5). The risk of allergy is low in people migrating from countries with lower to higher standards of living. First-generation immigrants have a lower prevalence of atopy compared to the native population, and a relatively low atopy risk has been shown in migrants moving from rural to urban areas. Lifestyle factors such as farming environment, smoking, family size, body weight, or frequency of colds significantly influenced the immunoglobulin (IgE) sensitization rate in adolescents. Early life risk factors influence the allergy risk in children. DNA methylation levels are believed to have a mediating role in the association between season of birth and allergic rhinitis. The mean methylation levels of the promoter regions of interferon (IFN-γ), were significantly high in children at six years of age with allergic rhinitis compared to those without allergic rhinitis (6). The association of high-sensitivity C-reactive protein (hs-CRP) with allergic disorders was studied, and it was found that there were no definite association between them.

The spectrum of allergens is highly diverse due to varied climate, flora, and food habits. Therefore, in order to facilitate an accurate diagnosis and to design vaccines for immunotherapy, proper identification, purification, and molecular characterization of allergy-eliciting molecules are essential. A meta-analysis found a sex difference for allergic rhinitis prevalence, with a male predominance in childhood and female predominance in adolescence worldwide except in Asia (7). A relationship between psychosocial factors and allergic or atopic diseases has been reported in several studies. The associations of psychosocial factors such as social status, depression, generalised anxiety, psychosocial stress, and type-D personality with the development of seasonal, perennial, and other allergies in adults are established in studies (8). An association of anxiety with seasonal allergies was also observed, whereas depression was associated with perennial allergies. Hence, allergic patients ideally require a psychological evaluation also. Allergic disorders showed an association with atopy, asthma, lower urinary tract infections, and irritable bowel disease.

Allergic rhinitis and allergic conjunctivitis are the most common allergic manifestations with a prevalence of 30%. Food allergy and atopic dermatitis are less frequent than respiratory allergy but are associated with a severe reduction in the quality of life. The most severe manifestation of allergy is anaphylaxis, which may be caused by sensitisation to allergens in food, insect venoms, and drugs.

PATHOGENESIS

An allergy occurs when the body's immune system becomes hyperreactive to a substance that could be harmless by itself, called antigen. The external substance that provokes allergies is called an allergen. The exposure to the allergens can occur as inhalation, ingestion, injections, or external contact with the eyes, airways, or skin. The immune response is not due to the noxious nature of the allergen, but rather to a misdirected recognition of the substance as harmful. Allergens constitute a diverse range of molecules with representatives of all the common polypeptide folds. Research suggests that allergy is driven by genetic and epigenetic factors, together with environmental factors such as microbiome and diet, leading to early-life disturbance in immunological development and disruption of immuno-inflammatory pathways. Variation in inherited susceptibility and exposures causes heterogeneity in manifestations of asthma and other allergic diseases. Asthma is a very common and complex disease that involves immune and respiratory dysfunction, and it is often associated with allergy. The increasing prevalence of asthma and allergy is related to changes in environment and lifestyle.

When epithelial cells are exposed to allergens, a cascade of signalling events are initiated that lead to IgE production by B cells. Circulating IgE binds to the receptors on the surface of the mast cells or basophils. Upon subsequent exposure, the allergens bind to the IgE and trigger the release of the contents of granules in the mast cells and basophils. These contents are histamine, heparin, proteases, cytokines, and other signalling molecules that are responsible for causing the symptoms of allergy. The immune system regulates itself to establish an appropriate immune response while tolerating harmless environmental antigens and self-antigens. Regulating Tcells play a central role in this balance through various mechanisms.

MAST CELLS AND IgE IN ALLERGY

Mast cells are key participants in allergic inflammation, containing a potent array of inflammatory mediators. Mast cells arise from the progenitor cells in the bone marrow and full maturation occurs in the peripheral tissue under the influence of various cytokines like stem cell factor, interleukins 3, 4, 6 and 9, and extracellular matrix factors (9). Mast cells express a great variety of stimulatory and inhibitory receptors. Antigen-specific mast cell degranulation can be induced by cross-linking of immunoglobulin free light chains. Antigen-independent mast cell activation can be established by various other receptors such as neurokinin receptors. Activated mast cells release their granules through exocytosis or by differential release of mediators without granulation. The triggering of mast cells plays an important role in eliciting the immediate phase of an allergic response, leading to acute local response such as oedema formation, tissue swelling, or bronchoconstriction. Through chemotactic and pro inflammatory mediators, mast cells also have an effect on late allergic response (10).

Immunoglobulin E antibodies, and mast cells have been closely linked to the pathophysiology of anaphylaxis and allergic reactions. IgE and mast cells are the key drivers of the long-term pathophysiological changes and tissue remodelling that is associated with chronic allergic inflammation. IgE can be produced locally by B cells in the gut or airway-associated lymphoid tissue, as well as in lymph nodes of individuals with food allergy, seasonal or perennial allergic rhinitis, and asthma (11). Antigen-dependent activation of the tissue mast cells that have specific IgE bound to their surface is the central event in the allergic reactions. IgE is thought to mediate biological functions primarily by binding to FcεR1, CD 23 and other receptors that are expressed on mast cells and other hematopoietic cells. The binding of antigen-specific IgE to FcεR1 sensitizes mast cells and other effector cells to release mediators in response to subsequent encounters with that specific antigen or with cross-reactive antigens. Binding of antigen-IgE immune complexes to CD 23 or FcεR1 can serve to amplify IgE-associated immune responses leading to the production of IgE to additional epitopes of the antigens that are contained in such immune complexes (11).

The induction of allergen-specific IgE antibodies is the first step in allergic sensitisation and is the prerequisite for the development of allergic disease. Children initially develop only clinically silent IgE sensitization without showing symptoms. IgE reactivity in sera of the children becomes detectable in the first few years of life until adolescence, whereas IgE reactivity profiles in adult allergic subjects showed that IgE reactivity pattern remained unchanged within a long observation period (12).

Children whose mothers had very high levels of allergen-specific IgG in their blood and transmitted the allergen-specific IgG to the children, didn't develop IgE response towards allergen in a 4–5-year follow-up period. IgE antibodies of allergic patients are directed primarily against conformational epitopes on properly folded allergens, whereas T cells recognize with their T-cell receptor short and unfolded allergen peptides which are entirely different from the epitopes recognized by IgE antibodies. The ability of mounting high allergen-specific antibody response may be controlled by genetic factors. In addition to hereditary predisposition, lifestyle factors such as farming environment, smoking, family size, body weight, or frequency of colds significantly influenced the IgE sensitization rate and pattern in adolescents (12). Several studies established the role of HLA genetic polymorphism on the immune response to some specific allergen components. A bidirectional relationship between psychosocial factors and allergic or atopic diseases has been reported in several studies. Epigenetic factors, microbiome, barrier function of respiratory and gut mucosa, as well as skin influence the allergen-specific immune response. Certain vaccines like BCG, which affect the Th1-Th2 balance, may have an influence on allergic sensitization. Respiratory infections, environmental factors such as climate, and manmade environmental changes may affect allergic sensitization (13). The potential contribution of the microbiota to the increasing rates of asthma and atopic dermatitis and food allergy has been increasingly reported. Research has proved the link of microbiota of the gastrointestinal tract, as well as those of the skin and respiratory tract to allergic diseases.

Allergic cascade has basically two arms, synthesis of IL-4 by the Th2 cell—which stimulates B cells to produce IgE—and synthesis of the lineage-specific eosinophil growth factor IL-5 by the Th2 cell. IgE and eosinophils are both important components of allergic inflammation that distinguish it from other forms of inflammatory diseases. IgE has a critical role both in the early and late phase of allergic inflammation. IgE influences the allergic inflammatory response by interacting with the high affinity IgE receptor (FcεR1) on mast cells and basophils and by binding to the low affinity IgE receptor (CD 23 or FcεR1) to augment cellular and humoral immune responses. IgE binds to the high affinity receptor on tissue mast cells. The cross-linking of IgE to FcεR1 by allergen then triggers mast cell degranulation and leads to the release of histamine and tryptase, the synthesis and release of lipid mediators such as leukotriene C4 and prostaglandin D2, and the transcription of numerous cytokines such as TNF (14). The binding of IgE to FcεR1 on basophil followed by cross-linking by allergen results in basophil degranulation with release of preformed inflammatory mediators and in the synthesis of lipid mediators and cytokines. IgE mediators with the CD23 receptor provides an important mechanism by which the allergen-specific IgE can augment cellular and humoral immune linking by allergen, resulting in basophil degranulation with release of preformed inflammatory mediators and in the synthesis of lipid mediators and cytokines. IgE mediators with the CD23 receptor provides an important mechanism by which the allergen response occurs in allergic inflammation. Regulatory T cells (Tregs) play a central role to keep the balance of immune system through various ways of actions. By means of molecule secretion and cell-cell contact mechanisms, Tregs may have the capacity to modulate effector T cells and suppress the action of pro-inflammatory cytokines. Abnormal regulatory T-cell function has been pointed to as a main cause in the development of allergic diseases.

Hygiene hypothesis: A different hypothesis has been postulated to explain the increase in the prevalence of allergy. The hygiene hypothesis postulates that improved hygiene through public health measures and the use of vaccines and antibiotics has reduced the incidence of infections that would normally stimulate the immune system. These infections would mature the immune system thereby protecting against the development of allergic responses to innocuous environmental substances (15). Modifications of the pattern of microbial exposure represent a critical factor underlying the rise in prevalence of atopic disorders. Children from large families and children attending day-care settings have a reduced risk of developing allergy and asthma. Exposure to farm animals in early life reduces the likelihood of developing allergy. A reduced activity of regulatory T cells and reduced immune deviation could explain the hygiene hypothesis (16).

ALLERGIC RHINITIS

After exposure to an allergen, atopic persons promptly respond by producing allergen-specific immunoglobulin E (IgE). IgE bind to IgE receptors on the mast cells in the respiratory mucosa and to basophils in peripheral blood. When the same antigen is subsequently inhaled, the IgE antibodies are bridged on the cell surface by antigen resulting in activation of the cell. Mast cells in the tissue release preformed and granules associated chemical mediators, which leads to the symptoms of allergic rhinitis.

The expression of allergic disease of the upper airways reflects an autosomal dominant pattern of inheritance with incomplete penetrance. The inheritance pattern is manifested as a propensity to respond to inhalant allergens exposure by producing high levels of allergen-specific IgE. The IgE response is controlled by immune response genes located within the major histocompatibility complex on chromosome-6.

ANAPHYLAXIS

Anaphylaxis represents the most severe type of allergic reactions, often a medical emergency and is due to the massive degranulation of mast cells releasing histamine. The allergic reaction is type-1 hypersensitivity dependent on the presence of specific IgE. Other reactions may mimic the clinical symptoms but without involvement of IgE. The usual clinical features include generalized urticaria and angioedema involving face, lips, tongue, and larynx. Patient may develop bronchospasm and stridor, hypotension with loss of consciousness and gastrointestinal symptoms. Onset is usually rapid after exposure, within minutes. Drugs and venoms give the fastest reactions, whereas agents like foods and latex may lead to a slower reaction. Systemic anaphylaxis is life threatening and may lead to death.

In anaphylaxis, IgE-mediated hypersensitivity reaction and the release of mediators are responsible for bronchoconstriction, increased airway mucus secretion, stimulation of gut smooth muscle, increased vascular permeability, and vasodilation leading to hypotension and urticarial rashes. The other mediators include mast cell tryptase and chemotactic factors for eosinophils. Mast cells on activation produce prostaglandins and leucotrienes, which reinforce the effect of smooth muscles. Platelets are activated by the platelet activating factor (PAF) that leads to the release of histamine and serotonin, which influence the vascular tone and permeability. Complement and kinin systems are also activated. Bradykinin, C3a and C5a act as smooth muscle constrictors and also increase vascular permeability (17). These cascades of events in a person with underlying atopy increases the risk of developing serious allergic reactions.

FOOD ALLERGY

Food allergy includes any abnormal reaction after the ingestion of food or food additives. Food allergy is due to factors inherent in food such as toxic contaminants or it may be due to unique physiologic characteristic of the host, like metabolic disorders. Food allergy is a serious health problem that affects between 1% and 10% of the population in developing countries. Food allergy can be due to an IgE- or non-IgE-mediated immune mechanism. IgE-mediated food allergy is more common and is characterized by the presence of antigen-specific serum IgE antibodies. Cow milk, egg, peanut, soya, wheat, and fish account for more than 85% of food allergies in children. But peanut, tree nuts, fish, and shellfish are the usual cause of food allergy among adults. About 2% of children have an allergy to cow's milk but this is less common in adults (18). The most common types of food allergy prevailing among the Indian population include legume allergy, prawn allergy, egg allergy, and milk allergy.

SKIN ALLERGY

Allergic diseases result from the subversion of the innate immune system by allergens and their associated chemical constituents to promote sensitization. Transcutaneous sensitization to allergens is a critical step in the pathogenesis of atopy. Primary human keratinocytes release preformed IL 13-1B and IL-18 cytokines that are secreted in response to activation of the Nlrp3 inflammasome. This inflammasome activation is very relevant to dust mite sensitization and dust mite-induced inflammation in the skin. Allergic skin disorders like urticaria and angioedema are IgE mediated, contact dermatitis is cell mediated and atopic dermatitis is mediated by both. The skin disorder that best fits the concept of systemic disease is atopic dermatitis. The interaction of dendritic cells leads to a T-cell response in the skin, initially of Th2 cell response and later Th1 response. This in turn initiates a systemic Th2 response inducing IgE synthesis and involvement of esoniophils. The common cytokines involved in atopic dermatitis are IL-5, IL-13, TNF-alpha, IL-17, and IL-31 (19). Restoration of the skin barrier is the main approach for treating and preventing atopic dermatitis.

ASTHMA AND ALLERGY

Asthma is a heterogeneous disorder that is characterized by chronic airway inflammation, airway hyperesponsiveness and variable obstruction. Specifically, airway inflammation is central to the other components. The processes that lead to asthma are complex and are not same for each individual patient. Asthma is one of the most common chronic non-communicable diseases in children and adults. Asthma triggers include allergic

and non-allergic stimuli, which produce a cascade of events leading to chronic airway inflammation. Atopy is present in 50–60% of adults and children with asthma, but is more common in severe asthma among children and adults with a history of childhood asthma. The chronic inflammation in asthma is predominantly eosinophilic, in which many cells and cellular elements play a role. The inflammatory reactions to inhaled allergens, occupational chemicals, and viral infections can heighten the airway responsiveness. Both T2 high endotype and a T2 low endotype exist in asthma. The T2 high endotype is mediated by the type 2 inflammatory pathways, which are characterized by the effects of the cytokines IL-4, IL-5, and IL-13, with elevated biomarkers, including fractional exhaled nitric oxide (FeNO), serum IgE, and blood and sputum eosinophil levels (20).

SUMMARY

The prevalence of allergy is increasing worldwide. Allergic reactions can range from mild itching and rhinitis to anaphylactic shock. Allergic disorders and its complications have also been reported to increase health care costs of the individual. Mast cell activation through FcεR1 is central to the pathogenesis of allergic diseases, including anaphylaxis, allergic rhinitis, and allergic asthma. Activation of FcεR1 by polyvalent allergen recognized by bound IgE leads to the initiation of an immediate hypersensitivity reaction, as well as a late-phase reaction.

REFERENCES

1. Rudolf V, Alexander K, Verena N, Pia G, Mariamma VH, Sabina F, et al. Molecular aspects of allergens and allergy. Adv Immunol 2018;138:195.

2. Nauta AJ, Engels F, Knippels LM, Garssen J, Nijkamp FP, Redegeld FA. Mechanisms of allergy and asthma. Eur J Pharmacol 2008;585:354–360.

3. Bhattacharya K, Sircar G, Dasgupta A, Gupta Bhattacharya S. Spectrum of allergens and allergen biology in India. Int Arch Allergy Immunol 2018;177 (3):219–237.

4. Dagmar S. Recent advances in clinical allergy and immunology. Int Arch Allergy Immunol 2019; 180:291–305.

5. Tham EH, Loo EX, Zhu Y, Shek LP. Effects of migration on allergic diseases. Int Arch Allergy Immunol 2019;178 (2):128–140.

6. Li Y, Rui X, Ma B, Jiang F, Chen J. Early-life environmental factors, IFN-γ methylation patterns, and childhood allergic rhinitis. Int Arch Allergy Immunol 2019;178 (4):323–332.

7. Pinart M, Keller T, Reich A, Fröhlich M, Cabieses B, Hohmann C, et al. Sex-related allergic rhinitis prevalence switch from childhoodto adulthood: A systematic review and meta-analysis. Int Arch Allergy Immunol 2017;172 (4):224–235.

8. Harter K, Hammel G, Krabiell L, Linkohr B, Peters A, Schwettmann L, et al. Different psychosocial factors are associated with seasonal and perennial allergies in adults: Cross sectional results of the KORA FF4 study. Int Arch Allergy Immunol 2019;179 (4):262–72.

9. Metz M, Grimbaldeston MA, Nakae S, Piliponsky AM, Tsai M, Galli SJ. Mast cells in the promotion and limitation of chronic inflammation. Immunol Rev 2007;217:304–328.

10. Takhar P, et al. Class switch recombination to IgE in the bronchial mucosa of atopic and nonatopic patients with asthma. J. Allergy Clin Immunol 2007;119:213–218.

11. Burton OT, Oettgen HC. Beyond immediate hypersensitivity: evolving roles for IgE antibodies in immune homeostasis and allergic diseases. Immunol Rev 2011;242:128–143.

12. Stemeseder T, Klinglmayr E, Moser S, Lang R, Himly M, Oostingh GJ, et al. Influence of intrinsic and lifestyle factors on the development of IgE sensitization. Int Arch Allergy Immunol 2017; 173 (2):99–104.

13. Alm JS, Lilja G, Pershagen G, Scheynius A. Early BCG vaccination and development of atopy. Lancet 1997;350 (9075):400–403.

14. Broide DH. Molecular and cellular mechanisms of allergic disease. J Allergy Clin Immunol 2001;108 (2):S65–71.

15. Strachan DP. Hay fever, hygiene, and household size. BMJ 1989;299:1259–1260.

16. Romagnani S. Coming back to a missing immune deviation as the main explanatory mechanism for the hygiene hypothesis. J Allergy Clin Immunol 2007; 119:1511–1513.

17. Karimi, K, Redegeld FA, Blom R, Nijkam FP. Stem cell factor and interleukin-4 increase responsiveness of mast cells to substance P. Exp Hematol 2007; 28:626–634.

18. Sampson HA. Update on food allergy. J Allergy Clin Immunol 2004;113:805–819.

19. Boguniewicz M, Leung DYM. Atopic dermatitis. J Allergy Clin Immunol 2006;117:S475–80.

20. Hargreave FE, Nair P. Opinions in allergy. Clin Exp Allergy 2009;39:1652–1658.

2 Allergic Rhinoconjunctivitis

Aratrika Das and Saibal Moitra

CONTENTS

INTRODUCTION

The term allergic rhinoconjunctivitis can be pronounced in the same breath from the pathophysiological point of view, but, in essence, they are two different illnesses as far as the clinical parameters are concerned. By definition, allergic rhinoconjunctivitis (AR) is typically an IgE mediated disorder, affecting the nose and eyes, thereby resulting in an eosinophilic inflammation of the inside lining of nose and conjunctival mucosa, and is usually chronic.

AR is elicited by environmental allergens combined with genetic priming. The symptoms persist for at least 1 hour a day for at least 2 consecutive days and become reversed spontaneously or with treatment. AR causes a significant burden to individuals and society at large. AR, which affects up to one-fifth of the world population can cause impairment in quality of life, sleep and work performance. At a societal level, AR can cause additional health costs in terms of healthcare utilization, a decrease in economic productivity and loss of school days, absence from work and early retirement. Ocular allergy, however, is a collection of ocular surface disorders with a prevalence of 10–30% in the general population. This also has a significant negative impact on quality of life and productivity.

PATHOPHYSIOLOGY

It is known that exposure to an airborne allergen in a genetically predisposed allergic individual activates the immune system with the subsequent generation of both allergen-specific IgE responses as well as allergen-specific T-cell responses (1, 2). Antigen-presenting cells such as dendritic cells strategically positioned on mucosal surfaces to rapidly interact with environmental antigens play a key role in the initiation of the allergic response by endocytosing and processing allergens they are exposed to in the mucosa and displaying these processed smaller fragments of allergen with human leukocyte class II molecules on their cell surface. Although the antigen presenting cell encounters an allergen on mucosal surfaces, the immune response it initiates occurs in local regional lymph nodes. This localization to lymph nodes of the antigen-presenting cell interaction with T cells increases the likelihood that the very small number of allergen-specific T cells will encounter that specific antigen-presenting cell presenting the processed allergen on its cell surface (3).

In regional lymph nodes, the antigen-presenting cell is exposed to the total circulating pool of T cells, which continuously traffic through regional lymph nodes to sample antigens presented on antigen-presenting cells. The repertoire of naive T cells that have never encountered antigens is estimated to comprise 25 million to 100 million distinct T-cell clones. When a naive CD4 T cell encounters an allergen, specific for its T-cell receptor displayed on an antigen-presenting cell, the interaction of the T cell with the antigen-presenting cell

DOI: 10.1201/9781003125785-2

induces clonal T-cell expansion with each T cell in the clone having the same allergen specificity. The allergen-specific CD4 T cells play a key role in orchestrating the subsequent allergic response by producing cytokines that regulate IgE synthesis (i.e., IL-4) and eosinophil proliferation (i.e., IL-5). The allergen-specific IgE antibodies that are generated by B cells during the initial phase of allergen sensitization circulate through the blood stream and tissues and affix to high-affinity IgE receptors expressed by tissue mast cells and circulating basophils. Subsequent re-exposure to the same allergen triggers cross-linking of allergen-specific IgE present on mast cells in the mucosa and induces rapid release of pre-formed cytoplasmic granule mediators (e.g., histamine and TNF) and newly generated lipid mediators (e.g., leukotriene C4 and prostaglandin D2 [PGD2]), as well as the transcription of cytokine genes that take several hours to be expressed (4, 5). The rapid release of histamine and TNF from mast cells within minutes of exposure to allergen is important in the immediate response. In addition, mediators released during the immediate response by mast cells such as TNF and histamine may contribute to the development of the late-phase inflammatory response by up-regulating adhesion molecules on endothelial cells in blood vessels to localize circulating leukocytes (eosinophils, basophils, and CD4 cells) to be recruited to tissue sites of allergic inflammation. Circulating leucocytes constitutively express adhesion molecules, whereas the interior of blood vessels is not associated with constitutive expression of adhesion molecules, unless stimulated with pro-inflammatory mediators (i.e., histamine) or cytokines (TNF, IL-1, or IL-4), which up-regulate expression of adhesion molecules on endothelium. Circulating leukocytes adherent to adhesion molecules expressed by endothelial cells then diapedese between endothelial cells, and in response to chemokines (released from epithelial cells as well as resident tissue inflammatory cells) migrate into the mucosa toward the surface epithelium. CC chemokines—in particular eotaxin, RANTES and monocyte chemotactic protein-1—are important in the chemotaxis of eosinophils from blood vessels into tissue sites of allergic inflammation. This improved understanding of the cellular and molecular mechanisms mediating the allergic inflammatory response has provided important insight into the contribution of individual mediators and cytokines to symptoms of allergic disease.

CLINICAL SYMPTOMS AND SIGNS

AR frequently starts in early childhood and continues in to adulthood. However, older children have a higher prevalence than younger ones, the peak being reached at 13–14 years of age. Onset of symptoms of rhinitis after the age of 20 years should raise the suspicion of non-allergic rhinitis (6). In the past AR was considered to be a disorder localized to the nose and nasal passages, but current evidence indicates that it may represent a component of systemic airways disease involving the entire respiratory tract (7).

The physiological, functional and immunological relationships between the upper and lower respiratory tracts represent a combined airway inflammatory disease, and this fact needs to be considered for optimal assessment and management of patients with AR.

Clinicians should make the clinical diagnosis of AR when patients present with a history and physical examination consistent with an allergic cause and one or more of the following cardinal symptoms: nasal congestion, runny nose, itchy nose and sneezing. The main signs on physical examination include clear rhinorrhea, nasal congestion and pale discoloration of nasal mucosa. The external assessment of nose, ears, sinuses, oropharynx, chest and skin is essential. The evidence of persistent mouth breathing, the horizontal nasal crease, frequent throat clearing and allergic propensity are suggestive of allergic rhinitis. The various other changes in the upper respiratory tract, as mentioned in the table, also point towards the diagnosis of AR.

Allergic conjunctivitis (AC), as mentioned earlier, is also frequently associated with AR and symptoms generally include redness and tearing and itching of the eyes. An evaluation of other associated parameters linked to the environment, drugs, family, comorbidities and response to previous interventions and over-the-counter medicines is highly recommended to determine the course and potential triggers of AR and AC. This is summarized in Table 2.1.

Allergic conjunctivitis is characterized usually by ocular itching, swelling and tearing but the more severe forms can present with photophobia and ocular pain. From redness of the conjunctiva to punctate keratitis and to ulcers and plaques of cornea, ocular presentation shows it all (8).

Most (80%) of patients with Seasonal Allergic Rhinitis (SAR) and Perennial Allergic Rhinitis (PAR) are under 30 years of age. Vernal Kerato Conjunctivitis (VKC) is a paediatric disease subsiding after puberty but Allergic Kerato

Table 2.1: Clinical Parameters to Be Checked in AR

History	Physical Examination
Personal	*Outward signs*
• Congestion • Nasal itch • Rhinorrhea • Sneezing • Eye involvement • Seasonality • Triggers	• Mouth breathing • Rubbing the nose/transverse nasal crease • Frequent sniffling and/or throat clearing • Allergic shiners (dark circles under eyes)
Family	
• Allergy • Asthma	*Nose*
Environmental	• Mucosal swelling, bleeding • Pale, thin secretions • Polyps or other structural abnormalities
• Pollens • Animals • Flooring/upholstery • Mould • Humidity • Tobacco exposure	
	Ears
Medication/Drug use	• Generally normal • Pneumatic otoscopy to assess for Eustachian tube dysfunction • Valsalva's maneuver to assess for fluid behind the ear drum
• Beta-blockers • ASA • NSAIDs • ACE inhibitors • Hormone therapy • Recreational cocaine use	
Quality of life	*Sinuses*
• Rhinitis-specific questionnaire	• Palpation of sinuses for signs of tenderness • Maxillary tooth sensitivity
Comorbidities	
• Asthma • Mouth breathing • Snoring ± apnea • Impaired smell or taste • Sinus involvement • Otitis media • Nasal polyps • Conjunctivitis	*Posterior oropharynx* • Postnasal drip • Lymphoid hyperplasia ("cobble stoning") • Tonsillar hypertrophy
Response to previous interventions	*Chest and skin*
• Avoidance measures • Saline nasal rinses • Second-generation oral • Antihistamines • Intranasal corticosteroids	• Atopic disease • Wheezing

Source: Adapted from Small et al. (7).

Conjunctivitis (AKC) mostly occurs between 30–50 years of age.

CLASSIFICATION OF ALLERGIC RHINITIS

AR is classified by the following criteria (9).

1. **The temporal pattern of exposure to an allergen trigger:**

   a. Seasonal—allergens develop only during specified periods of the year corresponding to pollination time of anemophilus plants or sporulation of mould.

   b. Perennial—adequate concentrations of allergens exist in the patient's immediate environment all year round. The main triggers include house dust mites, moulds, pet fur and cockroaches.

   c. Episodic—allergens are not normally present in the patients' environment like acid exposure while cleaning toilets. This form of AR is usually sporadic and short lasting.

2. **Frequency of symptoms:** This classification is easy for implementation in clinical practice and for choosing appropriate treatment.

   a. Intermittent AR—symptoms are less than 4 days per week or less than 4 weeks per year.

   b. Persistent AR—symptoms are more than 4 days per week or more than 4 weeks per year.

3. **Severity of symptoms:** According to this criterion, the AR symptoms are classified as

   a. Mild AR—the disease has no impact on the quality of life in spite of being symptomatic.

   b. Moderate AR—the disease affects the presence of 1–3 of all the 4 elements mentioned below.

   c. Severe AR—the disease impact is seen in all four elements.

   The elements defining quality of life are

   i. Daily activities and sports

   ii. School or workplace attendance

   iii. Sleep

   iv. The urgency of treatment, as reported by the patient

   The above severity classification is according to the modified ARIA classification (Figure 2.1).

4. **Disease pathophysiology:** This section has limited use in clinical practice.

   a. IgE mediated—this type is present in more than 90% patients of AR.

b. Non-IgE mediated—this type probably involves IgG antibodies, T lymphocytes or eosinophils.

The above classification has its limitations too. For example, the length of aeroallergen pollen season is dependent on geographic location and climatic conditions. As in temperate climates where pollen season is year round, it is difficult to distinguish between symptoms due to pollen from those due to perennial allergens like house dust mite. Again, many patients may have perennial rhinitis exacerbated by seasonal pollen exposure. In many patients with polysensitization the clinical implications of seasonal versus perennial are not clear. Patients of AR who have mixed rhinitis—i.e., allergic and non-allergic rhinitis—range from 44–87%.

Local AR

Local AR is a clinical phenotype that is characterized by localized allergic response (LAR) in the nasal mucosa in the absence of evidence of systemic atopy. These patients have a negative Skin Prick Test (SPT) and low specific IgE but direct nasal mucosal exposure to specific allergens elicit a positive response. There is a raised specific IgE in nasal mucosa. However, no evidence suggests that LAR is a precursor to AR evolution. Allergen immunotherapy (AIT) is of probable help in this case.

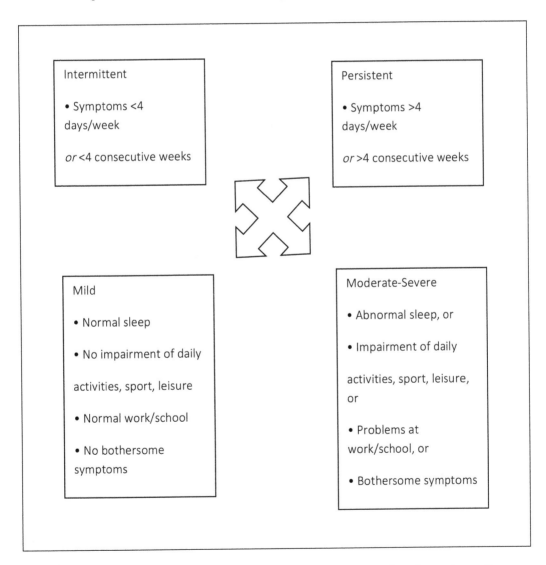

Figure 2.1 Classification of allergic rhinitis according to symptoms, duration and severity. [Adapted from Small et al. (7), Bousquet et al. (11).]

Another point to note is a seasonal AR symptom usually (60–90%) coexisting with symptoms of allergic conjunctivitis and it is this condition which is referred to as allergic rhinoconjunctivitis (ARC).

Allergic Conjunctivitis

It is classified classically into two groups:

a. Common allergic conjunctivitis, which includes seasonal and perennial forms (SAC and PAC)

b. Keratoconjunctivitis, including vernal and atopic forms (VKC and AKC)

SAC and PAC are mild to moderate allergic diseases, mostly associated with rhinitis involving an IgE mediated hypersensitivity response On the other hand, the more severe and rarer VKC and AKC involve a T helper mediated response.

DIAGNOSIS

Although a thorough history and physical examination are required to establish the clinical diagnosis of AR (Table 2.1), further diagnostic tests are necessary to confirm the allergens causing the rhinitis and conjunctivitis. There are in vivo and in vitro tests to pinpoint the allergens triggering AR.

In vivo tests include

a. Skin prick tests (SPT)

b. Organ challenge tests (OCT)

In vitro tests include the use of allergen-specific IgE tests (e.g., performed by immunosorbent assays) that provide a measure of a patient's specific IgE levels against particular allergens.

SPT is the primary, rapid, cost effective and most sensitive method of identifying specific allergen triggers. This is a bioassay performed by introducing a specific allergen into the patient's skin. In this method a drop of the commercial extract of the relevant allergens (e.g., pollen, dander, moulds, house dust mites) are placed on the skin of the forearm or back along with a positive control as histamine and negative control as normal saline. A needle is used to prick through the allergen drop to introduce it into the epidermis. After 20 minutes, a wheal and flare response will occur and positive or negative results are read as compared to the controls.

The in vitro tests are useful only if no normal skin is available for SPT or if the patient is on antihistamines. This knowledge of a specific causative allergen is needed for a target-oriented therapy. Even though allergy tests have risks and results are often inaccurate, the benefits over ride the harms rendered. So clinicians and patients should discuss costs, benefits and adverse effects of tests and the type of testing involved. However, SPT are generally considered to be more sensitive and cost effective than in vitro tests and provide physicians and patients with immediate results.

Sinonasal imaging should be routinely performed in patients of AR because there is a preponderance of benefit over harm. So as we see, while a trial of symptom driven pharmacotherapy may be a pragmatic and reasonable first step employed by the physician, severe symptoms or suboptimal therapeutic response warrant further specific investigations as stated above. Results of specific IgE reactivity not only confirm the presence of allergic disease but also help in directing environmental control interventions and determining whether a person may be a candidate for immunotherapy.

Apart from allergy tests, a growing number of articles on ocular allergy show an association between allergic conjunctivitis and keratitis and decreased tear film break up time (BUT). A few studies also assess meibomian gland morphology in different types of ocular allergy.

MANAGEMENT

For many years the algorithm for the treatment of AR has combined 4 basic modalities that often require concurrent application:

1. Education of patients and caregivers

2. Avoidance of allergens and irritants

3. Pharmacotherapy

4. Allergen immunotherapy, especially in SAR

The treatment goal is relief of symptoms and improvement of quality of life. Also, as mentioned earlier, AR and asthma appear to represent a combined airway inflammatory disease; and therefore, treatment of asthma is also an important consideration in patients with AR.

ENVIRONMENTAL MEASURES

The first-line treatment of AR involves the avoidance of relevant allergens and irritants in patients who have identified allergens correlated with clinical symptoms. For this, use of multiple avoidance techniques may be more effective than individual measures. The risks and benefits of the various methods need to be discussed with patients as they will be actively involved in all these treatment strategies.

A brief overview of the available methods is as follows:

- For grass, tree or weed pollen avoidance, windows of cars and homes should remain closed during pollen season and indoor air conditioners should be installed. HEPA filters are of particular importance here. Limiting the amount of time spent outdoors during pollen season is also helpful.

- In order to avoid dust mites, mattresses and pillows should be encased in impermeable plastic covers and the covers washed weekly in hot water. They should be kept in areas where relative humidity is below 50%.

- For individuals allergic to animal dander, removal of the pets is the best possible way to reduce allergens exposure from them. This usually results in a significant reduction of symptoms in 4–6 months.

- Moulds are ubiquitous both indoors and outdoors. So mould-allergic individuals should inspect and rectify humid areas in the house.

- A combination of these avoidance strategies can effectively improve the symptoms of AR. Of all these measures, removal of pets, acaricide use to kill dust mites and combination strategies evidently supports reduction of symptoms.

PHARMACOTHERAPY

The selection of pharmacological options suitable for a particular patient depends to a large extent on the form and clinical severity of AR, the patient's age, drug availability, cost and the patient's acceptance and satisfaction. There is also a step-up and a step-down approach to the treatment (10–13).

INTRANASAL CORTICOSTEROIDS (INCS)

Based on a number of randomised controlled studies, INCS are strongly recommended with minor limitations and a preponderance of benefit over harm. These form the first-line of therapy and the gold standard for the pharmacological therapy of allergic rhinitis. The active ingredients of INCS are beclomethasone, fluticasone, mometasone and budesonide. The medication should be prescribed by a doctor only after the first diagnosis of seasonal allergic rhinitis. A maximum daily dose of 200/400 microgram must be maintained. When used regularly and correctly, INCS effectively reduce inflammation of the nasal mucosa and improve mucosal pathology. INCS improve all nasal symptoms, including nasal congestion, rhinorrhea, itching

and sneezing. INCS are best started just prior to exposure to relevant allergens and—as the peak effect takes about 3 days to develop—they should be taken regularly.

The reported side effects are nasal burning and stinging, dryness and epistaxis occurring in 5–10% of the patients. Local atrophy with high potency topical corticosteroids has been known, but is extremely rare. These local effects can be prevented by aiming the spray away from the nasal septum. Systemic side effects, such as linear growth suppression, have also been minimal. A sensitive marker of HPA axis suppression has rarely been shown to be affected mainly by beclomethasone in long-term studies. In addition, no increase of bone fractures have been found in elderly people irrespective of the doses used.

In patients with persistent AR, INCS alone is recommended rather than a combination with oral antihistaminics, as in SAR by ARIA guidelines. ARIA guidelines also recommend that in patients with severe SAR a fixed combination of INCS and antihistaminic or INCS alone be used. In the initial two weeks the combination will work faster.

Other drug categories in the treatment of AR

- H1 receptor antagonists—second-generation oral and intranasal antihistaminics
- Antileukotrines
- Intranasal anticholinergics like ipratropium bromide
- Alpha sympathomimetics
- Intranasal normal saline solutions
- Biologics like omalizumab
- Cromones

The effects of these various drugs on AR and ocular allergy are shown in Table 2.2.

The oral and intranasal sympathomimetics act as decongestants and help in removing nasal congestion in AR. However, they are contraindicated in hypertensives and patients with severe coronary artery disease. They should not be used for more than 5 days because prolonged use will result in rhinitis medicamentosa or rebound nasal congestion.

Oral leukotriene receptor antagonists (LTRAs) are not recommended as primary therapy for patients with AR but they should be considered when oral antihistaminics, INCS individually or in combination are not well tolerated or found to be in effective. A recent meta-analysis of 11 published studies on the clinical effectiveness of LTRA concluded that

Table 2.2: Drug Categories Used in the Therapy of SAR and Their Effect on Nasal and Ocular Symptoms under Normal Exposure

Drug Category	SAR Symptoms and Ocular Symptoms					
	Sneezing	Itching	Watery Discharge	Nasal Blockage	Smell Disorders	Ocular Symptoms
Antihistamines (p.o.)	++	++	++	+/−	−	++
Antihistamines (i.n.)	++	+++	++	+	−	−
Ipratropium bromide (i.n.)	−	−	+++	−	−	−
α-sympathomimetics (i.n.)	−	−	−	++	+/−	−
α-sympathomimetics (p.o.)	−	−	−	+	−	+/−
Antileukotrienes (p.o.)	+	+	++	++	+	+
Glucocorticoids (i.n.)	+++	+++	+++	++	+	++
Glucocorticoids (p.o.)	+++	++	+++	++	+	+++
Anti-IgE (s.c.)	++	++	++	++	nd	++
Saline solutions (i.n.)	+	+	+	nd	−	−
Cromones (i.n.)	+	+	+	+/−	−	−

(i.n.) intranasal drugs, (p.o.) oral drugs, (s.c.) subcutaneous drugs, (−) no effect, (+/−) uncertain effect, (+) some effect, (++) strong effect, (+++) very strong effect, (nd) no data.

these agents had limited effectiveness in the treatment of AR, reducing mean daily symptom scores 5% more than with the placebo.

Allergic conjunctivitis can be treated by a variety of drugs such as topical antihistaminics (like cetrizine), ophthalmic mast cell stabilizers (like olopatadine), nonsteroidal anti-inflammatory drugs (like ketorolac), trimethamine drops and systemic and topical corticosteroids (like loteprednol etabonate). Care must be taken when using topical corticosteroids and pulsed regimens should be used to minimize side effects.

Omalizumab, a biologic specific against IgE, and ophthalmic decongestants (like tetrahydrozoline drops) are also helpful. Finally, ophthalmic lubricants (like artificial tears) complete the list.

ALLERGEN IMMUNOTHERAPY

This is the only treatment modality that can alter the natural history of allergic diseases. The process involves the subcutaneous administration of gradually increasing quantities of the patient's relevant allergens until a dose is reached that is effective in inducing immunologic tolerance to the allergen. This is also called subcutaneous immunotherapy or SCIT. The other form of allergen administration is via the sublingual route which is also called SLIT. The total duration of treatment is between 3 and 5 years. Preseasonal preparations are very useful for seasonal allergic rhinitis. Both forms of AIT, that is SCIT and SLIT, are contraindicated in severe asthma or

uncontrolled asthma or patients on beta-blockers. But anaphylaxis is hardly ever seen in sublingual form of AIT; hence, the sublingual form is considered to be safer than subcutaneous form of therapy.

Over the past decade studies of biologics used with AIT have shown promising results. Biologics appear as a promising approach to both asthma and AR as they decrease the onset and severity of AIT associated adverse events during induction phase and increase the efficacy of AIT itself.

A stepwise algorithm for treatment of AR is provided here (see Figure 2.2).

Current principles of drug selection in SAR: The pharmacotherapy of SAR is gradable. If the disease exacerbates, the treatment can be intensified by adding another medication (step-up approach). Conversely, if there is an improvement in symptom control, the therapy is reduced by discontinuing a couple of drugs (step-down approach) (14–16).

The current therapeutic algorithm for AR in MACVIA_ARIA guidelines using the Visual Analogue Scale or VAS includes one of the following in patients more than 12 years of age: Antihistaminic per oral (AHPO), Antihistaminic intranasal (AHIN), Glucocorticoid intranasal (GCIN), leukotriene receptor inhibitor (LTRI) and combination. VAS can be used at home to mark the severity of symptoms on a scale of 0–10. This is a precise and sensitive tool for assessment of AR and ocular symptoms, particularly in SAR.

One drug is chosen only in patients with VAS<2. However, in patients with VAS>5 with

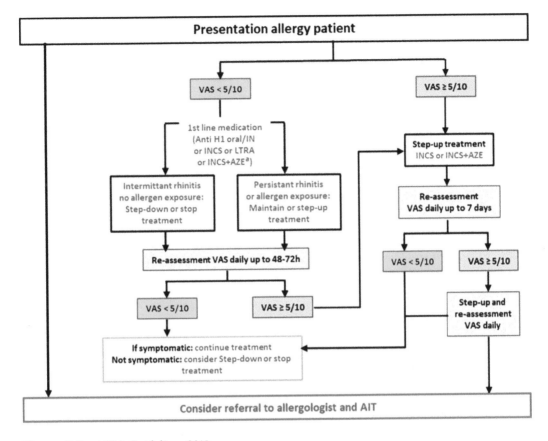

Figure 2.2 ARIA Guidelines 2019.

SAR treatment with GCIN or GCIN plus Azelastine (AZE) is preferred. VAS scoring should therefore be done on a daily basis and based on this treatment modification is done accordingly.

SURGICAL TREATMENT

Clinicians may refer to a surgeon for surgical reduction of the enlarged nasal inferior turbinate causing nasal obstruction. The surgery improves the symptoms and quality of life and results in a reduction of medication usage. Surgical treatment is also indicated in patients with severe deviated nasal septum (DNS), polyposis or chronic sinus disease that is refractory to medical treatment.

AR may worsen during pregnancy, and the treatment recommended in such conditions includes sodium cromoglycate and oral antihistaminics. AIT cannot be induced during pregnancy but maintenance doses are considered to be safe and effective.

COMPLEMENTARY AND ALTERNATIVE MEDICINES (CAM)

Various CAM have been used for the treatment of AR like acupuncture, homeopathy and herbal therapies of which acupuncture provides modest benefits for patients with AR. To date, with limited studies no recommendations have been illustrated regarding the use of herbal therapy in AR (6).

Treatment guidelines are not mandates. Adherence to these guidelines will not ensure successful outcomes in all situations. Therefore, clinicians will have to place the patient in light of circumstances presented by the individual patient and then determine the appropriate treatment.

The relationship between AR and comorbid conditions like otitis media and sinusitis should be determined.

In conclusion, it should also be determined whether different forms of allergy testing can provide clinically meaningful information. Studies are also needed to determine the effect of combined allergen formulations for AR that are standardized, tolerable and effectively dosed.

FUTURE DIRECTIONS

To date there are no FDA-approved sublingual immunotherapy or SLIT vaccines, even though they have been shown to be the most useful treatment for AR.

Allergoids (modified allergen extracts processed to preserve antigenicity while reducing allergenicity) and adjuvants (which increase the results of AIT) are other new formulations but none are FDA approved.

There is to date no cure for allergic rhinitis but, with newer diagnostic techniques and treatment regimens, a bright future of curing this disease is not far away.

REFERENCES

1. Broide DH. The pathophysiology of allergic rhino conjunctivitis. Allergy Asthma Proc 2007; 28 (4): 398–403.

2. Chaplin DD. Overview of the human immune response. J Allergy Clin Immunol 2006; 117:S430–S435.

3. Von Andrian UH, Mackay CR. T-cell function and migration. Two sides of the same coin. N Engl J Med 2000; 343:1020–1034.

4. Rosenwasser L. New insights into the pathophysiology of allergic rhinitis. Allergy Asthma Proc 2007; 28:10–15.

5. Hansen I, Kilmek L, Mosges R, et al. Mediators of inflammation in the early and the late phase of allergic rhinitis. Curr Opin Allergy Clin Immunol 2004; 4:159–163.

6. Textbook of allergy for the clinician: Edited By Pudupakkam K. Vedanthan, Harold S. Nelson, Shripad N. Agashe, Mahesh P A, Rohit Katial. Allergic Rhinitis-Edition: 1st Edition, 2014, eBook Published 19 April 2016 Pub. pp. 80–93 Boca Raton Imprint CRC Press DOI https://doi.org/10.1201/b16585.

7. Small P, Keith, PK, Kim H. Allergy. Asthma Clin Immunol 2018;14 (Suppl 2):51.https://doi.org/10.1186/s 13223-018-0280-7

8. Villani E, Rabbiolo G, Nucci P. Ocular allergy as a risk factor for dry eye in adults and children. Curr Opin Allergy Clin Immunol 2018;18 (5):398–403.

9. Emeryk A, Emeryk-Maksymiuk J, Janeczek K. New guidelines for the treatment of seasonal allergic rhinitis. Postepy Dermatol Alergol 2019;36 (3):255–260. https://doi.org/10.5114/ada.2018.75749.

10. Ludger Klimek, Claus Bachert, Jean Bousquet. ARIA guideline 2019: treatment of allergic rhinitis in the German health system. Allergo Journal International 2019; 28:255–276, https://doi.org/10.1007/s40629-019-00110-9

11. Bousquet J, Khaltaev N, Cruz AA, Denburg J, Fokkens WJ, Togias A, et al. Allergic rhinitis and its impact on asthma (ARIA) 2008 update (in collaboration with the World Health Organization, GA (2)LEN and Aller Gen). Allergy 2008; 63 (Suppl 86):8–160.

12. Scadding GK. Optimal management of allergic rhinitis. Arch Dis Child 2015; 100 (6):576–82.

13. Seidman MD, Gurgel RK, Lin SY, Schwartz SR, Baroody FM, Bonner JR, et al. Clinical practice guideline: allergic rhinitis executive summary. Otolaryngol Neck Surg 2015; 152 (1 Suppl):S1–S43.

14. Bachert C, Bousquet J, Hellings PW. Rapid onset of action and reduced nasal hyperreactivity: new targets in allergic rhinitis management. Clin Transl Allergy 2018; 8:25.

15. Bousquet J, Hellings PW, Agache I, Amat F, IAnnesi-Maesano I, Ansotegui IJ, et al. Allergic rhinitis and its impact on asthma (ARIA) Phase 4 (2018): Change management in allergic rhinitis and asthma multimorbidity using mobile technology. J Allergy Clin Immunol 2018;143 (3):864–69.

16. Bousquet J, Arnavielhe S, Bedbrook A, Bewick M, Laune D, Mathieu-Dupas E, et al. MASK 2017: ARIA digitally-enabled, integrated, person-centred care for rhinitis and asthma multimorbidity using real-world evidence. Clin Transl Allergy 2018; 8:45–66.

3 Atopic Dermatitis and Eczema

Bindu Cheriattil Govindan

CONTENTS

INTRODUCTION

Atopic dermatitis is a common cutaneous disorder that begins in infancy and follows a relapsing course with repeated exacerbations and remissions (1). The nomenclature for AD and eczema is widely varied. As early as 1892, prurigo diathesque was described. The condition was expressed using various terms like eczema infantum, asthmatic eczema, atopic dermatitis, endogenous eczema, extrinsic-intrinsic atopic eczema, IgE-mediated and non-IgE-mediated atopic eczema. In 2004 the world allergy organization reviewed the nomenclature and began using the term Atopic Eczema (AE). The terms AD, AE and eczema continues to be used interchangeably (1).

DEFINITION

It is difficult to define AD/AE effectively because it tends to show a wide variety of clinical features and there continues to be a lack of a definitive diagnostic test.

Indian Dermatology Expert Board Members (DEBM) prepared a set of evidence-based recommendations under the heading Guidelines on Management of AD in India. DEBM defined AD as a chronic, recurrent, inflammatory skin disease, having a childhood onset and characterised by variably pruritic eczematous lesions with flexural predilection, mostly seen in patients with history of atopic diathesis (1).

AE is an itchy, chronic or chronically relapsing inflammatory skin condition that often starts in early childhood (2).

DIAGNOSTIC CRITERIA

The diagnosis of AD is made clinically based on history and clinical features like age of onset, symptoms, morphology and distribution of lesions. Various groups have developed formal sets of criteria that aid the diagnosis of AD.

- Hanifin and Rajka proposed the earliest and most widely used criteria for diagnosis of AD based on vast clinical experience in 1980. To diagnose AD, the patient has to satisfy 3 of the 4 major criteria and 3 of the 23 minor criteria (3). This criteria helped in uniformity of diagnosis but. as the list was time consuming, it was not suitable for population-based studies.

- William et al in 1997 coordinated a UK Working Party's diagnostic criteria for AD, which proposed that in order to

DOI: 10.1201/9781003125785-3

make a diagnosis of AD one mandatory criteria and 3 of the 5 minor criteria need be fulfilled. An individual must have an itchy skin condition plus 3 or more of the following—onset of rash before the age of 2 years, history of flexural involvement, a history of atopic disease like asthma, a history of a generalised dry skin or visible flexural dermatitis (4). As the criteria are all noninvasive and less cumbersome, it was considered more suited for clinical and epidemiological studies and remains the most validated (5).

■ The American Academy of Dermatology proposed a criterion for the diagnosis of patients with atopic dermatitis. It includes four categories—essential, important, associated features and a set of exclusionary conditions (6).

• The *essential features* that must be present are pruritus and eczema. Pruritus is a cardinal symptom, and eczema—with typical morphology and age-specific patterns—must be present.

• *Important features* are early age of onset, history of atopy, dry skin and IgE response.

• *Associated features* are clinical associations that suggest a diagnosis of AD but are too non-specific to support the definition of AD. They include keratosis pilaris, palmar hyper-linearity, ocular changes, perioral excoriations, ichthyosis and lichenification.

• *Exclusionary conditions* are those that are important to rule out such as scabies, contact dermatitis, cutaneous T cell lymphoma, psoriasis, seborrheic dermatitis, immune deficiency diseases and erythroderma of other causes before confirming the diagnosis of AD (6).

EPIDEMIOLOGY

The prevalence of AD is estimated to be around 15–20% in children and 1–3% in adults. In industrialised nations the prevalence rate has increased 2-fold to 3-fold during the past few decades. The prevalence rate varies greatly in different countries and in regions within the nations (7).

The International Study of Asthma and Allergies in Childhood (ISAAC), phase 1 was a population-based study. The ISAAC conducted in 14 centres in India noted a 12-month period prevalence of AD to be from 2.4–6.1% (8). Prevalence of AD in the studied age groups i.e., 6–7 years and 13–14 years, in Indian centres participating in the study fell in the lower prevalence regions of less than 5% (9).

A large multicentric questionnaire-based study covering 8 countries concluded that among adults, prevalence was generally lower for males compared to females and it decreased with age. They noted that the point prevalence of adult AD in the overall/and treated population was 4.9%/3.9% in the United States, 3.5%/2.6% in Canada, 2.1%/1.5% in Japan and 4.4%/3.5% in the European Union. This study, one of the first to gather prevalence data in adults from the general population found a point prevalence of 2.1% in Japan and 8.1% in Italy, and it correlates with the point prevalence of 2–10% reported by the World Allergy Organisation (10).

Kabuabara et al. noted in a large sample size study that no significant difference was seen in AD prevalence in adolescence and early adulthood. This meta-analysis of 7 birth cohorts concluded that similar AD prevalence before and after childhood supports the fact that AD has a lifelong genetic predisposition to episodic skin disease (11).

AD persists from childhood through adolescence in around 40% of cases and this was predominantly noted in the female sex and those with asthma, rhino conjunctivitis or sensitised to inhalant or food allergens (12).

PATHOPHYSIOLOGY

The complex interplay of the immune system and genetic predisposition plays a major role in pathogenesis of AD (Figure 3.1). Although we are yet to have a complete understanding about the pathophysiology, various authors have identified epithelial barrier dysfunction

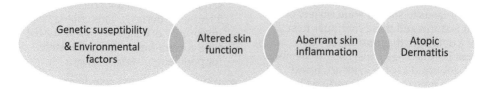

Figure 3.1 Pathophysiology of AD, schematic representation.

and immune dysregulation to play a major contributory role in the pathogenesis of AD.

Multiple factors, like epidermal gene mutations, skin barrier dysfunction, immune dysregulation, altered lipid composition and microbial imbalance contribute to the development of AD (13).

Genetic Factors

These play an important role in the expression of the atopic phenotype. The Filaggrin (FLG) is a major predisposing gene in atopic diseases (14). A mutation in the FLG gene causes a deficiency of FLG which in turn contributes to epithelial barrier defects and is critical to the pathogenesis of AD.

Barrier Dysfunction

Reduced expression of ceramide and FLG is the primary cause of barrier dysfunction and is associated with inflammation causing AD (1). This epithelial defect in combination with environmental factors and the effects of inflammatory cytokines result in the development of AD (15).

Immune Dysregulation

Allergen-specific Th2 cell seem to be critical in the pathogenesis of AD. An immunological bias towards Th2 response where cells tend to express IL-4, IL-5 and IL-13 in early lesions is noted in AD (2). The type of mutation in genes involved in skin barrier function along with adaptive immunity, usually the Th2 response, is highly likely to impact the incidence and severity of disease (15).

Hygiene Hypothesis

This hypothesis states that risk of developing AD could be less in children with repeated infections, exposure to pets or parasitic infestations due to the immunomodulatory effect. A case control study found no causal relationship between AD and infection in early life. The hygiene hypothesis may explain the rise in prevalence of AD in the past few decades. However, doubts remain if the hygiene hypothesis can be causally linked to AD (16).

Atopic March

Atopy is a personal or familial tendency to produce IgE antibodies in response to a low dose of allergen and to develop symptoms suggestive of asthma, rhino conjunctivitis or eczema (2). Atopic march is described when a progression occurs from AD in infants to allergic rhinitis and asthma in children. Vast evidence suggests the previous expression of AD as a prerequisite for the development of asthma and allergic rhinitis and specific sensitisation (17).

CLINICAL FEATURES
■ History

Most of the patients present with symptoms in childhood, usually before 2 years of age. The cardinal symptom of AD is pruritus, which is associated with chronic rashes. The itching is seen throughout the day, may be worse during night causing disturbances in sleep. The itch is aggravated by sweating, stress, warmth and woollen cloths. The clinical presentation of AD varies with age and 3 clinical stages are distinguished.

■ Clinical Features of the Infancy Phase

The first signs of AD are seen as early as in the second month of life. The lesions start on the face (Figure 3.2). Erythematous patchy lesions are seen on the cheek, which may turn papulovesicular. The perioral and perinasal areas are spared in the beginning. As the child begins to crawl, the extensor aspect of the elbows and knees are affected. Later both inner and outer surface of legs and hands are also affected. The diaper area is relatively spared (2).

The pruritis starts weeks later and the rubbing or scratching due to the itch causes crusty erosions (18). Lesion tends to become exudative and crusted. Secondary infection and lymphadenopathy are common in this age group. In infants around half of the cases of AD show no evidence of IgE-mediated sensitisation and are classified as nonatopic eczema (17).

■ Clinical Features of the Childhood Phase

Depending upon the skin type, the lesions of AD in children may be a mixture of hypo to hyperpigmented areas, erythema, crusting and warty lichenification. In 2 year-olds, lesions are classically seen in the elbow and knee flexures (2). The eczemas of the child's face will typically progress to involve the flexural areas mainly the antecubital fossa, wrist, ankle, the nape of neck and dorsum of hands and feet. These are either newly arising lesions or developing from preceding ones. Around 60% of the childhood eczema will disappear but sequalae like xerosis may remain (18).

■ Clinical Features of the Adolescent and Adult Phase

New eczematous lesions may arise or the lesions of infancy and childhood may persist

19

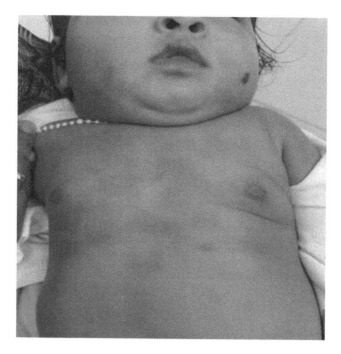

Figure 3.2 Erythematous skin lesions in an infant.

through adolescence. The skin lesions are seen typically in flexural regions, face, neck, palms and soles. The dryness of skin remains a problem. Eczema of adolescents is often associated with an infection known as Malassezia (18). Localised patches of AD are seen on the nipple especially in adolescents and young females. Involvement of the vermillion of the lips and adjacent skin is noted. The typical clinical features of AD in adolescents are eyelid dermatitis, and lesions localised to the forehead, perioral area, neck, upper part of chest and flexural areas. Adults with AD, in addition to skin manifestations, may also show photosensitivity.

Adolescents tend to develop problems in relationships with peers, anxiety, disturbed sleep and frustration. Significant psychological impact due to depression and isolation causing reduced quality of life is commonly seen in this age group.

DIFFERENTIAL DIAGNOSIS

- Contact dermatitis—The lesions tend to occur in areas where there is frequent contact with the allergen, especially the extremities.

- Seborrheic dermatitis—This is seen in infants less than 1 year of age. Pruritus is minimal. Erythematous, scaling and greasy lesions are noted in intertriginous parts like the diaper area, retro auricular skin and scalp.

- Psoriasis—The extensor surfaces of knee and elbow is involved. Scaling of scalp and pitting of nails and erythematous plaques with thick silvery scales are seen. Pruritus is less common.

- Scabies—Papules and linear burrows are seen in interdigital paces, wrist flexures and groin.

- Tinea corporis—Lesions are often annular with a central clearing, and pruritus is often absent

CLASSIFICATION OF SEVERITY

There are many scoring systems for assessing the severity of AD. Three scoring systems have been tested and validated (1, 2). The commonly used criteria are SCORAD (scoring SCOR atopic dermatitis AD). SCORAD incorporates both objective physician estimates of extend and subjective patient assessment of itch and sleep loss (1).

The other severity scoring system commonly used are EASI (Eczema Area and Severity Index) and POEM (patient-oriented eczema measure).

Controlling Factors Responsible for Exacerbation of AD (Figure 3.3)

- *Food allergy*: The common food allergens identified that trigger AD are milk products, peanuts, eggs, soy, wheat and shell fish.

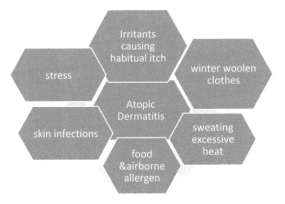

Figure 3.3 Triggering factors of AD.

A food allergy is diagnosed by clinical symptoms and signs after suspected intake and it should be reproducible. This helps to avoid a broad panel allergy testing. The DEBM recommendation is no empirical food restriction. Food should be restricted only on the basis of clinical experience and food diagnostic procedures and is recommended only if a specific food trigger is identified (1).

- *Clothing*: Smooth, cotton clothing that have loose fitting are recommended. Nylon fabric and irritating woollen fibres can cause skin irritation.

- *Climate and environment*: A warm, humid climate which causes increased sweating can cause exacerbations. Patients need to be advised to avoid occupations or recreational activities in humid, high temperatures.

- *Allergens and irritants*: Exacerbations are caused by physical irritation including scratching, contact allergens and exposure to microbes and fungi. Exposure to allergens can be avoided. Bathing helps wash away components of sweat, dust, dirt, debris, pollens and microbes on the surface of the skin. Perfumes, cosmetic products, formaldehyde, nickel, preservatives and rubber chemicals are common irritants and these are to be avoided.

- *Dry skin*: Emollients can play a protective role as dry skin contributes to barrier dysfunction.

- *Stress*: AD aggravation is often noticed when patients are in situations of stress. Psychotherapeutic approaches and behaviour therapy are helpful in reducing stress and thereby controlling the disease. Psychological interventions help improve patient well-being and significantly improve the skin lesions (19).

Complications and Comorbidities

- *Bacterial and viral infections*: Patients with AD are prone to secondary bacterial infection. Staphylococcal, streptococcal and *Fulminant herpes* simplex are commonly seen.

- *Growth delay*: In children affected with severe forms of AD, growth delay is noted.

- *Psychosocial aspects*: Social isolation and depression is common in long-standing disease.

- *Ocular abnormalities*: Conjunctival irritation is common in atopic individuals and cataract and keratoconjunctivitis have been associated with AD. This may be due to combination of rubbing and the use of topical steroids

- *Asthma and allergic rhinitis*: AD is a risk factor for the development of allergic airway diseases.

MANAGEMENT

1. **Investigations**

   AD is diagnosed clinically as there is no reliable biomarker to confirm the diagnosis.

   - *Serum total IgE*: An elevated level of serum IgE is seen in around 80% of patients with AD, but in 20% of those affected IgE was not detected. Based on the presence of IgE, AD is classified into extrinsic and intrinsic AD. Routine monitoring of serum IgE level is not recommended (1).

   - *Allergen-specific IgE*: IgE antibodies specific to allergens like food, mites and pets are elevated in patients with AD. Routine testing of allergen-specific IgE is not recommended (1).

- *Peripheral eosinophil count*: Absolute eosinophil counts are elevated in allergic disorders. They have an inconsistent association with disease severity.

- *Serum level of CD30, IL-12, IL-16, IL-18, IL-31 can be monitored*: None of these tests have been proven reliable in diagnosis and monitoring [1].

- *Histopathology*: Skin biopsy shows spongiosis, perivascular lymphocytic infiltrates and parakeratosis. Routine skin biopsy is not recommended for the diagnosis of AD.

- *Atopic patch test (APT)*: Intradermal or epicutanous patch test is a tool to detect allergic sensitisation. APT done with protein allergen elicits a triphasic response. A wheal and flare are noted in 15 minutes, erythema and deeper oedematous reaction in 6 to 24 hours and a delayed response in 48 hours [1, 2]. APT is not useful when used in isolation. In combination with a good history, clinical examination, serum-specific IgE and skin prick test, it may provide a better understanding of the disease. [20].

2. **Assessment**

The initial assessment includes a detailed history and clinical assessment of skin involvement and severity of disease. The examination of other systems (i.e. respiratory and gastrointestinal) play a relevant role in management of AD.

- *History*: Comprehensive history of the patient's diseases, recognising trigger factors.

- *Examination*: Assessment of skin involvement and severity.

- *Diagnosis*: Confirmation is done clinically, after exclusion of differential diagnosis.

- *Assess severity*: Done both subjectively and objectively using scoring system.
  - Identify disease triggers.
  - Identify exacerbating factors.
  - Patient and family education.
  - Multidisciplinary opinion for comorbidities and disease associations.

3. **Treatment**

A step-ladder treatment has been recommended by DEBM [1]. Topical treatments and or systemic therapy is started based on the severity of AD. After remission is achieved, a step-down to maintenance therapy is done to reduce the number of flare-ups [1].

First-Line Therapy

The initial management includes health education of the patient and family. Advice on reduction of triggering factors has to be stressed. Bathing is soothing for most patients, with moisturiser to be applied soon after. Foaming soaps, which are skin irritants, are to be avoided. Instead, soap substitutes such as emollients can be used for cleaning.

- *Moisturisers/Emollients*: Regular use of emollients plays a critical role as it helps reduce the barrier dysfunction. It softens the skin and reduces the itch. Regular use of emollients, even during remission helps in reducing the frequency of flare. Moisturisers are advised twice a day, preferably to be applied within 3 minutes after bathing. During acute flares, the frequency of use of moisturisers can be increased as they provide symptomatic relief.

- *PEDs or prescription emollient devices*: Are a newer class of topical agents used to target defects in skin barrier functions. They are more expensive but DEBM says they may be helpful in selective cases [1].

- *Topical suppression of inflammation*: Topical corticosteroids are the predominant treatment for inflammation in severe cases. The strength and mode of application depends on the severity of disease, age of the patient and site to be treated. Local side effects like telangiectasia and stria can be minimised if an appropriate dose is used. If not abused, topical corticosteroids are relatively safe and effective drugs.

- *Topical calcineurin inhibitors*: Pimecrolimus and tacrolimus are safe and effective in the treatment of AD and can be used in children and adults with active disease. TCI can be used as a first-line therapy, along with moisturisers, and they have a significant effect in both long-term and short-term treatment of AD [1]. TCI are recommended for maintenance therapy also. A Tacrolimus ointment of 0.1% for adults and 0.3% in children is used in moderate to severe AD that does not respond to adequate dose of topical steroids. Tacrolimus can be used in moderate to severe cases, especially in AD affecting sensitive skin areas [21]. Pimecrolimus is effective in mild to moderate AD.

- *Antihistamines*: Pruritus continues to be the most difficult symptom to treat. Oral sedating H1 receptor antagonists given 1 hour before sleep can be useful in patients with severe nocturnal itch. Although there are no specific anti-pruritic treatments, controlling inflammation has been found most effective.

- *Oral corticosteroids*: Steroids in the dose of 0.5 mg/kg body weight has a limited but definitive role in management of acute exacerbations. It acts rapidly and is well tolerated and valued in patients having repeated flares.

- *Antibiotics*: The majority of patients with AD have colonization of skin with various bacteria. Oral antibiotics are given if there is evidence of infection since these events can act as exacerbating factors. Regular use of topically applied medication may help but it is not advised as the possibility of the emergence of drug resistance strains increases.

- *Antivirals*: Herpes simplex infection may warrant the use of effective antivirals.

Second-Line Therapy

- *Reassess*: Patients not responding to first-line treatment have to be reassessed. The commonest cause is lack of adherence. Other causes are persistence of trigger factors and the presence of recurrent antibiotic-resistant infection.

- *Intensive topical treatment*: The potency of topical steroids can be increased for a short period for an outpatient. The severe flare-up may respond to same treatment given to an inpatient.

- *Wet Wrap technique*: This technique is an effective treatment for the control of severe AD. A generous quantity of low potency topical steroids is applied on the skin, and two layers of absorbent tubular bandage are applied overnight. The inner layer of the wet wrap is pre-soaked in warm water and the outer layer is dry. Localised areas of severe lichenification can be treated with occlusive colloid dressings.

- *Cyclosporin A* (CsA): Is an oral calcineurin inhibitor that supresses the activation of T cells. It is now recommended as the first choice among systemic immunomodulators in patients unresponsive to conventional topical treatment methods (1). CsA can be recommended in both adults and children

above the age of 2 years as an effective and safe second-line therapy, especially in cases of AD of moderate to severe severity. It can be given safely in daily divided doses of 3–5 mg/kg/day in adults and children for a long duration of 1–2 years (22).

Third-Line Therapy

- *Phototherapy*: Is effective in treatment of AD both as monotherapy and in combination with emollients and topical agents. Phototherapy may decrease the need for topical steroids and immunomodulators. Broad band ultra violet B (UVB), narrow band UVB (NB-UVB), UVA1 and psoralens and ultra violet A (PUVA) are effective treatments in severe AD. Acute flares need to be treated with intense treatment prior to subjecting for phototherapy. Narrow band phototherapy and UVB are the preferred options. NB-UVB is effective in children with severe AD. The treatment is well tolerated and complete clearance or minimal residual activity has been seen. Studies have shown a median length of remission of 3 months with phototherapy (23).

- *Azathioprine*: This is an immunosuppressant that is considered as an effective second-line agent in adult patients of AD not responding to, or with a contraindication to and side effects with CsA.

- *Mycophenolate mofetil (MMF)*: A DEBM consensus statement recommends mycophenolate mofetil in dose of 1.5 g/day as a safe alternative immunomodulator for long-term use in patients not responding to or having side effects with CsA (1). MMF has been found to be effective and safe for use in adult and paediatric AD. Monitoring for infections that may occur in patients on long-term therapy is necessary (24).

- *Methotrexate*: This has been shown to be well tolerated and safe for long-term treatment of moderate to severe AD. It has been found to be effective in adults and children above 8 years of age (25).

Fourth-Line Therapy: Biologics and Newer Therapies

- *Dupilumab*: This is a human monoclonal antibody directed against IL-4 and IL-13 that reduces the TH2-mediated inflammation seen in moderate to severe AD. Dupilumab produces a reduction in pruritus and skin lesions and thereby is an effective control of the disease. Patients treated with dupilumab had significant rapid improvement and no significant side effects other than headache and nasopharyngitis (26).

- *Omalizumab:* This helps to reduce the levels of free serum IgE level, but the efficacy of omalizumab in treatment of AD is doubtful. DEBM consensus states that omalizumab is not recommended in treatment of AD (1).

- *Other biologics*: Newer immunomodulators like Nemolizumab, Lebrikizumab, Tralokinumab, Ustekinumab and Apremilast have shown promising results. More data is needed to confirm their usefulness and safety in treating AD.

- *Tofacitinib*: This JAK inhibitor that acts by blocking Th2 pathway has shown promise in the treatment of AD. More studies are required to confirm its efficacy (27).

- *Crisaborole:* This is a PDE inhibitor ointment. It is effective in reducing pruritus and skin inflammation in cases of AD and can be used in children above the age of 2 years (28).

MAINTENANCE THERAPY

The majority of patients respond to treatment and go into remission. Avoidance of the trigger factors and continuous use of emollients play an important role in maintenance therapy. A weekender approach for topical steroids use and mid-week use of topical calcineurin inhibitors helps in significantly reducing the relapse rate. The DEBM consensus statement says that proactive treatment with TCS and Tacrolimus ointment during the long-term follow-up period helps to reduce the AD flares effectively (1).

DISEASE COURSE, PROGNOSIS AND OCCUPATIONAL ADVICE

The natural history of AD is favourable in that the majority of children affected undergo spontaneous resolution. An Indian experience suggests that disease when started in infancy undergoes a reduction in severity in a step-wise manner and heals completely by the age of 15 years. The true clearance rate may not be accurate as many may relapse later in adulthood. Poor prognostic factors noted are early onset, severe disease in childhood and a family history of atopy (29).

Young adults with AD should avoid occupations where there is risk of skin exposure to chemicals, irritants and physical trauma. Occupations with excessive hand involvement in wet work, exposure to irritants like mechanics, hair dressing and catering are to be avoided

as much as possible (2). Since atopic patients remain at risk for occupational dermatitis, avoidance of irritants may play a significant role in the course of the disease and prognosis.

REFERENCES

1. Rajagopalan M, De A, Godse K, et al. Guidelines on management of atopic dermatitis in India: an evidence -based review and an expert consensus: Indian J Dermatol 2019 May–Jun; 64(3): 166–81. https://doi.org/10.4103/ijd.IJD_683_18

2. Michael R. Ardern -Jones, Carsten Flohr, Nick Rooks, Colin A. Holden. Atopic dermatitis, Chapter 41: Rooks Textbook of dermatology, 9E 2016 Kenit (1). John Wiley ans sons, Ltd. P1263-1296.

3. Rudzki E, Samochoci Z, Rebandel P, et al. Frequency and significance of the major and minor features of Hanifin and Rajka among patients with atopic dermatitis. Dermatology 1994;189:41–6.

4. Williams HC, Burnery PG, Hay RJ, et al. The U.K. Working Party's diagnostic criteria for atopic dermatitis. I. Derivation of a minimum set of discriminators for atopic dermatitis Br J Dermatol 1994; 131(3):383–96. https://doi.org/10.1111/j.1365-2133.1994.tb08530.x

5. Brenninkmeijer EEA, Schram ME, Leeflang MMG, Bos JD, Spuls PI. Diagnostic criteria for atopic dermatitis: a systematic review. Br J Dermatol 2008; 158(4):754–65. https://doi.org/10.111/J.1365-2133

6. Eichenfield LF, Tom WL, Chamlin SL, et al. Guidelines of care for the management of atopic dermatitis: section 1. Diagnosis and assessment of atopic dermatitis. J Am Acad Dermatol 2014; 70(2):338–51.

7. Nurten S. Atopic dermatitis: global epidemiology and risk factors. Ann Nutr Metab 2015;66 (Suppl 1):8–16 https://doi.org/10.1159/000370220

8. Strachan DP, Sihbald B, Weiland SK. Ait-Khaled. Worldwide variation in prevalence of symptoms of asthma, allergic rhino conjunctivitis and atopic eczema ISAAC. Lancet 1998; 351:1225–32. (PubMed)

9. Kanwar AJ, De D. Epidemiology and clinical features of atopic dermatitis in India. Indian J Dermatol 2011; 56(5);471–5. https://doi.org/10.4103/0019-5154.87112

10. Barbarot, S., Auziere, S., Gadkari, A., Girolomoni, G., Puig, L., Simpson, E. L., ... Eckert, L.. Epidemiology of atopic dermatitis in adults: Results from an international survey. Allergy June 2018;73(6):1284–93. doi:10.1111/all.13401

11. Abuabara K, Yu AM, Okhovat J-P, Allen IE, Langan SM. The prevalence of atopic dermatitis beyond childhood: A systematic review and meta- analysis of longitudinal studies. Allergy 2018;73 (3): 696–704. https://doi.org/10.111/all.13320

12. Ricci G, Bellini F, Dondi A, Patrizi A, Pession A. Atopic dermatitis in adolescence. Dermatol Reports 2011; 4(1):e1. https://doi.org/10.4081/dr.2012.e1

13. Kim J, Kim BE, Leung DYM. Pathophysiology of atopic dermatitis: Clinical implications. Allergy Asthma Proc 2019; 40(2):84–92. https://doi.org/10.2500/aap.2019.40.4202

14. Sandilands A, Sutherland C, Irvine AD, McLean WH. Filaggrin in the front line: role in skin barrier function and disease. J Cell Sci 2009;122(9):1285–94. https://doi.org/10.1242/jcs.033969

15. Kaufman BP, Guttman-Yassky E, Alexis AF. Atopic dermatitis in diverse racial and ethnic groups—Variation in epidemiology, genetics, clinical presentation and treatment. Exp Dermatol 2018;27(4):340–57. https://doi.org/10.1111/exd.13514

16. Gibbs S, Surridge H, Adamson R, Cohen B, Benetham G, Reading R. Atopic dermatitis and the hygiene hypothesis: a case-control study. Int J Epidemiol 2004; 33(1)199–207. https://doi.org/10.1093/ije/dyg267

17. Bantz SK, Zhu Z, Zheng T. The atopic march: Progression from atopic dermatitis to allergic rhinitis and asthma. J Clin Cell Immunol 2014; 5(2):202. Published online 2014 Apr 7. https://doi.org/10.4172/2155-9899.1000202

18. Bieber T. Atopic dermatitis. Ann Dermatol 2010; 22(2):125–37. https://doi.org/10.5021/ad.2010.22.2.125

19. Arndt J, Smith N, Tausk F. Stress and atopic dermatitis. Curr Allergy Asthma Rep 2008; 8(4):312–317. https://doi.org/10.1007/s11882-008-0050-6

20. Vaidyanathan V, Sarda A, De A, Dhar S. Atopy patch test. Indian J Dermatol Venerol Leprol 2019; 85(3):338–41.

21. Reda AM, Elgendi A, Ebraheem AI, Aldraibi MS, Qari MS, Abdulghani MMR, et al. A practical algorithm for topical treatment of atopic dermatitis in the Middle East emphasising the importance of sensitive skin areas. J Dermatolog Treat 2019; 30(4):366–73. https://doi.org/10.1080/09546634.2018.1524823

22. Prezzano JC, Beck LA. Long term treatment of atopic dermatitis; Dermatol Clin 2017;35(3): 335–49.

23. Clayton TH, Clark SM, Turner D, Goulden V. The treatment of severe atopic dermatitis in the childhood with narrowband ultra violet B phototherapy. Clin Exp Dermatol 2007;32:28–33.

24. Phan K, Smith SD. Mycophenolate mofetil and atopic dermatitis: Systemic review and meta-analysis. J Dermatolog Treat 2020;31(8): 810–14.

25. Shah N, Alhusaven R, Walsh S, Shear NH. Methotrexate in the treatment of moderate to severe atopic dermatitis: A retrospective study: J Cutan Med 2018;22(5):484–7. https://doi.org/10.1177/1203475418781336

26. Beck LA, Thaçi D, Hamilton JD, et al. Dupilumab treatment in adults with moderate-to-severe atopic dermatitis. N Engl J Med 2014; 371:130–9. https://doi.org/10.1056/NEJMoa1314768

27. Bissonnette R, Papp KA, Poulin Y, et al. Topical tofacitinib for atopic dermatitis: A phase II a randomized trial. Br J Dermatol 2016;175:902–11. https://doi.org/10.1111/bjd.14871

28. Paller AS, Tom WL, Lebwohl MG, et al. Efficacy and safety of crisaborole ointment, a novel, nonsteroidal phosphodiesterase 4 (PDE4) inhibitor for the topical treatment of atopic dermatitis (AD) in children and adults. J Am Acad Dermatol 2016;75:494–503.e6. https://doi.org/10.1016/j.jaad.2016.05.046

29. Dhar S, Banerjee R. Atopic dermatitis in infants and children in India. Indian J Dermatol Venerol Leprol 2010; 76(5):504–13. https://doi.org/10.4103/0378-6323.69066

4 Urticaria

Venugopal Panicker and Arjun Suresh

CONTENTS

INTRODUCTION

Skin is one of the largest immunological organs and is often a target for allergic and immunological response.[1] Urticarias are pruritic, edematous, erythematous plaque lesions of variable size that blanch under pressure and often have a pale centre. Wheals are transient, and, in most types of urticaria, last for less than 24 hours.[1,2] The lesions are round, polymorphic or serpiginous and can rapidly grow and coalesce.[3] Incidence has been reported to be around 8.8%.[4] Angioedema is due to local increase in vascular permeability, often notable in the face, oropharynx, genitalia and, less frequently, in the gastrointestinal tract. These swellings are painful but rarely itchy. Wheals primarily affect the superficial skin layers (papillary dermis), whereas angioedema can involve the submucosa, the deeper reticular dermis and subcutaneous tissues. Wheals and angioedema can occur together or alone. Urticaria occurs alone in around 50% of cases, with angioedema in 40% of cases and angioedema occurs alone in 10% of cases.

ACUTE URTICARIA

Acute urticaria is defined as having wheals occurring for less than 6 weeks; however individual lesions usually last only 24 hours.[2,4] Acute urticaria is usually seen in young children and around 30% of cases may progress to chronic urticaria[3,4]. Acute urticaria is idiopathic in about 50% of patients (acute spontaneous urticaria-ASU), following respiratory tract infections in 40%, in response to drugs in 9%, and to foods in 1% of cases.[4–6] Up to 36% of patients with ASU can progress to chronic spontaneous urticaria (CSU)[6]. Foods, β-lactam antibiotics, insects, contact with an external agent or parasites usually cause IgE-dependent acute urticaria. Drugs like opioids, muscle relaxants, radio-contrast agents and vancomycin cause mast cell degranulation and pro-inflammatory mediator release. Complement-mediated acute urticaria can be triggered by serum sickness, transfusion reactions and viral or bacterial infections. Acetylsalicylic acid (aspirin) and NSAIDs can cause urticaria through their effects on the metabolism of arachidonic acid.[2,4,5] Common foods that cause urticaria are milk, eggs, peanuts, fish and shellfish. Urticaria due to mycoplasma pneumonia and parasitic infections has been commonly reported in children, while due to viral hepatitis and infectious mononucleosis are seen usually in adults.[7–10]

CHRONIC URTICARIA

Chronic urticaria is defined as the presence of daily or almost daily wheals or angioedema for more than 6 weeks with individual lesions lasting for 4–36 hours.[2,6,11] Prevalence is estimated to be 0.5–5%.[3] Women are more commonly affected, with peak age of onset occurring between 20 and 40 years.[4,11–13]

Though cause is often elusive, chronic spontaneous urticaria (CSU) has been consistently associated with respiratory infections in 25–50% of patients. Viral infections such as hepatitis A and B; and infection of the

 DOI: 10.1201/9781003125785-4

nasopharynx also have been associated. CSU has been associated with *Helicobacter pylori* and has been shown to remit with elimination and relapse with reinfection.[6,8]

Psychosocial factors may play a role, as evidenced by a higher percentage of mood disorders, anxiety and personality disorders in patients with CSU. However, it is still uncertain if these are a consequence of CSU.[11,14–16]

Patients with food allergies usually have intermittent symptoms that present often within an hour of food intake.[4] Among food allergy detected by skin prick testing in about, 25–30% of cases, aeroallergen positivity has been reported to be as high as 60%.[10,17,18] Common food allergens seen were hazelnut, potato, apple, oatmeal, pork, beef and seafood.[11] In contrast, a study in Kerala showed that 98% of patients with chronic urticaria had some form of food allergy. Common offending food allergens were wheat (28%), garlic (22%), ground nut (20%), cashew nut (18%), prawns (17%), ginger (16%), peas (12%) and black pepper (10%).[24]

Pseudo allergens (e.g., food additives and some spices) are believed to be the cause of CU but this remains controversial, and few studies have shown less than 30% resolution 10 to 14 days after removal of the pseudo allergens from the patients' diets.[19–21] Drugs, especially NSAID and ACE inhibitors, are associated with CSU. NSAID can precipitate or exacerbate CSU. ACE inhibitors cause CSU by non-immunological bradykinin accumulation and often resolve by stopping the drug, though symptoms can persist in some patients for months.[22–24,30]

In around 45% of patients, circulating immunoglobulin G (IgG) autoantibodies that recognise IgE antibodies or the alpha subunit of the high-affinity IgE receptor on dermal mast cells and basophils are seen. Their presence in turn leads to chronic stimulation of these cells and the release of histamine and other inflammatory mediators that cause urticaria and angioedema. CSU is also associated with antithyroid antibodies in approximately 27% of cases; however, antibodies do not correlate with thyroid function.[12,25,26,2]

CLASSIFICATION OF CHRONIC URTICARIA

Urticaria may be classified according to etiology (Table 4.1).

CHRONIC INDUCIBLE URTICARIA
Dermographic Urticaria/Immediate Symptomatic Dermatographism

Wheals appear after stroking or scratching the skin (skin writing), which causes shearing forces. Wheals appear within 5 minutes and subside within 5–30 minutes and are usually intensely pruritic. Young adults usually in the 2nd or 3rd decade of life are commonly affected, with a mean duration of around 6.5 years. It is the most common form of physical urticaria.[27,28]

Delayed Pressure Urticaria/ Delayed Dermatographism

Wheals that are painful appear around 4–8 hours after exposure to pressure, and lesions lasts 24–48 hours. This commonly affects males in their 30s. Mean duration is 6–9 years. Palms, soles and buttocks are commonly affected areas.[6,8,27]

Cold urticaria occurs on exposure to firm cold bodies, cold fluids or even cold air. Disease is more common in women and has a mean duration of 4.2 years. Disease can occur as a result of infection, neoplasia or autoimmune diseases. However, in most patients it is idiopathic[8].

Heat urticaria occurs on exposure to warm solids or air, while solar urticaria occurs on exposure to light in wavelengths ranging from 280 to 760 nm, with UV light being implicated in the majority of cases.

Cholinergic urticaria is caused by increased body temperature after physical exercise and/ or emotional stress and is common in young adults, usually in the age group of 16–35 years. Pin-sized wheals surrounded by erythema are characteristic.[6–8]

Adrenergic urticaria presents with wheals with a white halo, often in response to stress. The disease responds to treatment with the beta-adrenoreceptor-blocker, propranolol.[29]

Contact urticaria is defined by the appearance of wheals at sites where chemical substances have come into contact with skin. The disease can be strictly confined to the areas of contact, like with nettles (urtica urens or urtica dioica), but generalised systemic symptoms can occur, especially in IgE-mediated allergic contact urticaria. Common eliciting factors are food, plants, drugs, cosmetics, industrial chemicals, animal products and textiles.[8]

Aquagenic urticaria can be further classified as classical, wherein water acts as a carrier for epidermal antigens or salt dependent, where osmotic pressure changes induce urticaria.[11]

Urticaria may occur in association with certain syndromes (Table 4.2). Mastocytosis (also known as mast cell disease) is divided into cutaneous mastocytosis (CM) and systemic mastocytosis. CM includes urticaria pigmentosa (UP), mastocytoma of the skin and diffuse CM.

Hereditary alpha tryptasemia is an autosomal dominant genetic trait in which the person carries extra copies of the alpha tryptase gene (TPSAB1), which can be derived from

Table 4.1: Classification of Chronic Urticaria[8,12]

1. Chronic Spontaneous Urticaria
2. Chronic Inducible Urticaria

2a. Physical Urticaria

1. *Dermographic Urticaria (urticaria factitial)*	"Skin writing", mechanical shearing forces (wheals arising after 1–5 min)
2. *Delayed pressure Urticaria*	Vertical pressure (wheals arising with a 3–8 h latency
3. *Cold Contact Urticaria*	Cold air/water/wind
4. *Heat Contact Urticaria*	Localised heat
5. *Solar Urticaria*	UV and/or visible light
6. *Vibratory Urticaria*	Vibratory forces, e.g., pneumatic hammer

2B. Special Types

1. *Cholinergic*	Due to a brief increase of the body core temperature often secondary to exercise, passive heat or spicy food
2. *Adrenergic*	Elicited by stress
3. *Aquagenic*	Exposed to water
4. *Contact*	

3. Diseases related to urticaria for historical reasons, and syndromes that present with hives and/or angioedema

Urticaria pigmentosa	
Urticarial vasculitis	
Bradykinin-mediated angioedema (e.g., HAE)	
Cryopyrin-associated periodic syndromes (CAPS)	Familial cold auto-inflammatory syndrome (FCAS), Muckle-Wells syndrome (MWS) or neonatal-onset multisystem inflammatory disease (NOMID).
Schnitzler's syndrome	Recurrent urticarial rash and monoclonal gammopathy, recurrent fever attacks, bone and muscle pain, arthralgia or arthritis and lymphadenopathy
Bullous pemphigoid (prebullous stage)	
Well's syndrome	Granulomatous dermatitis with eosinophilia/eosinophilic cellulitis
Gleich's syndrome	Episodic angioedema with eosinophilia
Exercise-induced anaphylaxis	

Table 4.2: Various Clinical Syndromes Associated with Urticaria

Cutaneous Urticarial Syndromes

Urticarial dermatitis
Contact dermatitis
Papular urticaria
Mastocytosis
Exanthematous drug eruption
Autoimmune bullous disorders

- Bullous pemphigoid
- Gestational pemphigoid
- Linear IgA dermatosis
- Dermatitis herpetiformis
- Epidermolysisbullosaacquisita

Pruritic urticarial papules and plaques of pregnancy

Rare cutaneous urticarial syndromes

- Autoimmune progesterone/estrogen dermatitis
- Wells syndrome
- Interstitial granulomatous dermatitis
- Neutrophilic eccrine hidradenitis
- Urticaria like follicular mucinosis

Systemic Urticarial Syndromes

Vasculitides

- Urticarial vasculitis
- Other vasculitides

Immunologic disorders

- Connective tissue diseases
- SLE, Sjogren syndrome, dermatomyositis
- Juvenile rheumatoid arthritis

Hematologic diseases

- Waldenstrom macroglobulinemia
- Schnitzler syndrome
- Hypereosinophilic syndromes
- Polycythemia vera
- Non-Hodgkin lymphoma (B cell)

Autoinflammatory syndromes

- Hereditary periodic fever syndromes
- Cryopyrin-associated periodic syndromes
- Other autoinflammatory syndromes

parents and are usually duplications on a single chromosome. However, if both parents carry the duplication, the child can have up to 4 copies. This results in elevated levels of tryptase (>8 ng/ml). Some develop allergic-like symptoms such as skin itching, flushing, hives and even anaphylaxis; gastrointestinal symptoms such as bloating, abdominal pain, diarrhoea and/or constipation (frequently diagnosed as irritable bowel syndrome or IBS), heartburn, reflux and difficulty swallowing; connective tissue symptoms such as hypermobile joints and scoliosis; cardiac symptoms such as a racing or pounding heartbeat or blood pressure swings—sometimes with fainting; as well as anxiety, depression, chronic pain, panic attacks, and other symptoms. They together make up what is called hereditary alpha tryptasemia syndrome.

PATHOPHYSIOLOGY[4,6,8,12]

Mast cells and basophils are the major effector cells involved in the development of urticarial lesions. Degranulation releases preformed vasoactive mediators, primarily histamine.[12,26]

Mast cells can be activated by immunological (especially IgE-mediated immediate hypersensitivity reaction) or non-immunological mechanisms. Histamine and other mediators, such as platelet-activating factor (PAF) and cytokines released from activated skin mast cells, result in sensory nerve activation, vasodilatation and plasma extravasation, as well as cell recruitment to urticarial lesions.

IgE-mediated mechanisms are believed to be less important in chronic urticaria as evidenced by a lack of co-relation between disease severity and IgE levels. Though around 30–50% patients may have anti-IgE or high affinity IgE receptors, the significance is not known. Anti-IgE is also seen in atopic dermatitis and several autoimmune diseases.

Non-immunological degranulation is believed to be induced by reactive oxygen species or compliment systems (C3a, C4a and C5a), which can act as an anaphylatoxin.

MAST CELL INDEPENDENT URTICARIA

Pathogenesis is believed to be due to prostaglandin release from the epidermis rather than histamine from mast cells. Common examples include development of contact urticaria to sorbic acid, cinnamic acid, cinnamic aldehyde, methyl nicotinate or dimethyl sulfoxide. These patients do not respond to antihistamines, but rather to acetylsalicylic acid and NSAIDs.[6,8,12]

Causes of urticaria may be summarised as in Table 4.3.

Table 4.3: Causes of Urticaria[3,8,12,30]

Immunoglobulin E (IgE) mediated
Aeroallergens
Contact allergen
Food allergens
Insect venom
Medications
Parasitic infections

Non IgE immunologically mediated
Aeroallergens (proteases)
Autoimmune disease
Bacterial infections
Cryoglobulinemia
Fungal infections
Lymphoma
Vasculitis
Viral infections

Non-immunologically mediated
Contact allergen
Elevation of core body temperature
Food pseudo allergens
Light
Mastocytosis
Medications (direct mast cell degranulation)
Physical stimuli

DIAGNOSIS

Diagnosis is primarily based on history and clinical examination while investigations may be usually supportive or confirmatory in some cases (Table 4.4). A detailed history is taken regarding onset, duration, associated symptoms, location, severity, potential triggers, recent infection, drug intake, illicit drug use, occupation, stress, response to prior therapy, family history of atopy, sexual history and so on.[3,8,11,12,25]

With chronic urticaria, or in acute cases a nonspecific workup including a complete blood count with differential, erythrocyte sedimentation rate and/or C-reactive protein testing, liver enzymes and thyroid-stimulating hormone measurement may be done to rule out underlying causes (Table 4.5). When history is suggestive of a physical urticaria, challenge testing with standardised physical stimuli can confirm the diagnosis. Concomitant autoimmune disorders, thyroid dysfunction, and acute or chronic bacterial (e.g., *Helicobacter pylori*), viral (e.g., hepatitis virus), parasitic (e.g., Anisakis simplex), or fungal infections need to be evaluated. Allergy testing is not recommended unless there is specific indication of an allergic cause.[3,4,12]

Table 4.4: Clues from History and Clinical Examination

Urticaria-Associated History and Physical Examination Findings with Possible Etiologies

Clinical clue	Possible etiology
Abdominal pain, dizziness, hypotension, large erythematous patches, shortness of breath, strider, tachycardia	Anaphylaxis
Dermatographism, physical stimuli	Physical urticaria
Food ingestion temporally related to symptoms	Food allergy
High-risk sexual behaviour or illicit drug use history	Hepatitis B or C (cryoglobulinemia) virus, human immunodeficiency virus
Infectious exposure, symptoms of upper respiratory tract or urinary tract infections	Infection
Joint pain, uveitis, fever, systemic symptoms	Autoimmune disease
Medication use or change	Medication allergy or direct mast cell degranulation
Pregnancy	Pruritic urticarial papules and plaques of pregnancy
Premenstrual flare-up	Autoimmune progesterone dermatitis
Smaller wheals (1 to 3 mm); burning or itching; brought on by heat, exercise, or stress	Cholinergic urticaria
Thyromegaly, weight gain, cold intolerance	Hypothyroidism
Travel	Parasitic or other infection
Weight loss (unintentional), fevers, night sweats	Lymphoma
Wheals lasting longer than 24 hours, nonblanching papules, burning or other discomfort, residual hyperpigmentation, fevers, arthralgias	Urticarial vasculitis

Table 4.5: Diagnostic Tests for Urticaria

Type	Subtype	Routine Test	Differential Diagnosis Tests
Spontaneous Urticaria	Acute urticaria	None	None
	Chronic urticaria	CBC, ESR, TSH	Test for infections, thyroid function test thyroid antibodies, functional autoantibodies, skin biopsy
Inducible Urticaria	Cold urticaria	CBC, ESR, cold provocation test	Test for cryoproteins
	Pressure urticaria	CBC, ESR, pressure test (dermographometer, fric test)	None
	Heat urticaria	CBC, ESR, heat provocation test	None
	Solar urticaria	CBC, ESR, UV and visible light threshold test	Rule out other light-induced dermatoses
	Symptomatic dermographism	CBC, ESR Dermographometer-threshold testing	None
	Vibratory angioedema	Test with vortex	None
	Aquagenic urticaria	Wet clothes at body temperature for 20 minutes	None
	Cholinergic urticaria	Exercise and hot bath provocation	None
	Contact urticaria	Cutaneous provocation tests	None

(ESR: erythrocyte sedimentation rate; CBC: complete blood count; TSH: thyroid-stimulating hormone; CSU: chronic spontaneous urticaria; UV: ultraviolet.)

With an autologous serum skin test (ASST) done by an intradermal injection of the patient's own serum, a positive response can be used an indicator for circulating autoantibodies to the high-affinity IgE receptor on the mast cell in CU patients. The autologous plasma skin test (APST) proposed recently has a greater positive predictive value than ASST and correlated well with antinuclear antibody positivity and angioedema.[31]

Basophil activation test (BAT) is an in vitro test that assesses the histamine upregulation

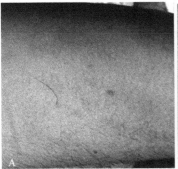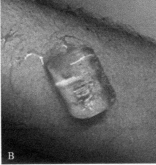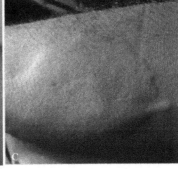

Figure 4.1 Cold-induced urticaria demonstrated by provocation test. Normal skin (A), provocation done by ice cube (B) and development of urticaria (C).

or release of activation markers of donor basophils following stimulation from CSU patients' serum and helps to co-assess disease activity in CSU patients. Patients with negative BAT had a better response to omalizumab. Indirect BAT is a safe and reliable diagnostic tool but is usually not routinely available in daily clinical practice.[31]

Routine skin biopsy is not recommended but may be done to rule out vasculitis or in resistant cases. Biopsy may show a neutrophilic infiltrate or an eosinophilic infiltrate or a mixed pattern. Neutrophilic infiltrates often correlate with poor response to antihistaminics.[32,33]

Cold urticaria can be diagnosed by a provocation test, which includes an ice cube challenge test in which an ice cube, melting in a see-through plastic bag, is placed on the skin for 5 minutes. 10 minutes after removal of the cube a local wheal will develop (Figure 4.1) A shorter or longer provocation time may be used e.g., 30 seconds (in patients who are very sensitive or afraid of strong reactions) and up to 20 minutes (in patients with a positive history but no reaction after 5 minutes).[33–35]

Other methods include testing with cool packs or cold-water baths (e.g., an arm can be submerged in cold water at 5–10°C for 10 minutes) and Temp*Test*® measurements. Because of the risk of causing systemic reactions, cool packs, and cold-water baths should be used with caution. Temp*Test*® is a Peltier effect-based cold provocation device that allows exposure of the skin to thermal elements with defined temperature and hence may be used in cold as well as heat urticaria. Heat urticaria can also be diagnosed by skin testing with metal or glass cylinders filled with warm water or a warm water bath for 5 minutes. Urticaria appears after 10 minutes. Usually temperatures between 45°C and 36°C are tested.[34–36]

Urticaria factitia can be diagnosed by using dermographometer, which can be used to apply a shearing force from 20 to 60 gm/mm². [34,36]

Solar urticaria can be diagnosed by applying UV-A (6 J/cm²), UV B (60 mJ/cm²) and visible light from 10 centimetres for 10 minutes, which results in wheal and flare reaction.[37,38]

Delayed pressure urticaria can be diagnosed by applying different weights to the skin, which exert a defined pressure on the skin surface. Dermographometer can be used, applying vertically to the back skin a pressure of 100 g/mm² for 70 seconds. Results recorded after 6 hours is considered as positive, if a delayed red palpable swelling occurs.[34,36]

Contact urticaria can be diagnosed by a patch test (open application or with occlusion), which is applied for 20 minutes on healthy and on previously damaged skin. The area should be examined after 30 minutes and after 24 hours if protein contact dermatitis is suspected. A normal skin prick or patch test can be performed. Alternatively, the patient can be exposed in a controlled way. Finally, specific IgE measurements may be helpful.[39,40]

TREATMENT

The therapeutic approach to CU involves

a. The identification and elimination of underlying causes

b. The avoidance of eliciting factors

c. Tolerance induction

d. Pharmacological treatment to prevent mast cell mediator release and/or the effects of mast cell mediators

In most cases of physical urticaria, agents can be avoided or exposure minimised by measures like using sunscreens in solar urticaria or lamps with a UV filter.

Plasmapheresis may be tried in severe cases with functional autoantibodies.

A pseudo allergen-free diet, containing only low levels of natural as well as artificial food pseudo allergens, has been tried and may be useful, at least partially, for many patients.

Inducing tolerance can be useful in some subtypes of urticaria. Examples are cold urticaria, cholinergic urticaria and solar urticaria, where a rush therapy with UV-A has been proven to be effective within 3 days.[12]

SYMPTOMATIC PHARMACOLOGICAL TREATMENT

Pharmacological management of urticaria involves antihistamines (Table 4.6), leukotriene antagonists, omalizumab, corticosteroids, immunosuppressants like cyclosporine, etc. If 4 times the regular dose of antihistaminics proves ineffective, leukotriene receptor antagonist may be added, but evidence does not suggest a significant benefit. Following which, a course of omalizumab may be tried, and, if there is no response after 6 months, a trial of cyclosporine (3–5 mg/kg/day) can be given. In severe cases oral prednisolone in doses of 20–50 mg can be used over short periods of time (14 days). Alternative options that have been found to be

Table 4.6: Usual Doses of Antihistaminics Commonly Used

Cetirizine	10–20 mg
Desloratadine	5 mg
Fexofenadine	120 mg
Loratadine	10 mg
Bilastine	20 mg
Rupatadine	10 mg

useful in severe refractory cases are sulfasalazine, dapsone, hydroxychloroquine, colchicine, mycophenolate mofetil, 5-aminosalicylic acid, intravenous immunoglobulin G (IVIg), rituximab, warfarin, etc. Danazol has been used in cholinergic urticaria.[3,4,6,8,12] An algorithm for management of chronic urticaria is given in Figure 4.2.

Angioedema, antithyroid antibodies, and the autologous serum skin test may be associated with a lack of response to antihistamines. Positive ASST has been associated with prolonged disease, which is poorly responsive to routine therapy, and a delayed response to omalizumab.[31]

Cold urticaria can be treated with cold desensitisation but requires the gradual exposure

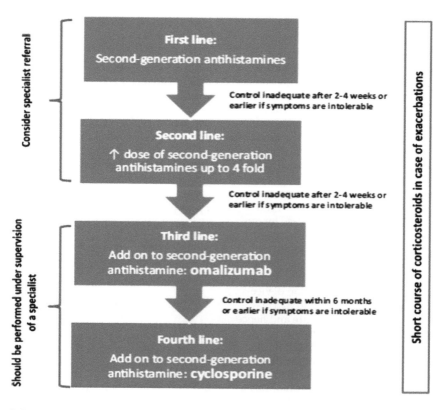

Figure 4.2 Treatment algorithm for chronic urticaria.[6]

of an increasing skin surface area to cold water above the threshold temperature and to be done daily to maintain a desensitised state.[41–43] Other treatment option includes second-generation antihistaminics which can be dosed up to 4 times the usual dosage.[12,44,45] Patients who achieve remission can have doses reduced to a minimum level that prevents symptoms. Patients who do not respond to the usual therapy can be treated with omalizumab, which can bring symptomatic relief with doses of around 300 mg every 4 weeks for a period of 12 months. When symptom remission occurs, antihistaminics can be tapered.[46–48] Other options includes cyclosporine.[49] Etanercept and benralizumab may be used in some selected cases.[50,51] Glucocorticoids may be used but are usually ineffective in most patients.[49] Montelukast may be useful in some patients.[52]

Solar urticaria can be treated with antihistaminics. Glucocorticosteroids—either topical or oral—can be used when antihistaminics alone are ineffective. Other treatment options include omalizumab, psoralen plus ultraviolet A (PUVA) radiation and narrow band UVB, plasmapheresis, cyclosporine. Plasmapheresis may be used alone or in conjunction with PUVA therapy. Intravenous immunoglobulin at doses ranging from 1.4 to 2.5 g per kg may be given over 2–5 days. Desensitization may be tried but effects usually last only a few days.[53,54]

Vibratory angioedema can be treated well with exposure prevention. Antihistamines are usually effective. Disease refractory to multiple antihistamines, antileukotriene agents, dapsone, cyclosporine, prednisone, and omalizumab may respond to ketotifen, a strong antihistamine and mast cell stabiliser, given at a dose of 1 to 2 mg twice daily.[55,56]

Aquagenic urticaria can be treated with antihistaminics. Omalizumab can be used. Some patients respond to propranolol at doses of 10 to 40 mg daily. Stanozolol was found effective in a patient with HIV infection, hepatitis C virus infection, and aquagenic urticaria, who had failed therapy with oral antihistamines. Barrier creams may be useful in some cases.[57,58]

Heat urticaria can be treated with combination of H1 and H2 antihistamines. Desensitisation with daily hot bath may be useful.[59,60]

Cholinergic urticarias can be treated with antihistaminics. However, in case the second-generation fails, hydroxyzine, a first-generation agent, can be attempted. Ketotifen, omalizumab and anabolic steroid, danazol have been reported to be effective.[66]

Delayed pressure urticaria often does not respond to antihistamines alone. Other agents that are effective include omalizumab, montelukast, dapsone, sulfasalazine and non-steroidal anti-inflammatory drugs. Oral steroids are the most effective treatment, but doses above 30 mg per day may be necessary; hence they are unsuitable for long-term use.[62]

TNF-α inhibitors (etanercept, infliximab, and adalimumab) may be effective in the treatment of CSU. Intravenous Ig (IVIg) may be used in treatment of antihistamine-refractory CSU due to its immunoregulatory effects. It acts by Fc receptor blockade (IVIg blocks FcεRI activity on mast cells, which prevents IgE binding and degranulation), inhibition of complement deposition, enhancement of regulatory T cells, inhibition or neutralisation of cytokines and growth factors, accelerated clearance of autoantibodies, modulation of adhesion molecules and cell receptors and activation of regulatory macrophages through the FcγRIIb receptor.[31]

Autologous whole blood and autologous serum injections are effective in some patients. Easy availability and lack of significant adverse effects make these options attractive but are currently limited by sparse evidence. However, available evidence suggest autologous whole blood may be slightly better than autologous serum and also that autologous serum therapy may have better results in patients who are ASST positive.[63]

CONCLUSION

Urticaria is a common disorder that often presents with angioedema. It can be generally classified as acute (lesions occurring for <6 weeks), chronic (lesions occurring for >6 weeks) and inducible (lesions result from a physical stimulus). A history and clinical examination and investigations may reveal a diagnosis in some, but no obvious cause can be identified in many patients. Treatment is often difficult due to varying response to therapy. Avoidance of agent-causing urticaria if known or desensitization strategies can be useful in some patients. Second-generation, non-sedating H1-receptor antihistamines represent the mainstay of therapy for both acute and chronic urticaria, and an up-dosing of these agents can result in better control for some individuals. Severe chronic urticaria may be treated by omalizumab and cyclosporine. Short courses of oral corticosteroids can provide temporary benefits, but long-term use is discouraged. Other newer therapies like rituximab, IVIg may be useful in some cases.

REFERENCES

1. Fonacier LS, Dreskin SC, Leung DYM. Allergic skin diseases. J Allergy Clin Immunol 2010;125(2):S138–49.

2. Poonawalla T, Kelly B. Urticaria. Am J Clin Dermatol 2009;10(1):9–21.

3. Schaefer P. Acute and chronic urticaria: evaluation and treatment. Am Fam Physician 2017;95(11):717–24.

4. Powell RJ, Leech SC, Till S, Huber P a. J, Nasser SM, Clark AT. BSACI guideline for the management of chronic urticaria and angioedema.Clin Exp Allergy 2015;45(3):547–65.

5. Yadav S, Bajaj AK. Management of difficult urticaria. Indian J Dermatol 2009;54(3):275–9.

6. Kanani A, Betschel SD, Warrington R. Urticaria and angioedema. Allergy Asthma Clin Immunol 2018;14(2):59.

7. Wedi B, Raap U, Wieczorek D, Kapp A. Urticaria and infections. Allergy Asthma Clin Immunol 2009;5(1):10.

8. Zuberbier T. Urticaria. Allergy 2003;58(12):1224–34.

9. Williams KW, Sharma HP. Anaphylaxis and urticaria. Immunol Allergy Clin North Am 2015;35(1):199–219.

10. Kulthanan K, Chiawsirikajorn Y, Jiamton S. Acute urticaria: etiologies, clinical course and quality of life. Asian Pac J Allergy Immunol 2008;26(1):1–9.

11. Antia C, Baquerizo K, Korman A, Bernstein JA, Alikhan A. Urticaria: a comprehensive review: Epidemiology, diagnosis, and work-up. J Am Acad Dermatol 2018;79(4):599–614.

12. Zuberbier T, Aberer W, Asero R, Latiff AHA, Baker D, Ballmer-Weber B, et al. The EAACI/GA²LEN/ EDF/WAO guideline for the definition, classification, diagnosis and management of urticaria. Allergy 2018;73(7):1393–1414.

13. Sussman G, Hébert J, Gulliver W, Lynde C, Waserman S, Kanani A, et al. Insights and advances in chronic urticaria: a Canadian perspective. Allergy Asthma Clin Immunol 2015;11(1):7.

14. Uguz F, Engin B, Yilmaz E. Axis I and Axis II diagnoses in patients with chronic idiopathic urticaria. J Psychosom Res 2008;64(2):225–9.

15. Staubach P, Eckhardt-Henn A, Dechene M, Vonend A, Metz M, Magerl M, et al. Quality of life in patients with chronic urticaria is differentially impaired and determined by psychiatric comorbidity. Br J Dermatol 2006;154(2):294–8.

16. Ben-Shoshan M, Blinderman I, Raz A. Psychosocial factors and chronic spontaneous urticaria: a systematic review. Allergy 2013;68(2):131–41.

17. Liutu M, Kalimo K, Uksila J, Kalimo H. Etiologic aspects of chronic urticaria. Int J Dermatol 1998;37(7):515–9.

18. Malanin G, Kalimo K. The results of skin testing with food additives and the effect of an elimination diet in chronic and recurrent urticaria and recurrent angioedema. Clin Exp Allergy J Br Soc Allergy ClinImmunol 1989;19(5):539–43.

19. Zuberbier T, Chantraine-Hess S, Hartmann K, Czarnetzki BM. Pseudoallergen-free diet in the treatment of chronic urticaria. A prospective study. Acta Derm Venereol 1995;75(6):484–7.

20. Magerl M, Pisarevskaja D, Scheufele R, Zuberbier T, Maurer M. Effects of a pseudoallergen-free diet on chronic spontaneous urticaria: a prospective trial. Allergy 2010;65(1):78–83.

21. Di Lorenzo G, Pacor ML, Mansueto P, Martinelli N, Esposito-Pellitteri M, Lo Bianco C, et al. Food-additive-induced urticaria: a survey of 838 patients with recurrent chronic idiopathic urticaria. Int Arch Allergy Immunol 2005;138(3):235–42.

22. Tan EKH, Grattan CEH. Drug-induced urticaria. Expert Opin Drug Saf 2004;3(5):471–84.

23. Nielsen EW, Gramstad S. Angioedema from angiotensin-converting enzyme (ACE) inhibitor treated with complement 1 (C1) inhibitor concentrate. Acta Anaesthesiol Scand 2006;50(1):120–2.

24. Scalese MJ, Reinaker TS. Pharmacologic management of angioedema induced by angiotensin-converting enzyme inhibitors. Am J Health-Syst Pharm AJHP Off J Am Soc Health-Syst Pharm 2016;73(12):873–9.

25. Maurer M, BindslevJensen C, Gimenez-Arnau A, Godse K, Grattan CEM, Hide M, et al. Chronic idiopathic urticaria (CIU) is no longer idiopathic: time for an update. Br J Dermatol 2013;168(2):455–6.

26. Bernstein JA, Lang DM, Khan DA, Craig T, Dreyfus D, Hsieh F, et al. The diagnosis and management of acute and chronic urticaria: 2014 update. J Allergy Clin Immunol 2014;133(5):1270–7.e66.

27. Bhute D, Doshi B, Pande S, Mahajan S, Kharkar V. Dermatographism. Indian J Dermatol Venereol Leprol 2008;74(2):177.

28. Nobles T, Schmieder GJ. Dermatographism [Internet]. In: StatPearls. Treasure Island (FL): StatPearls Publishing; 2019 [cited 2019 Jun 30]. Available from: http://www.ncbi.nlm.nih.gov/books/NBK531496/

29. Shelley W, Shelley ED. Adrenergic urticaria: a new form of stress-induced hives. The Lancet 1985;326(8463):1031–3.

30. Antia C, Baquerizo K, Korman A, Bernstein JA, Alikhan A. Urticaria: a comprehensive review. J Am Acad Dermatol 2018;79(4):599–614.

31. Mandel VD, Alicandro T, Pepe P, Bonzano L, Guanti MB, Andreone P, Pellacani G Chronic spontaneous urticaria: a review of pathological mechanisms, diagnosis, clinical management, and treatment. Eur. Med. J 2020 [cited 2020 Oct 27]. Available from: https://www.emjreviews.com/dermatology/article/editors-pick-chronic-spontaneous-urticaria-a-review-of-pathological-mechanisms-diagnosis-clinical-management-and-treatment/

32. Fine LM, Bernstein JA. Guideline of chronic urticaria beyond. Allergy Asthma Immunol Res 2016;8(5):396–403.

33. Schoepke N, Doumoulakis G, Maurer M. Diagnosis of urticaria. Indian J Dermatol 2013;58(3):211–8.

34. Deacock SJ. An approach to the patient with urticaria. Clin Exp Immunol 2008;153(2):151–61.

35. Siebenhaar F, Staubach P, Metz M, Magerl M, Jung J, Maurer M. Peltier effect–based temperature challenge: an improved method for diagnosing cold urticaria. J Allergy Clin Immunol 2004;114(5):1224–5.

36. Siebenhaar F, Weller K, Mlynek A, Magerl M, Altrichter S, Santos RV dos, et al. Acquired cold urticaria: clinical picture and update on diagnosis and treatment. Clin Exp Dermatol 2007;32(3):241–5.

37. Chong W-S, Khoo S-W. Solar urticaria in Singapore: an uncommon photodermatosis seen in a tertiary dermatology center over a 10-year period. Photodermatol Photoimmunol Photomed 2004;20(2):101–4.

38. Güzelbey O, Ardelean E, Magerl M, Zuberbier T, Maurer M, Metz M. Successful treatment of solar urticaria with anti-immunoglobulin E therapy. Allergy 2008;63(11):1563–5.

39. Wakelin SH. Contact urticaria. Clin Exp Dermatol 2001;26(2):132–6.

40. Gimenez-Arnau A, Maurer M, De La Cuadra J, Maibach H. Immediate contact skin reactions, an update of contact urticaria, contact urticaria syndrome and protein contact dermatitis – "A Never Ending Story." Eur J Dermatol 2010;20(5):552–62.

41. Black AK, Sibbald RG, Greaves MW. Cold urticaria treated by induction of tolerance. Lancet Lond Engl 1979;2(8149):964.

42. von Mackensen YA, Sticherling M. Cold urticaria: tolerance induction with cold baths. Br J Dermatol 2007;157(4):835–6.

43. Tannert LK, Skov PS, Jensen LB, Maurer M, Bindslev-Jensen C. Cold urticaria patients exhibit normal skin levels of functional mast cells and histamine after tolerance induction. Dermatology 2012;224(2):101–5.

44. Siebenhaar F, Degener F, Zuberbier T, Martus P, Maurer M. High-dose desloratadine decreases wheal volume and improves cold provocation thresholds compared with standard-dose treatment in patients with acquired cold urticaria: a randomized, placebo-controlled, crossover study. J Allergy Clin Immunol 2009;123(3):672–9.

45. Krause K, Spohr A, Zuberbier T, Church MK, Maurer M. Up-dosing with bilastine results in improved effectiveness in cold contact urticaria. Allergy 2013;68(7):921–8.

46. Metz M, Altrichter S, Ardelean E, Kessler B, Krause K, Magerl M, et al. Anti-immunoglobulin E treatment of patients with recalcitrant physical urticaria. Int Arch Allergy Immunol 2011;154(2):177–80.

47. Metz M, Ohanyan T, Church MK, Maurer M. Omalizumab is an effective and rapidly acting therapy in difficult-to-treat chronic urticaria: a retrospective clinical analysis. J Dermatol Sci 2014;73(1):57–62.

48. Le Moing A, Bécourt C, Pape E, Dejobert Y, Delaporte E, Staumont-Sallé D. Effective treatment of idiopathic chronic cold urticaria with omalizumab: report of 3 cases. J Am Acad Dermatol 2013;69(2):e99–101.

49. Marsland AM, Beck MH. Cold urticaria responding to systemic ciclosporin. Br J Dermatol 2003;149(1):214–5.

50. Gualdi G, Monari P, Rossi MT, Crotti S, Calzavara-Pinton PG. Successful treatment of systemic cold contact urticaria with etanercept in a patient with psoriasis. Br J Dermatol 2012;166(6):1373–4.

51. Maurer M, Altrichter S, Metz M, Zuberbier T, Church MK, Bergmann K-C. Benefit from reslizumab treatment in a patient with chronic spontaneous urticaria and cold urticaria. J Eur Acad Dermatol Venereol JEADV 2018;32(3):e112–3.

52. Bonadonna P, Lombardi C, Senna G, Walter Canonica GW, Passalacqua, G. Treatment of acquired cold urticaria with cetirizine and zafirlukast in combination. J Am Acad Dermatol. 2003 Oct;49(4):714-6. PubMed

53. Botto NC, Warshaw EM. Solar urticaria. J Am Acad Dermatol 2008;59(6):909–20.

54. Hughes R, Cusack C, Murphy GM, Kirby B. Solar urticaria successfully treated with intravenous immunoglobulin. Clin Exp Dermatol 2009;34(8):e660–2.

55. Lawlor F, Black AK, Breathnach AS, Greaves MW. Vibratory angioedema: lesion induction, clinical features, laboratory and ultrastructural findings and response to therapy. Br J Dermatol 1989;120(1):93–9.

56. Ting S, Reimann BE, Rauls DO, Mansfield LE. Nonfamilial, vibration-induced angioedema. J Allergy Clin Immunol 1983;71(6):546–51.

57. Rothbaum R, McGee JS. Aquagenicurticaria: diagnostic and management challenges. J Asthma Allergy 2016;9:209–13.

58. Pawar H, Kanichai Francis N. Aquagenic urticaria: a review of literature and case reports. J Turk Acad Dermatol 2014;8.

59. Irwin RB, Lieberman P, Friedman MM, Kaliner M, Kaplan R, Bale G, et al. Mediator release in local heat urticaria: protection with combined H1 and H2 antagonists. J Allergy Clin Immunol 1985;76(1):35–9.

60. Daman L, Lieberman P, Ganier M, Hashimoto K. Localized heat urticaria. J Allergy Clin Immunol 1978;61(4):273–8.

61. Feinberg JH, Toner CB. Successful treatment of disabling cholinergic urticaria. Mil Med 2008;173(2):217–20.

62. Kobza-Black A. Delayed pressure urticaria. J Investig Dermatol Symp Proc 2001;6(2):148–9.

63. Brewer DD. A systematic review of autohemotherapy as a treatment for urticaria and eczema. Cureus [Internet] 2014; 6(12) [cited 2020 Oct 27] Available from: https://www.cureus.com/articles/2722-a-systematic-review-of-autohemotherapy-as-a-treatment-for-urticaria-and-eczema

5 Hereditary Angioedema

Sailal Mohanlal

CONTENTS

INTRODUCTION

Angioedema is the swelling of deep dermis, subcutaneous, or submucosal tissue due to vascular leakage. Angioedema can occur with or without urticaria. Urticaria or hives presents as transient pruritic wheals with pale, central swelling and surrounding epidermal erythema anywhere in the body. Urticaria is of varying size and resolves within 24–48 hours without scarring.

Angioedema may be classified into histamine-mediated and non-histamine-mediated angioedema. Histamine-mediated angioedema can be allergic, pseudo allergic or idiopathic. Non-histamine mediated angioedema is largely driven by bradykinin and can be hereditary, acquired or drug-induced, such as with angiotensin-converting enzyme inhibitors.[1]

Hereditary angioedema (HAE) is associated with recurrent episodes of angioedema, without urticaria or pruritus, affecting the skin or mucosa of the respiratory and gastrointestinal tract. Though self-limited and resolving within 2–5 days, laryngeal angioedema if present may cause asphyxia and even death.

The prevalence of HAE is estimated at approximately 1 individual per 60,000.[2] There are no sex or ethnicity predilections. Forty percent of attacks occur before 5 years of age: frequency of attacks may increase after puberty. Prior to availability of effective therapy, mortality was around 30% due to laryngeal oedema.

CLINICAL FEATURES

Many subjects have prodromal symptoms including fatigue, nausea, myalgia and flu-like symptoms. Dermatological manifestation may include serpentine, mottled, and or "chicken-wire" pattern of erythematous discolouration and erythema marginatum. Face, genitals and extremities are most commonly affected. Angioedema may be painful, non-pruritic, nondependent and non-pitting. An episode usually starts with tingling or sensation of fullness and irritation followed by swelling and a sense of tightness over the next 2–3 hours, peaking by 24 hours and subsiding by about 48–72 hours.

UPPER AIRWAY ATTACKS

Laryngeal oedema alone or associated swelling of the lips, tongue, uvula, and soft palate can occur. Prodromal symptoms may include sore, scratchy, or itchy throat, sensation of tightness or lump in the throat, dysphagia, voice changes such as hoarseness or roughness of voice, and "barky" cough. Laryngeal attacks wane over period of time and is less common above 45 years.

GASTROINTESTINAL SYMPTOMS

This may include abdominal colic, nausea, vomiting and diarrhoea. Symptoms are due to bowel wall oedema.

DOI: 10.1201/9781003125785-5

Suspicion of angioedema arises with:

1. Recurrent episodes of angioedema **without urticaria** or pruritus, lasting 2–5 days (without treatment)

2. Unexplained recurrent episodes of self-limited, colicky, abdominal pain with or without cutaneous angioedema

3. Unexplained laryngeal oedema

4. Angioedema in the absence of angiotensin-converting enzyme (ACE) inhibitors, nonsteroidal anti-inflammatory drugs (NSAIDs), or allergic triggers

5. Family history of angioedema

6. Low complement component 4 (C4) level in a patient with angioedema

Most angioedema patients might have received multiple courses of antihistamine and corticosteroids. A trial of non-sedating antihistamines at higher doses, 2–4 times the usual doses, or in combination is usually performed to differentiate the condition from histaminergic acquired angioedema.

PATHOGENESIS

Bradykinin-mediated increased vascular permeability—unlike a histamine-mediated allergic reaction—plays the major role in hereditary angioedema (HAE). Serum bradykinin levels are up to 7 times normal values, and the lack of response to antihistamines distinguishes it from urticaria (Figure 5.1).

There are three recognised types of hereditary angioedema (see Table 5.1).[3]

C1-inhibitor (C1-INH) is a serine protease inhibitor for multiple steps in the classical and lectin complement pathways, intrinsic coagulation, fibrinolytic pathways and kinin generating pathways. Deficient C1-INH causes elevated bradykinin. C1-INH normally plays a role in limiting bradykinin production by inhibiting both kallikrein and active factor XII. C1-INH deficiency or dysfunction causes low C4 because the C1 complex normally cleaves C4 as part of the classical complement pathway. Low C4 level is a sensitive screening tool for C1-INH deficiency. The C1-INH gene is located in the long arm of chromosome 11.[4] Predominantly an autosomal dominant disease, 25% of cases are due to de novo mutations.

INVESTIGATION

Low complement levels were tested 1 month apart. Low C1-INH protein levels are the foundation for diagnosing HAE. However, associated urticaria, response to antihistamine

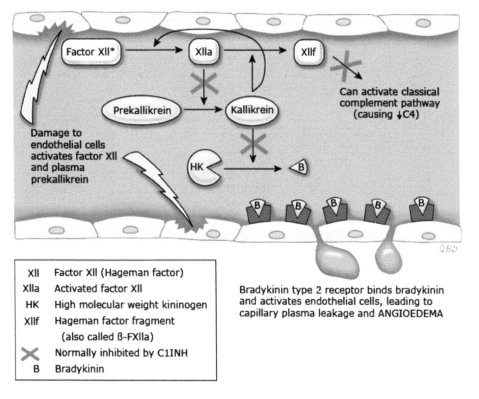

XII	Factor XII (Hageman factor)
XIIa	Activated factor XII
HK	High molecular weight kininogen
XIIf	Hageman factor fragment (also called β-FXIIa)
✕	Normally inhibited by C1INH
B	Bradykinin

Bradykinin type 2 receptor binds bradykinin and activates endothelial cells, leading to capillary plasma leakage and ANGIOEDEMA

Figure 5.1 Pathogenesis of angioedema.[5,6]

Table 5.1: Types of Hereditary Angioedema

Type of Hereditary Angioedema	Prevalence	Characteristics
Type 1	Constitutes 85% (most common)	Deficient C1-INH with less than 30% of normal. Genetic mutation of SERPING1 gene
Type 2	Constitutes 15%	Dysfunctional C1-INH with normal or elevated C1-INH, but low activity
Type 3	Constitutes <1%	Normal C1-INH and complement levels, probable variants in factor XII, gene for angiopoietin-1 (*ANGPT1*), gene for plasminogen. It is a diagnosis of exclusion and may require trial of high dose antihistamines

Source: Cicardi M et al.

and normal C1-INH make the diagnosis unlikely. If the likelihood is low, C4 level is used as a screening test; if this is inconclusive, further testing with C1-INH is warranted. Some patients may have hypergammaglobulinemia. An algorithm for the diagnosis of HAE is given in Figure 5.2.

Complement studies are prone to errors. Fresh or frozen serum that is less than 4 hours' old should be tested. Testing C4 and C1-INH protein levels are more reliable than C1-INH function. A C4 level <50% or <10 mg is pathological. A strong family history influences the decision making.

DIFFERENTIAL DIAGNOSIS

1. Acute and chronic urticaria, anaphylactic reactions

   Acuteness of onset, presence of trigger factors like aeroallergens, food allergens, drugs, insect bite provide vital clues, Evaluation for tryptase levels may be done after stabilisation, in case of laryngeal oedema or anaphylaxis

2. Allergic contact dermatitis

   Associated triggers, presence of microvesiculation in skin with deep erythema provides insight to this condition. Patch test may be useful.

3. Idiopathic angioedema

4. Drug-induced angioedema

   NSAIDs and ACEI are well known to cause angioedema. A proper drug history is vital.

5. Connective tissue disorders

   Many of the autoimmune diseases like SLE, scleroderma, and polymyositis may show low complement and oedema.

6. Acquired angioedema

   This is seen in B cell lymphoproliferative disorders in some patients is seen in older patients.

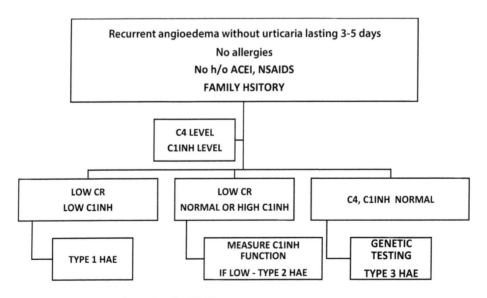

Figure 5.2 Diagnostic algorithm for HAE.

ACUTE TREATMENT

Laryngeal oedema may be experienced by 50% of susceptible individuals and this may be life threatening. Cutaneous and gastrointestinal manifestations are more common. Angioedema in HAE does not respond to antihistamine, corticosteroids or epinephrine. In case of laryngeal oedema, priority would be in stabilising the airways.

First-Line Therapies

1. Plasma-derived C1-INH concentrate (pdC1-INH)

2. Recombinant human C1-INH synthetic bradykinin B-receptor antagonist, Ecallantide, which is a recombinant plasma kallikrein inhibitor

Second-Line Therapies

1. Solvent/detergent-treated plasma (lower risk of transmission of infectious diseases)

2. Fresh frozen plasma

ACUTE LARYNGEAL ANGIOEDEMA

Intubation and airway management may be difficult due to distorted anatomy. Cricothyroidotomy and tracheostomy may be required in some cases. C1 inhibitors like icatibant or ecallantide should be administered as early as possible in the attack.

Icatibant and ecallantide may be given subcutaneously. Gastrointestinal symptoms are managed more with supportive care. Plasma can be administered. Butyl scopolamine, metoclopramide, or prochlorperazine can be helpful for cramping, nausea and vomiting. Cutaneous attacks are managed based on location of involvement, duration of attack and number of sites.

Human plasma, referred to as plasma-derived C1-INH or pdC1-INH is administered intravenously as the preferred treatment for an acute attack as a slow infusion. In few cases (1%) patients may require a second dose. Adverse events may include headache or infectious disease transmission. Recombinant human C1-INH (rhC1-INH) has a similar protease inhibitory activity but a shorter half-life. The dose is 50 units/kg with maximum of 4200 units. Ecallantide is a genetically engineered recombinant plasma kallikrein inhibitor that is a first-line acute therapy for laryngeal angioedema and gastrointestinal attacks. The adult dose is 30 mg.[7]

PROPHYLAXIS

Short-term prophylaxis is used before invasive procedures, and long-term prophylaxis involves regular administration for maintaining an acceptable quality of life. Planned action is needed to educate the patient, test family members, identify and avoid possible triggers, and manage HAE attacks.

EDUCATION

Education should focus on triggers, risk factors, and the early treatment of HAE attacks. The genetics of HAE and the need for testing family members has to be stressed. Treatment options should be discussed.

TESTING OF FAMILY MEMBERS

With autosomal dominant inheritance and variable penetrance, 50% of first-degree relatives may have an abnormal gene, but remain asymptomatic. Mortality has been shown to be lower with crisis management and when asymptomatic relatives have been previously warned.

AVOIDANCE OF TRIGGERS

Usual triggers include drugs like estrogen, ACE inhibitors, trauma, dental and oral infections.

CONCLUSION

Angioedema is the swelling of deep dermis, subcutaneous, or submucosal tissue due to vascular leakage. Angioedema may be classified into histamine-mediated and non-histamine-mediated angioedema. Histamine-mediated angioedema can be allergic, pseudo allergic or idiopathic. Bradykinin mediated increased vascular permeability; plays the major role in hereditary angioedema Laryngeal oedema may be experienced by 50% of susceptible individuals and this may be life threatening. Cutaneous and gastrointestinal manifestations are more common. Planned action is needed to educate patient and family members. Education should focus on triggers, risk factor, and the early treatment of HAE attacks. The genetics of HAE and the need for testing family members has to be stressed. Treatment options should be discussed.

REFERENCES

1. Kaplan AP, Joseph K. The bradykinin-forming cascade and its role in hereditary angioedema. Ann Allergy Asthma Immunol. 2010; 104(3):193.

2. Nordenfelt P, Nilsson M, Björkander J, Mallbris L, Lindfors A, Wahlgren CF. Hereditary angioedema in Swedish adults: report from the National Cohort. Acta Derm Venereol. 2016; 96(4):540.

3. Cicardi M, Aberer W, Banerji A, Bas M, Bernstein JA, Bork K, Caballero T, Farkas H, Grumach A, Kaplan AP, Riedl MA, Triggiani M, Zanichelli A, Zuraw B. Classification, diagnosis, and approach to treatment for angioedema: consensus report from the Hereditary Angioedema International Working Group. Allergy. 2014 May; 69(5):602–16. Epub 2014 Mar 27.

4. Pappalardo E, Cicardi M, Duponchel C, Carugati A, Choquet S, Agostoni A, Tosi M. Frequent de novo mutations and exon deletions in the C1inhibitor gene of patients with angioedema. J Allergy Clin Immunol. 2000; 106(6):1147.

5. Morgan PB. Hereditary angioedema—therapies old and new. N Engl J Med. 2010; 363:581.

6. Longhurst H, Cicardi M. Hereditary angio-oedema. Lancet. 2012; 379:474.

7. Bowen T, Cicardi M, Farkas H, Bork K, Longhurst HJ, Zuraw B, Aygoeren-Pürsün E, Craig T, Binkley K, Hebert J, Ritchie B, Bouillet L, Betschel S, Cogar 2010 International consensus algorithm for the diagnosis, therapy and management of hereditary angioedema. Allergy Asthma Clin Immunol. 2010; 6(1):24. Epub 2010 Jul 28.

6 Food Allergy

Mahesh P Anand

CONTENTS

INTRODUCTION

Food Allergy is a potentially life-threatening disease which can involve multiple systems and is due to an abnormal response to exposure to food antigens, usually IgE mediated. Studies have observed an increasing prevalence of food allergy in the world, which is being called the second allergy epidemic (1, 2). The first report of food allergy is believed to have come from Hippocrates, but rapid strides in understanding of food allergy came about after the introduction of double-blind placebo-controlled studies by Charles May nearly five decades ago (2). The highest prevalence has been observed in young children, but now, increasingly, adolescents and young adults also suffer from food allergy (3). Food allergy causes significant morbidity and poor quality of life and occasional mortality and it presents a large public health burden, especially in more developed countries (4). With increasing westernization, the emerging economies are likely to suffer from a greater prevalence of food allergy (3).

Many food allergy cases persist over time, and the prevalence has been gradually increasing in many countries across the globe. Since oral food challenge (OFC) testing is very difficult and time- consuming to perform, there is a lack of findings that have confirmed food allergy in population- based studies except for a few such as Europrevall (5). Population studies have used surrogate markers, such as a strong history and markers of sensitization, such as the skin prick test or serum-specific IgE, which is not as strong as an oral food challenge test (6, 7). Other studies have evaluated emergency room visits for food allergy and food-related anaphylaxis (3). These are not reliable for various reasons; access to medical services may be variable as is patient health seeking behavior, and the population that visits hospitals is not generally representative of the general public (3). Similarly, assessing a self-reported food allergy is not reliable and overestimates actual food allergy by many-fold, since self-reports tend to classify food intolerance or food aversion as food allergy (3). Objective measurements along with history are useful, but it is important to note that a majority (around 50–70%) of the individuals sensitized to serum-specific IgE can consume the foods without any food allergy (8). Therefore, one must be cautious when interpreting food sensitization results.

EPIDEMIOLOGY

The prevalence of food allergy varies with geographical location, ethnicity, level of westernization and type of outcome measures used in the study. It also varies with age, with a higher prevalence among younger children. Overall, the prevalence is between 5–10% in developed countries and around 7% in South Korea and China. The HealthNuts study (8) from Australia observed that an oral challenge

DOI: 10.1201/9781003125785-6

confirmed a food allergy of over 10% in 1-year-old children. The highest percentage was to eggs at 8.8%, followed by peanuts at 3%. A milk food challenge was not performed. Another Australian study observed a food allergy (without oral food challenge confirmation) prevalence of 1.3% in adults 20–45 years of age. Prawn (0.9%) and peanut (0.4%) were common culprits. The self-reported prevalence of food allergy in adults is around 4–5%, but again this is likely to be an overestimation. In a period of 10 years, anaphylaxis related to food leading to hospital admission in the United States doubled (9), while a >60% increase was observed in New Zealand (3). In less than 15 years, there was a 4-fold increase (from 2–8.2 per lakh population) in food related anaphylaxis in Australia, which was the highest increase over time reported in the world (10). The highest rates were observed in the young 0–4-year-old children where an increase from 7.3 to 30.2 per lakh population was observed (10). Ethnicity plays an important factor in the prevalence of food allergy. In an Australian study, East Asian children had higher food allergy than Caucasian children (11). Food allergy has been increasing over time in countries such as China, where over a 10-year period the prevalence increased from 3.5% to 7.7% (12).

DEFINITIONS

Various definitions (12–15) are needed for clinical characterization and to understand the therapeutic effect of various interventions. The EAACI guideline on allergen immunotherapy for food allergy is a detailed document evaluating the current evidence of the role of various allergen immunotherapies for foods.

Food allergy is defined as an adverse reaction to foods mediated by an immunologic mechanism involving specific-IgE, cell-mediated or mixed mechanisms. It is a specific immune response that occurs reproducibly to any given food. The dose of food allergen that can cause a food allergic reaction can be varied and sometimes very small. It generally involves the skin, GIT or the respiratory tract.

Sensitization is defined as having detectable IgE antibodies by a skin prick test or serum-specific IgE. If a person is sensitized to an allergen, it does not confirm clinical reactivity. Sensitization is known as an 'intermediate phenotype' in the course of allergic diseases. A genetically predisposed person, during the course of their life, becomes initially sensitized to allergens and may develop clinical reactivity later. Not all sensitized subjects develop clinical reactivity in their lifetime. It is not clear yet how many of the food allergen life time sensitized subjects develop clinical food allergy in their lifetime.

Class I food allergen is defined as those allergens that cause sensitization to proteins that are resistant to digestion and heat (cooking). Sensitization occurs through the gastrointestinal tract. These food allergens retain their conformational identity.

Class II food allergens are defined as those allergens that cause reactions due to cross-reactivity to aeroallergens to which the subject has been previously sensitized.

Food intolerance is an adverse reaction to a food, food additive, beverage or compound present in foods that produces untoward symptoms in any of the organ systems. It is generally non-IgE mediated and can be delayed.

Pseudo food allergy is similar to food allergy but is due to very different causes as compared to the IgE-mediated food allergy. For example, food rich in histamines (egg plant, certain fish and shellfish) can incite similar clinical symptoms on consumption.

Oral allergy syndrome (OAS) is an adverse reaction limited to the oral mucosa, tongue and throat to raw foods due to previous sensitization to aeroallergens such as pollens. Most of these patients have co-existent allergic rhinitis. It is also known as pollen-food allergy syndrome (PFAS).

Allergen immunotherapy is defined as the introduction of repeated allergen exposure of known quantities by the sub-cutaneous, sub-lingual or oral routes at regular intervals to modulate the immune response. This modulation of the immune response results in decreased symptoms and reduced medication requirements and prevents the development of new allergies.

Desensitization is an increase in the threshold at which a person reacts to the food allergen when the subject is receiving food allergen immunotherapy. It includes situations where the subject is protected from accidental ingestion. It is limited for use only during the course of allergen immunotherapy and requires months of allergen immunotherapy to achieve desensitization.

Remission is a temporary state of non-responsiveness to the food allergen in which the subject is not on immunotherapy currently, but has completed allergen immunotherapy. There is no clinical reaction on exposure to the food allergen.

Oral tolerance is an absent clinical reactivity to the food allergen and is due to natural occurrence rather than as a result of treatment with an allergen immunotherapy. It does not need continued exposure to the food allergen to continue the non-responsive state.

Sustained un-responsiveness is an absence of clinical reaction to foods after discontinuing immunotherapy. Many years of allergen immunotherapy are necessary to achieve this clinical state. The subject may need to continue the exposure to foods to maintain the non-responsive state, similar to how aspirin desensitization is maintained with continued exposure.

PATHOGENESIS

Risk Factors

The key risk factors for the development of food allergy are genetic and environmental, and gene-environment interactions leading to epigenetic changes that influence the onset of food allergy. Studies have observed that siblings of a child with food allergy have a higher risk of food allergy than the general population (16). Peanut allergy-specific loci were observed in the HLA-DR and HLA-DQ gene regions (17). Epigenetic studies on DNA methylation observed associations with genes involved in the Th2 pathways; *IL1RL1, IL5RA, STAT4, IL4* and CCL18 (18).

The environmental risk factors have been classified into a different hypothesis (19) (Figure 6.1), which has evolved over time. It is still not clear which of them are more important than others, as the evidence for each of them is still evolving. The oldest hypothesis is the 'Hygiene hypothesis' first postulated by Strachan for respiratory allergies. It is also called 'Microbial exposure hypothesis' or 'Old friends hypothesis' This postulates that reduced exposure to the microbes which are harmless and potentially useful to us due to excessive cleanliness, sterilization and disinfection leads to altered immune regulatory responses such as allergies. It is important to learn that out of all the cells in the human body, only 10% are human cells and the rest are bacterial cells! The highest concentrations of these are present in the gut. How these bacteria affect the human cells, 'switching on' and 'switching off' certain genes are the subjects of meta-genomics. Unlike asthma, there is limited evidence regarding 'Hygiene hypothesis' and food allergy. Prebiotics and probiotics have not shown to reduce or prevent food allergy. It is my suspicion that it is unlikely to create an impact. The gut microbiome is a colony of a very large number of bacteria which needs to be very diverse for it to be the most beneficial to the host. Attempting to replenish it with only 1 group of bacteria is unlikely to work. Imagine a city full of only 1 profession; for example, a city in which all the citizens are doctors. The city is unlikely to thrive! Similarly, the diverse bacteria support one another and are critical for their proposed immunomodulatory effect. The evidence that delivery by caesarean section or taking antibiotics in the first year of life increases food allergy is limited. Few studies of gut microbiome have yielded any conclusive evidence that changes in the microbiota increase the risk of food allergy. Unlike in asthma, pet exposure is not seen to be protective against food allergy.

The other hypotheses include 'Dual allergen exposure hypothesis', 'Allergen avoidance hypothesis' and the 'Nutritional immunomodulation hypothesis'. The 'Dual allergen exposure hypothesis' (19) suggests that exposure to the allergen via the skin, especially when the skin barrier is affected—as in atopic

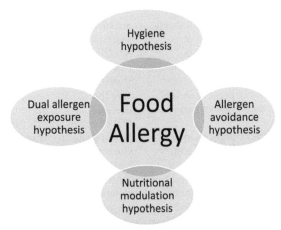

Figure 6.1 Various hypotheses for the development of food allergy.

dermatitis—overrides the tolerance developed due to oral exposure. There is a fairly strong evidence now that the early introduction of foods such as peanuts prevents food allergy to peanuts in high risk children (Leap Study). If the allergenic food is introduced late, does it increase the risk of food allergy? The evidence here is not that strong. The 'Allergy avoidance hypothesis' (19) suggests that early avoidance of allergens, for example in the maternal diet avoiding peanuts, may reduce peanut allergy in the offspring. However, the evidence is limited for recommendation to avoid food allergens in the maternal diet as a routine measure to prevent food allergy in children. Evidence regarding the use of hypoallergenic infant formula which contains partial or extensively hydrolyzed proteins to reduce the risk of food allergy is also not encouraging. The 'Nutritional immunomodulation hypothesis' (19) suggests that certain foods in the maternal diet or early childhood could help reduce the risk of food allergy. The foods studied include anti-oxidants, folate, omega 3 fatty acids and vitamin D. There is no good evidence that any of them are useful in reducing the incidence of food allergy in children.

The barrier function of the skin and intestinal epithelium is critical for the development of tolerance or sensitization. This epithelium performs the key barrier functions for the entry of the allergens. Epithelium is also responsible for the secretion of several important cytokines that are critical for the development of food allergy such as Thymic Stromal Lymphopoietin (TSLP), IL-25 and IL-33 commonly called alarmins. Epithelial dysregulation is critical for the development of food allergy and gene mutations and polymorphisms in barrier relevant genes filaggrin, SPINK5 and SERPINB7 are linked to food allergy. The key factors maintaining skin barrier integrity are the genetic mutations, immune responses such as an increase in type 2 cytokines, impaired keratinocytes, skin microbiome and use of detergents. Skin is an important route for sensitization to food allergens which are commonly present in the house dust that a child comes regularly in contact with.

Many children outgrow food allergies to some foods such as wheat, egg, milk and soy, but allergies to peanuts, seafood and tree nuts are generally life-long. Studies have observed a differential immunologic response in children who outgrow their allergies to common food allergens such as milk and egg. Mapping of the allergenic epitopes, the areas that the subject's IgE binds to help us to understand the immunologic

reasons for these differences (2). Children who continued to have persistent food allergies had IgE antibodies to sequential linear epitopes, while children who outgrew their allergies had IgE antibodies to conformational epitopes that are important for the 3-dimensional structure (2). Further, studies observed that subjects whose IgE binds to several different allergenic epitopes were more likely to have more severe reactions, as compared to subjects whose IgE could bind to fewer allergenic epitopes (20, 21).

CROSS-REACTIVE FOOD ALLERGENS AND ORAL ALLERGY SYNDROME

It is very important to consider cross-reactive food allergens when evaluating a patient with food allergy (19). One of the most common food allergens in the world is peanut, which cross reacts with other legumes, but the risk is low at 5%. The cross-reactivity of tree nuts is higher with other tree nuts at 35%. The risk is even higher than 35% for walnut with pecan and cashew nuts with pistachio. Cross-reactivity between cow's milk and goat and sheep milk is the highest among all foods and is greater than 90%. However, cow's milk has only a 5% cross-reactivity with mare's milk and a 10% cross-reactivity with beef. Other foods with high cross-reactivity include shellfish with other shellfish (75%) and fish with other fish (50%). Grains have lower cross-reactivity with other grains (20%). The key reason for cross-reactivity is that the IgE binds to other homologous proteins in other foods or pollens (oral allergy syndrome). Foods also cross react with aeroallergens, and many of these are known to cause the oral allergy syndrome. Grasses cross react with apples, peaches and tomatoes; some weeds cross react to bananas, kiwis, peaches and melons and trees such as birch to nuts, vegetables and fruits.

Cross-reactivity between food and aeroallergens is well known. It was first described in 1942 and defined as oral allergy syndrome in 1987 (15). The prevalence of OAS is around 10% of children with allergic diseases. Studies focused on pollen allergic individuals note that 20–70% of subjects with pollen allergies have experienced OAS. It is seen in 45% of subjects with seasonal allergies and 34% of subjects with eosinophilic esophagitis (15). The most common symptoms of OAS are oral and pharyngeal itching on consumption of food, especially raw food. Most of these patients tolerate the same food when it is cooked. Tightness in the throat, ear or nasal itching, change in voice and nausea are common. Rarer manifestations include systemic symptoms (3%) and anaphylaxis

Table 6.1: Cross-Reactive Food Allergens with Other Pollens for the Oral Allergy Syndrome

Profilin Family		Lipid Transfer Proteins		PR-10 Family	
Aeroallergens	Food Allergens	Aeroallergens	Food Allergens	Aeroallergens	Food Allergens
Bermuda grass (Cyn d 12)	Almond (Pru du 4)	Artemesia (Art v 3)	Almond (Pru du 3)	Alder (Aln g 1)	Carrot (Dau c 1)
Prosopis (Pro j 2)	Apple (Mal d 4)	Latex (Hev b 12)	Apple (Mal d 3)	Birch (Bet v 1)	Apple (Mal d 1)
Artemesia (Art v 4)	Banana (Mus a 1)	Ragweed (Amb a 6)	Banana (Mus a 3)	White Oak (Que a 1)	Chest nut (Cas s 1)
Amaranthus (Ama r 2)	Celery (Api g 4)		Celery (Api g 2,6)		Celery (Api g 1)
Timothy grass (Phl p 12)	Hazelnut (Cor a 2)		Hazelnut (Cor a 8)		Hazelnut (Cor a 1)
	Orange (Cit s 2)		Orange (Cit s 3)		Walnut (Jug r 5)
	Pineapple (Ana c 1)		Pomegranate (Pun g 1)		Raspberry (Rub i 1)
	Strawberry (Fra a 4)		Strawberry (Fra a 3)		Strawberry (Fra a 1)
	Tomato (Sola l 1)		Tomato (Sola l 3,6,7)		Tomato (Sola l 4)
	Watermelon (Citr l 2)		Lentil (Len c 3)		Soybean (Gly m 4)

(1.7%) (15). Upon physical examination, swelling of the pharyngeal mucosa, uvula, periorbital region and urticaria in the perioral region have been described. Rarely, subjects will present with wheezing, dyspnea and low blood pressure. Foods that cross react with pollens and are associated with systemic reactions, include celery, lentils, tomato, peach, plum, almond and apricots (15).

More than 60% of food allergens derived from plant sources belong to 1 of the 3 protein super-families. These include the pathogenesis-related (PR) family, Cupin family and the Prolamin family, which is further subdivided into lipid transfer proteins (LTP) and the 2S albumin sub-families (15). LTPs are present in many plant sources and are one of the 'pan-allergens' due to their ubiquitous nature. LTPs are generally resistant to both heat and digestion and retain their conformational structure as to elicit an IgE reaction, even after heating at 90°C for 20 minutes (example, Mal d 3 from apple) (15). LTPs can cross react with one another and are known to elicit severe food allergy reactions. Some common LTPs include Mal d 3 (apple), Pru p 3 (Peach), Gly m 1 (soy), Jug r 3 (walnut), Ara h 9 (peanut) and Tri a 14 (wheat) (15). LTPs cross react with aeroallergens and examples can be found in Table 6.1. The PR family is very important for oral allergy syndrome. These pathogen-related proteins were evolutionarily developed to protect the plants against invasion by pathogens. These are important Class II allergens and have significant cross-reactivity with aeroallergens.

These proteins are heat and digestion labile unlike LTPs. Some common examples include, Mal d 1 (apple), Api g 1 (celery), Ara h 8 (peanut). Gly m 4 (soy) and examples of cross-reactivity can be found in Table 6.1. Profilins are also called pan-allergens due to their ubiquitous nature and are also labile and easily denatured due to heat and digestion. Both PR-10 proteins and profilins therefore most commonly cause the oral allergy syndrome, especially when foods are consumed raw and are less associated with very severe reactions unlike the LTPs. Some examples of Profilins include Ana c 1 (pineapple), Ara h 5 (peanut) and Dau c 4 (carrot). Their cross-reactivity to aeroallergens are listed in Table 6.1. The 2S families are important food allergens, but no cross-reactivity to aeroallergens have been demonstrated as yet. Similarly, for the Cupin family, mainly in terms of the 7S and 11S food allergens (the seed storage proteins), no cross-reactivity to aeroallergens has been yet identified.

CLINICAL FEATURES

The clinical features of food allergic reactions are quite varied. It depends on whether they are purely IgE mediated, mixed IgE and non-IgE mediated or purely non-IgE mediated or cellular reactions (2). The common presentations of IgE mediated food allergic reactions are urticaria, angioedema, itching and flushing involving the skin, cough, wheezing, bronchitis, dyspnea, chest tightness, hoarseness, laryngeal edema, rhinitis, nasal congestion, sneezing, conjunctivitis and periorbital edema involving the eyes and respiratory tract, oral allergy syndrome with itching or even swelling of the lips, tongue and palate, acute gastrointestinal spasm with colicky abdominal pain, diarrhea, nausea, vomiting, involving the GIT, dizziness, fainting, palpitations, hypertension, hypotension, anaphylaxis, food associated exercise-induced anaphylaxis involving the cardiovascular system and others such as uterine cramping and contractions, metallic taste, anxiety, feeling of doom or death. The clinical presentations of mixed IgE and non-IgE food allergic reactions include atopic dermatitis, asthma, eosinophilic esophagitis, eosinophilic gastritis, eosinophilic gastroenteritis. Cellular, or purely non-IgE mediated, reactions include celiac disease, food protein–induced procto-colitis syndrome, food protein–induced entero-colitis syndrome, food protein–induced enteropathy syndrome, food protein–induced pulmonary hemosiderosis (Heiner's syndrome), contact dermatitis and dermatitis herpetiformis.

DIAGNOSIS

The most important diagnostic tools for evaluating food allergy are a detailed history, skin prick testing to the relevant allergens and serum-specific IgE. Component resolved diagnostics are useful but not easily available

in most parts of the world. The gold standard test for the diagnosis of food allergy remains the double-blind placebo-controlled challenge (DBPCFC) test. The key points to be noted in the history are listed in Table 6.2. A correlation between history and the investigations such as SPT and serum-specific IgE (ssIgE) are critical for the correct identification of the offending allergen. It is common for patients to relate their symptoms to food allergy, but when questioned in detail, it becomes quite likely that the symptoms are not related to the food. It is useful to select the antigens for testing both for the SPT as well as ssIgE based on the history, rather than using a large standard panel for testing.

Skin Prick testing is the most common and accepted screening test for food allergy. It is easily performed as an outpatient procedure and results are immediately available. It is less expensive and technically demanding as compared to a ssIgE. Skin prick testing is always preferred over ssIgE unless there are absolute contraindications for SPT, such as anaphylaxis or the unavailability of normal skin, among others. The reason for this is that, SPT is considered as 2 tests in 1. To get the same information in a ssIgE test, we need to have both the measurements of the ssIgE and the basophil histamine release

Table 6.2: Relevant Points in the Diagnosis (History Taking, Skin Prick Testing and Serum-Specific IgE) in Food Allergy

History

Timing	Most food allergies occur within 2 hours of consumption. Severe food allergies are generally seen within 30 minutes. The most severe allergies may occur in minutes after consumption.
Exposure	Most food allergies occur after consuming the food. Some subjects may complain of itching in the hands when they touch the raw food before cooking. Very severe allergic subjects will complain of severe symptoms, including anaphylaxis, even on inhaling the food particles, though they have not consumed the food themselves (example, a friend has opened a bag of peanuts near them)
Cooking/Raw	Some subjects have food allergy when they consume the food in raw or partially cooked forms, which may disappear after strong heating. For example, milk and eggs might be tolerated when baked but not in other forms; or cooked fruits cause no reaction, but raw fruits do.
Dose	Dose is important in food allergy. It is not uncommon to note a particular threshold beyond which food allergy occurs. What is important for the clinician to elicit in the history is that every time that threshold is reached the patient should have a clinical reaction. For example, if a subject has hives upon eating 10 peanuts, but not less than that, every time he eats 10 or more peanuts, he should have a reaction.
Repeatability	It is important to ask questions that confirm repeatability of clinical reactions to the same food. "Was there any time, you consumed the food and did not have a reaction?" is a useful question to ask.
Situation	Some foods cause reactions only when ingested immediately before or after exercise. Only exercise or only food consumption without exercise will not cause a reaction. Other factors that could incite a reaction are co-consumption of alcohol or drugs such as NSAIDs.

Skin Prick Test and Serum-Specific IgE

Test is negative when there is a strong history	It is possible that the skin prick test could be negative. The key reason is that some food proteins can be labile and denatured during preparation of the SPT solution. Similarly, the reagent solution may not contain the offending protein (which is lost during processing) for developing the serum-specific IgE. That the reaction is not IgE mediated should be kept in mind.

assay. SPT tests the presence of specific IgE attached to the mast cells and basophils in the appropriate configuration (2 IgE molecules close to one another binding to the allergen) and its degranulation on exposure to the allergen via skin puncture. Serum-specific IgE measures free IgE which is not bound to the mast cells and basophils. How much of it is bound to the mast cells and basophils and the configuration of binding is unknown. Most studies in the world find that prevalence of a positive ssIgE (>0.35 KUI/L) is much higher than a positive SPT (>3 mm) to the same allergen. A large Europrevall study (6) in India, China and Russia observed that while the serum-specific IgE positive rates were very high, the positive SPT was quite low and the actual probable food allergy even lower. The highest sensitivity of SPT to common food allergens is to peanuts (95%), followed by eggs (92%) and milk (88%). The highest specificity of SPT is to wheat (73%), followed by milk and soy (68%).

Serum-specific IgE, similar to SPT, detects sensitization but does not confirm clinical food allergy. Many populations in the world (India, China and Africa) have a high rate of sensitization to foods with very low prevalence of food allergy (6). The highest sensitivity of ssIgE to common food allergens is to peanut (96%), followed by egg (93%) and milk (87%). The highest specificity of ssIgE is to peanut (59%), followed by egg (49%) and milk (48%) (19). Studies have identified certain cut-offs for some foods. It may not be ideal for all populations and care should be exercised in interpretation. In children above 2 years of age if the ssIgE is above 7 KUI/L (egg), 15 KUI/L (milk) and 14 KUI/L (peanut), then 95% of subjects would react to an oral food challenge; therefore, the clinician can make the judgement to avoid the oral food challenge (19). For children less than 2 years of age, when ssIgE is greater than 2 KUI/L for egg and 5 KUI/ L for milk, approximately 95% of children would react positively to a food challenge and thus, it can be avoided (19).

Component resolved diagnostics (CRD) is a very useful tool in the diagnosis of clinical food allergy. Foods contain stable proteins and labile proteins. Stable proteins are most likely to cause food allergy. Stability to gastric acids or heat (cooking) are important characteristics of food allergens. CRD can help to identify IgE to stable allergens, and this increases the chances that the subject has a clinically important food allergy. Stable allergens for various important allergenic foods include Ara h1, Ara h2, Ara h3, Ara h6, Ara h9 for peanuts, casein for milk, Tri a 19 for wheat, Ovomucoid for egg, and

Gly m5, Gly m6, Gly m8 for soy. Two platforms are commonly available to test for component resolved diagnostics. One is the ImmunoCAP ISAC chip platoform that tests 112 components and the other is the AllergyExplorer (ALEX) that tests 125 components.

Oral Food Challenge (OFC) Testing

Oral food challenges are one of the most intensive tests in the diagnosis of food allergy and testing the development of tolerance. Oral food challenges are mainly indicated when the in vivo (SPT) and/or in vitro (ssIgE) are inconsistent with the patient's history to assess whether additional foods can be introduced in the diet in subjects with multiple food restrictions, to assess tolerance to cross-reactive foods, whether a certain food processing can impact tolerance to that food and whether the food associated with atopic dermatitis can cause immediate reactions (22). The foods chosen must have an important value to the patient. If the food is rarely consumed and can nutritionally be substituted with other choices, oral food challenges to that food can be avoided. It is important to remember that in highly sensitized subjects oral food challenges can cause a very severe reaction, leading to hospitalization, need for ICU care or even death in exceptional circumstances. Only 1 death has been reported in the United States after OFC in nearly half a century (22). The contraindications for OFCs are similar to those for allergen immunotherapy. Situations like uncontrolled asthma, severe atopic dermatitis, cardiovascular disease, pregnancy and beta-blocker therapy would make resuscitation difficult. In some situations when these are reversible, such as in the presence of an acute viral illness and fever or with the use of medications that will interfere with the OFCs, the test may be rescheduled (22). The commonly used second-generation antihistamines (cetirizine, loratadine and fexofenadine) will need to be avoided for at least 5 days before OFCs. The first-generation antihistamines such as cyproheptadine and clemastine will need to be avoided longer for up to 11 days (22, 23). Antidepressants, tricyclic antidepressants and benzodiazepines may need to be avoided for 3–7 days, except imipramine which should be avoided for more than 10 days (23). The other drugs that may have to be avoided since they interfere with the interpretation of the OFCs are ACE inhibitors, beta-blockers, bronchodilators, NSAIDs and Proton pump inhibitors. NSAIDs such as aspirin and diclofenac, which are short-acting, need to be avoided for 1 day and longer-acting

Table 6.3: Summary of the Oral Food Challenge

Confirm indication and contraindications	The risk benefit for the patient has to be carefully evaluated before scheduling for the OFC.
Medication history	Several medications need to be avoided (please refer to text). If they have been consumed, the test needs to be rescheduled.
Setting and emergency preparation	OFCs must always be performed at a hospital with the ICU care readily available under the supervision of a physician/pediatrician trained in OFC and acute care management. All emergency medications, IV lines, fluids, airway management, oxygen, nebulizers should be at the ready. In case of non-responsiveness, the subject may be shifted to an acute care facility.
Time to be allotted for OFC	Usually, OFC testing may take 3–6 hours. In case there is a reaction, at least 4 hours of additional observation is needed.
Choice of food matrix for OFC	It is useful to have multiple choices. For example, for cow's milk, it could be in the form of cow's milk, yoghurt, or even ice cream.
Last food consumption	Avoid food for at least 4 hours before a food challenge. This helps to confirm that the reaction is due to the food being tested. Fasting enhances the food allergen absorption. A hungry child is likely to co-operate with the consumption of the food during an OFC.
Masking agents for DBPCFC	The challenge vehicle preferred is a critical component. The use of capsules is not preferred due to the following: • they may be difficult for children to swallow, a sufficient food allergen may not be used, allergenicity may be altered due to processing (dehydration of food) • oral and pharyngeal symptoms will be missed (since a capsule bypasses it) oral cavity and pharynx • early warning signs may be missed (due to delayed absorption of food after which the next dose may be given) For the test and the placebo for a DBPCFC, the sensory properties of both the agents have to be similar. Examples of recipes can be found in Bird et al (Ref 22)
Protocol	4-dose protocol or 6-dose protocol can be used. 4-dose protocol follows: 1/12, 1/6, 1/4 and 1/2 of the total serving for the 4-challenge doses 6-dose protocol follows: 1%, 4%, 10%, 20%, 30% and 35% of the total serving for the 6 challenge doses Doses are typically given 30 minutes apart The doses used for important foods have been reviewed extensively in Bird et al (Ref 22).
Definitions in a DBPCFC	The highest tolerated dose is the amount of food allergen consumed without any clinical reaction. The reactive dose or eliciting dose is the dose at which the objective reaction to food was observed.
Stopping the OFC	If any 1 of the following signs are present, OFC should be stopped immediately: • Respiratory: wheezing, stridor, dysphonia, repetitive cough • Cardiovascular: hypotension • GIT: vomiting, severe abdominal pain lasting >3 minutes • Skin: >3 urticarial rash, confluent erythema, angioedema

NSAIDs such as naproxen avoided for 3–4 days, but piroxicam needs to be avoided for at least 10 days before OFC. There is no need to avoid intranasal and inhaled corticosteroids, montelukast, topical steroids, tacrolimus and selective serotonin reuptake inhibitors (22). It is important to understand that alcohol, drugs such as ACE inhibitors and NSAIDs and antacids can potentiate the severity of the reaction on OFC. Anti-IgE omalizumab will blunt the severity of the food reaction or avoid it altogether. Foods where extreme caution is needed when performing OFCs are peanuts, tree nuts, fish and shellfish, which can be associated with severe and near-fatal reactions. The summary of OFCs, preparation, protocol, initiation, settings and stopping the OFCs are presented in Table 6.3.

MANAGEMENT OF FOOD ALLERGY

One of the cornerstones of the management of food allergy is avoidance of the food allergen. Given the societal constraints, especially in children, it is very difficult to avoid accidental ingestion of foods. This causes a significant deterioration in quality of life for the sufferer, as well as their caregivers. The lack of appropriate food labelling is a cause for concern in many countries, and there is a need for legislation mandating labelling foods when they contain possible food allergens. The other important tool for the clinician is to use food allergen immunotherapy, which has been rapidly developing over the last two decades and has been found to be quite effective in many studies. It is important to confirm that the food related symptoms are indeed due to IgE mediated food allergy, and preferably conduct an oral food challenge to confirm the current levels of clinical reactivity (13). One also needs to carefully consider whether there is a possibility of spontaneous resolution for some of these food allergies such as cow's milk and egg. A good clinical history that the child is reacting less to these foods as compared to the previous years and a reducing wheal size on SPT and serum-specific IgE on serial testing are useful markers that spontaneous resolution may be possible. They can be used as oral (OIT) immunotherapy, sublingual (SLIT) immunotherapy and epicutaneous (EPIT) immunotherapy. Current evidence regarding the three forms are discussed.

Oral Immunotherapy (OIT)

This is the most promising form of immunotherapy for foods. It involves daily consumption of the allergen in powder form mixed with other foods. The powder form of the allergen contains not only the proteins, but also the carbohydrates and lipids of the offending food. Similar to other forms of immunotherapy, OIT involves exposure to increasing doses of the food allergen (build-up) and maintenance with regular doses of immunotherapy. The mechanisms of action are similar for other forms of immunotherapy; the switch from the Th2 to Th1 pathway with a reduction in allergen-specific IgE and an increase in allergen specific IgG4, reduced basophil activity and increased T 'regulatory' cells. Of the three forms of immunotherapy for food allergy, the best response so far has been obtained with OIT. Studies on peanut and egg have been encouraging. For peanut allergies, Vickery (24) studied subjects <4 years with a maintenance dose of 300 mg and observed high rates of desensitisation. In an earlier study (25), they had observed children and adolescents <16 years of age with a maintenance dose of 4000 mg and up to 5 years of OIT, a 50% sustained unresponsiveness was observed for a peanut oral food challenge of 5000 mg. In a randomized placebo-controlled trial for peanut allergy, OIT was better than SLIT in improving the threshold for clinical reactivity (26). For egg allergy, studies included children 1–16 years

of age with a duration of 22 to 60 months with a maintenance dose of 0.3–1.6 grams. It was observed that 57–75% of children passed the oral food challenge for 8–10 gm of egg (27–29). Randomised placebo-controlled trials for milk allergy included either 150–200 ml of milk or 500–4000 mg of milk protein as a maintenance dose, and the study duration varied from 4 months to 1 year. Rates of desensitization/tolerance varied from 36% to 90% (30–32). Some OIT studies have also used concomitant omalizumab, especially for rapid desensitization in individuals at high risk for milk and peanut and encouraging results were found (33, 34). Studies have also found encouraging results with multi-food OIT in children who have more than one food allergy (35).

Sublingual Immunotherapy (SLIT)

SLIT involves the administration of glycerinated or tablets of allergen extracts in the sublingual region to be held for 2 minutes before swallowing. It is generally administered daily over many years. It is commonly used for aeroallergens but has been used for food as well. It has very few side effects, mostly limited to the oropharynx (mild itching or tingling), that in most cases reverse spontaneously. It has been studied for peanut, milk and hazelnut (26, 36, 37) and has been found to be useful in improving the oral food challenge threshold 20–40 times the initial tolerated dose. One study observed that 70% of the subjects responded to SLIT, compared to 15% of subjects receiving placebo (36). Subjects were studied between ages 2–53 years in different studies.

Epicutaneous Immunotherapy (EPIT)

EPIT involves the application of allergen patches to the skin, usually in the upper arm or in the back and changed every day. It has been studied with some success for peanut and milk but it induced only modest changes immunologically and is possibly less effective than SLIT or OIT. It has minimal side effects with irritation of the skin at the patch site. It has been tested primarily in younger children and, to date, no severe reactions were noted. A more than 10-fold increased tolerance for milk (38) (over 3 months) and peanuts (39) (over 1 year) were observed.

The contraindications of food allergen immunotherapy are similar to those for aeroallergen immunotherapy. Active malignancy, active autoimmune disorders, poor adherence, severe asthma, uncontrolled asthma in spite of adequate treatment, eosinophilic esophagitis, gastrointestinal eosinophilic disorders, pregnancy, severe systemic illness, significant cardiovascular or other vital organ diseases, thyroiditis even when in remission, uncontrolled atopic dermatitis, certain drugs such as beta-blockers and ACE inhibitors, chronic urticaria and mastocytosis are some of the contraindications.

Management of Oral Allergy Syndrome (Pollen-Food Allergy Syndrome)

Management of oral allergy syndrome rests on the avoidance of the foods. A prescription of epinephrine may be given when there is a history of severe reactions to these foods, such as laryngeal swelling, wheezing or low blood pressure. Immunotherapy to the offending aeroallergen has been found to be beneficial (40).

PREVENTION OF FOOD ALLERGY

Various studies have confirmed the benefits of early introduction (4–6 months) of solid allergenic foods such as peanuts, as evidenced from well controlled studies, such as the LEAP (Learning Early about Peanut) study, LEAP-ON and EAT studies (3). In the LEAP study (41), children less than 1 year of age (4–11 months) with a high risk of peanut allergy (pre-existing atopic dermatitis with or without egg allergy), were randomized to peanut consumption or avoidance. All children had SPT to peanut with a wheal size equal to or less than 4 mm. The children who were sensitized to peanuts and were exposed to peanuts developed peanut allergy in 10.6% of cases, while children who avoided peanuts developed peanut allergy in 35.3% of cases. In children who were not sensitised to peanuts, peanut allergy was seen in 1.9% (exposed to peanut) and 13.7% (avoided peanut). The EAT study (42, 43) evaluated early the introduction of 6 allergenic foods in young infants before 6 months of age and found that early introduction of foods helped to prevent food allergy. While the standard food introduction group had a prevalence of food allergy of 34.2%, the early introduction group had a food allergy prevalence of 19.2%. This is an important step in reducing the overall food allergy prevalence among children. Some countries, such as Australia, recommend that solid allergenic foods should be introduced around 6 months of age but never before 4 months (www.allergy.org.au). Breastfeeding for a minimum of 6 months is recommended by all countries. There is no evidence that using hydrolysed formula has no benefit in food allergy prevention (44).

The current recommendations (19) for introduction of peanut depends on the presence and severity of atopic dermatitis and egg allergy. For children with no atopic dermatitis or food allergy, peanut can be introduced as per family preference and cultural practices. For children with mild to moderate atopic dermatitis, peanut introduction is recommended at 6 months of age. For children in the highest risk category of developing peanut allergy (severe atopic dermatitis with or without egg allergy), peanut introduction should ideally be started at 4–6 months, after confirming that the child does not already have a peanut allergy. This recommendation is based on the findings from the LEAP study. Evidence on egg and milk are not as strong as for peanut. Delayed introduction of milk may increase the risk of milk allergy (45) and for egg, studies have shown both protection (46) and increased risk of egg allergy (47) with early introduction. It is possible that many infants may have already developed egg allergy by 4–6 months (19).

The HealthNuts study observed 11.5 times higher odds of developing peanut allergy and 3.7 times higher odds of developing egg allergy in vitamin D-deficient infants (48). The role of vitamin D supplementation in deficient infants and its protective effect on food allergy is still being evaluated. Moisturizing the skin, due to its protective effect on food allergy and atopic dermatitis by improving the skin barrier (49), could be useful, but further studies are needed. The practice in Asian countries of applying oil to infants every day needs to be evaluated further. There is as of yet no strong evidence whether or not probiotics can be useful, though one study observed a reduced risk for developing another allergy with *Lactobacillus rhamnosus* (50).

CONCLUSION

The understanding of food allergy has grown by leaps and bounds over the last two decades. However, much remains to be understood. The diagnosis of food allergy needs to be simplified for the medical practitioner. Novel methods of prevention and treatment of food allergies are urgently needed to improve the quality of life of food allergy sufferers.

REFERENCES

1. Iweala OI, Choudhary SK, Commins SP. Food allergy. Curr Gastroenterol Rep 2018 Apr 5; 20(5):17.

2. Sampson HA. Food allergy: past, present and future. Allergol Int 2016 Oct; 65(4):363–9.

3. Tang MLK, Mullins RJ. Food allergy: is prevalence increasing?: food allergy prevalence time trends. Intern Med J 2017 Mar; 47(3):256–61.

4. Renz H, Allen KJ, Sicherer SH, Sampson HA, Lack G, Beyer K, et al. Food allergy. Nat Rev Dis Primers 2018 Jun 7; 4(1):17098.

5. Schoemaker AA, Sprikkelman AB, Grimshaw KE, Roberts G, Grabenhenrich L, Rosenfeld L, et al. Incidence and natural history of challenge-proven cow's milk allergy in European children—EuroPrevall birth cohort. Allergy 2015 Aug; 70(8):963–72.

6. Li J, Ogorodova LM, Mahesh PA, Wang MH, Fedorova OS, Leung TF, et al. Comparative study of food allergies in children from China, India, and Russia: the EuroPrevall-INCO Surveys. J Allergy Clin Immunol Pract 2019 Dec; S2213219819310323.

7. Mahesh PA, Wong GWK, Ogorodova L, Potts J, Leung TF, Fedorova O, et al. Prevalence of food sensitization and probable food allergy among adults in India: the EuroPrevall INCO study. Allergy 2016 Jul; 71(7):1010–9.

8. Osborne NJ, Koplin JJ, Martin PE, Gurrin LC, Lowe AJ, Matheson MC, et al. Prevalence of challenge-proven IgE-mediated food allergy using population-based sampling and predetermined challenge criteria in infants. J Allergy Clin Immunol 2011 Mar; 127(3):668–676.e2.

9. Rudders SA, Arias SA, Camargo CA. Trends in hospitalizations for food-induced anaphylaxis in US children, 2000–2009. J Allergy Clin Immunol 2014 Oct; 134(4):960–962.e3.

10. Mullins RJ, Dear KBG, Tang MLK. Time trends in Australian hospital anaphylaxis admissions in 1998–1999 to 2011–2012. J Allergy Clin Immunol 2015 Aug;136(2):367–75.

11. Koplin JJ, Peters RL, Ponsonby A-L, Gurrin LC, Hill D, Tang MLK, et al. Increased risk of peanut allergy in infants of Asian-born parents compared to those of Australian-born parents. Allergy 2014 Dec;69(12):1639–47.

12. Burks AW, Sampson HA, Plaut M, Lack G, Akdis CA. Treatment for food allergy. J Allergy Clin Immunol 2018 Jan;141(1):1–9.

13. Pajno GB, Fernandez-Rivas M, Arasi S, Roberts G, Akdis CA, Alvaro-Lozano M, et al. EAACI Guidelines on allergen immunotherapy: IgE-mediated food allergy. Allergy 2018 Apr;73(4):799–815.

14. Koleilat A. Food Intolerance. BJSTR [Internet]. 2017 Jul 13 [cited 2020 Nov 24]; 1(2). Available from: http://biomedres.us/fulltexts/BJSTR.MS.ID.000190.php#/

15. Carlson G, Coop C. Pollen food allergy syndrome (PFAS): a review of current available literature. Ann Allergy Asthma Immunol 2019 Oct;123(4):359–65.

16. Gupta RS, Walkner MM, Greenhawt M, Lau CH, Caruso D, Wang X, et al. Food allergy sensitization and presentation in siblings of food allergic children. J Allergy Clin Immunol Pract 2016 Sep; 4(5):956–62.

17. Hong X, Hao K, Ladd-Acosta C, Hansen KD, Tsai H-J, Liu X, et al. Genome-wide association study identifies peanut allergy-specific loci and evidence of epigenetic mediation in US children. Nat Commun 2015 May; 6(1):6304.

18. Hong X, Ladd-Acosta C, Hao K, Sherwood B, Ji H, Keet CA, et al. Epigenome-wide association study links site-specific DNA methylation changes with cow's milk allergy. J Allergy Clin Immunol 2016 Sep; 138(3):908–911.e9.

19. Sicherer SH, Sampson HA. Food allergy: a review and update on epidemiology, pathogenesis, diagnosis, prevention, and management. J Allergy Clin Immunol 2018 Jan; 141(1):41–58.

20. Flinterman AE, Knol EF, Lencer DA, Bardina L, den Hartog Jager CF, Lin J, et al. Peanut epitopes for IgE and IgG4 in peanut-sensitized children in relation to severity of peanut allergy. J Allergy Clin Immunol 2008 Mar;121(3):737–743.e10.

21. Shreffler WG, Beyer K, Chu T-HT, Burks AW, Sampson HA. Microarray immunoassay: Association of clinical history, in vitro IgE function, and heterogeneity of allergenic peanut epitopes. J Allergy Clin Immunol 2004 Apr;113(4):776–82.

22. Bird JA, Leonard S, Groetch M, Assa'ad A, Cianferoni A, Clark A, et al. Conducting an oral food challenge: an update to the 2009 Adverse Reactions to Foods Committee Work Group Report. J Allergy Clin Immunol Pract 2020 Jan; 8(1):75–90.e17.

23. Sampson HA, Gerth van Wijk R, Bindslev-Jensen C, Sicherer S, Teuber SS, Burks AW, et al. Standardizing double-blind, placebo-controlled oral food challenges: American Academy of Allergy, Asthma & Immunology–European Academy of Allergy and Clinical Immunology PRACTALL consensus report. J Allergy Clin Immunol 2012 Dec; 130(6):1260–74.

24. Vickery BP, Berglund JP, Burk CM, Fine JP, Kim EH, Kim JI, et al. Early oral immunotherapy in peanut-allergic preschool children is safe and highly effective. J Allergy Clin Immunol 2017 Jan;139(1): 173–181.e8.

25. Vickery BP, Scurlock AM, Kulis M, Steele PH, Kamilaris J, Berglund JP, et al. Sustained unresponsiveness to peanut in subjects who have completed peanut oral immunotherapy. J Allergy Clin Immunol 2014 Feb;133(2):468–475.e6.

26. Narisety SD, Frischmeyer-Guerrerio PA, Keet CA, Gorelik M, Schroeder J, Hamilton RG, et al. A randomized, double-blind, placebo-controlled pilot study of sublingual versus oral immunotherapy for the treatment of peanut allergy. J Allergy Clin Immunol 2015 May; 135(5):1275–1282.e6.

27. Vickery BP, Pons L, Kulis M, Steele P, Jones SM, Burks AW. Individualized IgE-based dosing of egg oral immunotherapy and the development of tolerance. Ann Allergy Asthma Immunol 2010 Dec; 105(6):444–50.

28. Jones SM, Burks AW, Keet C, Vickery BP, Scurlock AM, Wood RA, et al. Long-term treatment with egg oral immunotherapy enhances sustained unresponsiveness that persists after cessation of therapy. J Allergy Clin Immunol 2016 Apr;137(4):1117–1127.e10.

29. Burks AW, Jones SM, Wood RA, Fleischer DM, Sicherer SH, Lindblad RW, et al. Oral immunotherapy for treatment of egg allergy in children. N Engl J Med 2012 Jul 19; 367(3):233–43.

30. Skripak JM, Nash SD, Rowley H, Brereton NH, Oh S, Hamilton RG, et al. A randomized, double-blind, placebo-controlled study of milk oral immunotherapy for cow's milk allergy. J Allergy Clin Immunol 2008 Dec;122(6):1154–60.

31. Narisety SD, Skripak JM, Steele P, Hamilton RG, Matsui EC, Burks AW, et al. Open-label maintenance after milk oral immunotherapy for IgE-mediated cow's milk allergy. J of Allergy Clin Immunol 2009 Sep;124(3):610–2.

32. Keet CA, Frischmeyer-Guerrerio PA, Thyagarajan A, Schroeder JT, Hamilton RG, Boden S, et al. The safety and efficacy of sublingual and oral immunotherapy for milk allergy. J Allergy Clin Immunol 2012 Feb;129(2):448–455.e5.

33. Wood RA, Kim JS, Lindblad R, Nadeau K, Henning AK, Dawson P, et al. A randomized, double-blind, placebo-controlled study of omalizumab combined with oral immunotherapy for the treatment of cow's milk allergy. J Allergy Clin Immunol 2016 Apr;137(4):1103–1110.e11.

34. Schneider LC, Rachid R, LeBovidge J, Blood E, Mittal M, Umetsu DT. A pilot study of omalizumab to facilitate rapid oral desensitization in high-risk peanut-allergic patients. J Allergy Clin Immunol 2013 Dec;132(6):1368–74.

35. Bégin P, Winterroth LC, Dominguez T, Wilson SP, Bacal L, Mehrotra A, et al. Safety and feasibility of oral immunotherapy to multiple allergens for food allergy. All Asth Clin Immun 2014 Dec; 10(1):1.

36. Fleischer DM, Burks AW, Vickery BP, Scurlock AM, Wood RA, Jones SM, et al. Sublingual immunotherapy for peanut allergy: a randomized, double-blind, placebo-controlled multicenter trial. J Allergy Clin Immunol 2013 Jan; 131(1):119–127.e7.

37. Enrique E, Pineda F, Malek T, Bartra J, Basagaña M, Tella R, et al. Sublingual immunotherapy for hazelnut food allergy: a randomized, double-blind, placebo-controlled study with a standardized hazelnut extract. J Allergy Clin Immunol 2005 Nov; 116(5):1073–9.

38. Dupont C, Kalach N, Soulaines P, Legoué-Morillon S, Piloquet H, Benhamou P-H. Cow's milk epicutaneous immunotherapy in children: a pilot trial of safety, acceptability, and impact on allergic reactivity. J Allergy Clin Immunol 2010 May; 125(5):1165–7.

39. Jones SM, Sicherer SH, Burks AW, Leung DYM, Lindblad RW, Dawson P, et al. Epicutaneous immunotherapy for the treatment of peanut allergy in children and young adults. J Allergy Clin Immunol 2017 Apr;139(4):1242–1252.e9.

40. Asero R. How long does the effect of birch pollen injection SIT on apple allergy last? Allergy 2003 May; 58(5):435–8.

41. Du Toit G, Roberts G, Sayre PH, Bahnson HT, Radulovic S, Santos AF, et al. Randomized trial of peanut consumption in infants at risk for peanut allergy. N Engl J Med 2015 Feb 26; 372(9):803–13.

42. Perkin MR, Logan K, Marrs T, Radulovic S, Craven J, Flohr C, et al. Enquiring About Tolerance (EAT) study: feasibility of an early allergenic food introduction regimen. J Allergy Clin Immunol 2016 May;137(5):1477–1486.e8.

43. Perkin MR, Logan K, Bahnson HT, Marrs T, Radulovic S, Craven J, et al. Efficacy of the Enquiring About Tolerance (EAT) study among infants at high risk of developing food allergy. J Allergy Clin Immunol 2019 Dec;144(6):1606–1614.e2.

44. Boyle RJ, Ierodiakonou D, Khan T, Chivinge J, Robinson Z, Geoghegan N, et al. Hydrolysed formula and risk of allergic or autoimmune disease: systematic review and meta-analysis. BMJ 2016 Mar 8; i974.

45. Onizawa Y, Noguchi E, Okada M, Sumazaki R, Hayashi D. The association of the delayed introduction of cow's milk with IgE-mediated cow's milk allergies. J Allergy Clin Immunol Pract 2016 May; 4(3):481–488.e2.

46. Natsume O, Kabashima S, Nakazato J, Yamamoto-Hanada K, Narita M, Kondo M, et al. Two-step egg introduction for prevention of egg allergy in high-risk infants with eczema (PETIT): a randomised, double-blind, placebo-controlled trial. The Lancet 2017 Jan;389(10066):276–86.

47. Bellach J, Schwarz V, Ahrens B, Trendelenburg V, Aksünger Ö, Kalb B, et al. Randomized placebo-controlled trial of hen's egg consumption for primary prevention in infants. J Allergy Clin Immunol 2017 May;139(5):1591–1599.e2.

48. Allen KJ, Koplin JJ, Ponsonby A-L, Gurrin LC, Wake M, Vuillermin P, et al. Vitamin D insufficiency is associated with challenge-proven food allergy in infants. J Allergy Clin Immunol 2013 Apr; 131(4): 1109–1116.e6.

49. Simpson EL, Chalmers JR, Hanifin JM, Thomas KS, Cork MJ, McLean WHI, et al. Emollient enhancement of the skin barrier from birth offers effective atopic dermatitis prevention. J Allergy Clin Immunol 2014 Oct;134(4):818–23.

50. Berni Canani R, Di Costanzo M, Bedogni G, Amoroso A, Cosenza L, Di Scala C, et al. Extensively hydrolyzed casein formula containing Lactobacillus rhamnosus GG reduces the occurrence of other allergic manifestations in children with cow's milk allergy: 3-year randomized controlled trial. J Allergy Clin Immunol 2017 Jun;139(6): 1906–1913.e4.

7 Drug Allergy

Rajesh Venkitakrishnan

CONTENTS

INTRODUCTION

An adverse drug reaction (ADR) has been defined as an appreciably harmful or unpleasant reaction, resulting from an intervention related to the use of a medicinal product, which predicts hazard from future administration and warrants prevention or specific treatment, alteration of the dosage regimen, or withdrawal of the product.[1] Adverse drug reactions constitute a serious hazard in clinical practice and account for substantial morbidity and health care costs.[2] As per the US Food and Drug Administration, a drug is defined as a substance or product intended to be used in the diagnosis, cure, mitigation, treatment, or prevention of disease and intended to affect the structure or any function of the body of humans or animals. The reported rates of ADR vary. Distinguishing a true allergic drug reaction from its close mimics is challenging for the less experienced physician. The present review attempts to equip the practitioner with updated knowledge on the diagnosis and approach to drug allergy.

INCIDENCE AND RISK FACTORS

The reported occurrence of drug reactions varies in different published series. The variations in severity of occurrence, patient perceptions, difference in definitions, and reporting bias account for these wide ranges. In general, adverse reactions affect 10–20% of hospitalized patients and as much as 25% of out-patients.[2-4] Type A reactions account for the vast majority. Type B reactions are less frequent, with an estimated occurrence of 10–15% of all adverse drug reactions.[5] The commonest drugs causing hypersensitivity reactions are β-lactam antibiotics and non-steroidal anti-inflammatory drugs (NSAIDs).[6] Other common causes include radio-contrast media, neuromuscular blocking agents, and antiepileptic drugs. Immediate hypersensitivity to local anaesthetics is distinctly rare, despite common complaints.

Factors increasing the risk of developing an ADR have been previously reviewed.[7-9] These include patient-related aspects (age, gender, genetic factors, and some viral infections) and factors directly related to the agent (frequency of exposure, route of administration, or molecular weight). Drug allergy classically occurs in middle-aged adults, and is more frequent in women. Genetic polymorphisms in HLA, as well as viral infections (HIV and the EBV), lead to increased risk of developing ADR.[10] Susceptibility to drug allergy is dictated in some cases by genetic polymorphisms in

DOI: 10.1201/9781003125785-7

Table 7.1: Risk Factors for Drug Allergy

Factor Link	Risk Factor	Example
Patient related	Female Sex	Gemifloxacin Rash
	HLA association	HLA-B allelle
	Viral infections	HIV (sulfonamide allergy)
	EBV infection	Amoxycillin
	Atopic state	Reactions tend to be severe
	Prior history of reaction	Reactions common, fast onset and severe
	Multiple drug allergies	Increased chance
Disease related	Immunodeficiency states	Repeated drug administration
	Multiple diseases needing polypharmacy	Drug interactions causing reaction
Drug related	Impurity, preservatives, diluents	
	Dose, frequency and duration	Repeated doses, prolonged therapy
	Route	Maximum with IV route; least oral
	Polymerization, haptenization	

drug metabolism. Topical, intramuscular, and intravenous routes of administration are more likely to cause allergic drug reactions than oral administration. Prolonged high doses or frequent doses of medication are more likely to cause ADR than a large single dose. Large macromolecular drugs (e.g., insulin or horse antisera) or agents that bind to haptens (such as penicillin) are associated with a greater likelihood of causing hypersensitivity reactions (Table 7.1). Although atopic patients do not have an increased risk for drug allergy, they are at increased risk[11] for serious allergic reactions.

CLINICAL SIGNIFICANCE

Adverse drug reactions are a major hazard in clinical practice and account for sizeable morbidity and health care costs.[2] ADRs are associated with

a. Small but significant rates of mortality

b. Hospitalization with attendant costs

c. Loss of productive days

d. Impaired quality of life until the reaction wears off

e. Delay in optimal treatment of the primary condition

f. Performance of additional investigations

Hence, the cost of ADR to the health system is substantial. A study from Britain reported that 0.32% of serious ADRs were fatal, whereas another study reported that 18% of all hospital deaths during a period of audit could be directly or indirectly attributed to one or more drugs.[12] Another study of subjects who died of anaphylaxis revealed that out of 164 deaths, 39% were drug-induced. The incidence of serious ADR is also increasing, which probably could be multifactorial (increasing drug usage, better awareness and improvement in reporting). Between 1998 and 2005 serious ADEs increased 2.6-fold.[13]

CLASSIFICATION AND MECHANISMS

The classification (Table 7.2) and evaluation of ADRs is difficult because, for many drugs, the underlying mechanism is not elucidated. Although different classifications systems are in vogue, adverse drug reactions may conveniently be divided into 2 broad subtypes.

- Type A reactions: which are predictable and are an extrapolation of pharmacologic properties of the drug

- Type B reactions: which are not predictable, unrelated to the pharmacological effect, usually not dose dependent and restricted to specific subpopulations.[3] Type B reactions may be subdivided into hypersensitivity, idiosyncratic, and exaggerated sensitivity (intolerance) drug reactions, based on the immune-pathogenesis of the reaction.

Hypersensitivity reactions are mediated by immunologic and/or inflammatory mechanisms that are unintentionally triggered by the drug. Idiosyncratic drug reactions and exaggerated sensitivity reactions are independent of the immune system or inflammatory cells. Idiosyncratic reactions may be the result of genetic differences in the patient (e.g., primaquine causing nonimmune haemolytic anaemia in patients with glucose-6-phosphate dehydrogenase deficiency).[14] Exaggerated sensitivity occurs at normal or sub-therapeutic doses due to altered drug metabolism or increased end-organ sensitivity.

Table 7.2: Classification of Adverse Drug Reactions

Type of Reaction	Clinical Event	Example	Feature
Type A	Overdose	Opiates causing respiratory depression	1. Predictable 2. Dose dependent 3. Occurs in larger number of exposed patients 4. Extension of pharmacologic action 5. Not unique to special populations
	Side effect	Tachycardia with beta-blockers	
	Collateral damage	Diarrhoea with antibiotics	
	Drug interactions	Azithromycin and HCQ causing QTc prolongation	
Type B	Intolerance	Single-dose aspirin causing tinnitus	Unpredictable, occurs in small populations only with specific risk factors, dose independent and not due to pharmacologic action
	Idiosyncracy	Primaquine causing hemolysis in G6PDD subjects	
	Allergy	Anaphylaxis with beta lactams	

Drug hypersensitivity reactions (DHRs) are the adverse effects of pharmaceutical formulations (including active drugs and excipients). The reactions clinically resemble allergy. The international consensus on drug allergy has reserved the term drug allergy when a drug-specific immune response is demonstrable.[15] The differentiation between idiosyncratic drug reactions and drug allergy can be difficult to discern clinically, but it is of considerable importance because diagnosis and management will differ. The term drug pseudo-allergy, used to describe allergic-like reactions, is no longer recommended.

The World Allergy Organization has suggested sub-classification to immediate and delayed reactions, which reflect the time of onset of the symptoms.[16] This distinction may be helpful in judging whether the immunologic mechanism is antibody (e.g., IgE) mediated or T-lymphocyte-mediated. Immediate DHRs are often due to an IgE mediated pathway and occur within 1–6 hours after drug dosing. Delayed DHRs may occur any time after 1 hour after administering the medication. They can occur after many days of therapy and are often associated with a T-cell-dependent mechanism. Mechanistically, immune-mediated reactions are classified according to the Gell and Coombs' classification system.

a. *Type 1*: Immediate-type reactions mediated by IgE antibodies

b. *Type 2*: Cytotoxic reactions mediated by IgG or IgM antibodies

c. *Type 3*: Immune-complex reactions (type III)

d. *Type 4*: Delayed-type hypersensitivity reactions mediated by T cell mediated cellular immune mechanisms. Increased understanding of the varied role of T cells has prompted subclassification of types reactions to 4a–4d by some authors.[15,17]

Much work has been done in elucidating the mechanisms and pathways contributing to ADR, but knowledge gaps exist. These gaps can be attributed, in part, to the lack of a validated animal model of drug allergy. Another challenge lies in identifying and isolating the antigenic components and metabolites of potential drug allergens. Two theories—the prohapten-hapten concept and the p-i concept have been put forward to explain the underlying mechanisms. A single drug, such as penicillin, can cause a variety of allergic reactions via different mechanisms.

THE PROHAPTEN-HAPTEN CONCEPT

Karl Landsteiner first proposed that multivalency is an essential requirement for the initiation of immune responses to foreign substances. Some macromolecules satisfy this need intrinsically by virtue of large molecular weight with multiple recurring epitopes. Some small molecules have multiple recurrences of a single epitope and thus become 'complete' allergens. There are two ways in which small chemicals can fulfil the requirement for multivalency. First, some of them have a covalent binding with cell membrane macromolecules to form multivalent hapten-carrier complexes. Second, immunologically inert drugs can be converted into reactive intermediates during drug metabolism. A number of complex stages ensue till a final effecter pathway for ADR develops.[18] These stages include

a. Formation of a complete antigen

b. Processing of the complete antigen by antigen-presenting cells

c. Recognition of the antigenic determinant by T lymphocytes

d. Generation of a drug-specific antibody or sensitized T cells

e. Elicitation of a clinical immune response

THE P–I CONCEPT

A distinct pathway for drug immunogenicity has been described by Pichler and colleagues.[19] P–I denotes pharmacological interaction of drugs with immune receptors. As per this concept, an inert drug, which is unable to covalently bind to peptides, can activate the immune system by binding directly to the T cell receptors. Subsequently, stimulation of T cells with cytokine production, proliferation, and cytotoxicity may ensue. This drug-T cell receptor interaction is similar to the interaction of drugs with other pharmacological receptors and is thus distinct from the recognition of processed hapten-carrier complexes by T cell receptors. However, the clinical picture is indistinguishable from the multivalent pathway.

DANGER HYPOTHESIS

Bacterial or viral products can interact with Toll like receptors on dendritic cells and promote antigen processing. A link between these 'danger signals' and immunogenicity has been recently shown for drugs causing contact dermatitis. The role of this pathway for drugs causing systemic reactions is far less established.

DRUGS IMPLICATED

The list of drugs that can potentially elicit an ADR is huge, and the preparation of an exhaustive list is challenging. In addition, serum sickness-like syndrome, drug-induced vasculitis, blood dyscrasia, and hypersensitivity reactions can be caused by many drugs (Table 7.3).

CLINICAL FEATURES

The clinical presentation of an ADR is variable, depending upon the agent implicated, the pathways involved, and patient factors. Although many organ systems can be affected, skin is by far the most common site affected.[20] The temporal association of reaction following drug intake aids in making a clinical diagnosis. In the most dramatic immediate IgE mediated reactions, manifestations occur minutes after the drug consumption. However, delayed cell mediated reactions may appear hours to days after drug exposure.

Cutaneous manifestation most commonly takes the form of a generalized maculopapular rash, having onset within hours to 3 weeks after drug exposure.[21] Lesions typically begin in the truncal area and later spread to the limbs. Urticaria and angioedema may occur. More severe forms of cutaneous reactions with secondary systemic consequences include Stevens–Johnson syndrome (SJS) and toxic epidermal necrolysis (TEN). SJS starts as a maculopapular rash and may extend as bullae, mucous membrane ulcerations, conjunctivitis, fever, sore throat, and fatigue. TEN has features similar to SJS, but it also results in widespread skin exfoliation resulting in a scalded skin appearance.

Anaphylaxis is the most dreaded and dramatic ADR. Multisystem manifestations include drug rash with eosinophilia and systemic symptoms (DRESS) syndrome, serum sickness, drug-induced lupus erythematosus (DILE), and vasculitis. DRESS manifests as widespread rash, fever, lymphadenopathy, and hepatic dysfunction. Peripheral blood eosinophilia is a hallmark. Serum sickness is an immunecomplex-mediated reaction that is characterised by fever, lymphadenopathy, arthralgia, and cutaneous lesions. The typical features of DILE include acute febrile episode and malaise; myalgia, arthralgia, and arthritis may also occur. Cutaneous involvement occurs in a minority. Serum sickness and DILE are usually self-limited, with features remitting spontaneously within a few weeks of drug discontinuation. However, the fate of DRESS is more unpredictable, even after drug discontinuation. Features may worsen or persist for weeks and even months.

DIFFERENTIAL DIAGNOSIS

Since the features of drug allergy are protean with regard to onset, organ involvement, and course, differentiation from other conditions that mimic drug-induced allergic reactions is crucial (Table 7.4).

Table 7.3: Common Drugs Implicated in Urticaria, Angioedema and Anaphylaxis

1.	Antiplatelet agents – Aspirin, Clopidogrel, Ticagrelol
2.	Antimicrobials – Penicillins, cephalosporins, clavulanic acid, vancomycin, fluoroquinolones
3.	Chemotherapy agents – Cisplatin, carboplatin, paclitaxel
4.	NSAIDs – Diclofenac, ketorolac, mefenamic acid
5.	Neuromuscular blockers – Atracurium, thiopentone, suxamethonium
6.	Intravenous iron preparations, desferoxamine
7.	Biological agents – Omalizumab, rituximab
8.	Anticonvulsants
9.	Chlorhexidene, Povidone iodine, excipients

Table 7.4: Common Differential Diagnoses of Adverse Drug Reactions

IgE-Mediated ADR	Non-IgE-Mediated ADR
Insect bite/stings	Psoriasis
Atopic dermatitis, asthma	Viral infections
Carcinoid syndrome	Streptococcal/staphylococcal infections
Food allergy	Insect bites/stings
Latex allergy	Still's disease
Parasitic disease	Kawasaki's disease
Mastocytosis, hematologic malignancies	Acute graft versus host disease
Viral hepatitis	

DIAGNOSIS

The diagnosis of drug allergy is often challenging because of the wide variations in presentation, concurrent polypharmacy, limitations of available tests, and uncertainties in the natural history of drug allergy. When supported by a consistent history and compatible findings, skin tests such as skin prick testing (SPT) and intradermal tests are useful for the diagnosis of IgE-mediated reactions. Biochemical or immunological markers that confirm the activation of particular immunopathologic pathways are often utilised. Solid-phase immunoassays (RAST, ELISA) have been established for a wide variety of drug allergies, using sera from skin test–positive patients for standardization. Definite diagnosis of drug allergy involves drug provocation testing (DPT), during which incremental doses of the offending drug are administered.

The international consensus position paper on drug allergy has given guidelines regarding when to further evaluate suspected ADR and when to avoid further evaluation.[15] Further evaluation is suggested when

1. The risk/benefit ratio is positive and the tests performs well

   a. For suspected allergy to β-lactam antibiotics, NSAIDs, and local anaesthetics

2. The drugs are required to be administrated

   a. An equally effective, structurally unrelated alternative does not exist

3. When there is a history of prior severe DHR for multiple drugs (the best way to protect the patient is to find the culprit agents).

Further evaluation or testing is not suggested when

1. Cases have a low chance of causalty

   a. Non-compatible clinical features

   b. Non-compatible chronology

   c. No reaction when drug repeatedly taken

   d. Reaction occurring even without drug administration

2. Alternative diagnosis reached (e.g., herpes virus eruption, chronic urticaria)

3. Drug provocation occurs; if the reaction was too severe, non-controllable or life threatening

SKIN TESTING

Demonstration of specific immune responses are immensely helpful but not sufficient for diagnosing drug allergy. They should be done 4–6 weeks after the reaction. The best body of evidence comes from penicillin skin testing.[21] Prick and intradermal skin testing for drug-specific IgE antibodies have been usefully applied to β-lactam antibiotics and a variety of other drugs, such as ciprofloxacin, trimethoprim, carboplatin and related drugs, neuromuscular blockers, thiobarbiturates, some anticonvulsants, and local anaesthetics. Cross-reactivity with penicillins and cephalosporins has been reported.[22] Positive intradermal skin tests have been reported for imipenem and other β-lactams, but validated skin test protocols are not available.

The technique, interpretation, and standardization of skin prick testing are described elsewhere in this textbook. For immediate DHRs, the prick test is initially preferred due to its simplicity, rapidity, low cost, and high specificity. Intradermal tests may be performed if skin prick tests are negative. Compared to skin prick tests, they have a better sensitivity for drug-specific IgE. Skin tests should be done with the intravenous formulation of the drug, whenever feasible.

The clinical implication of negative tests is well established only for penicillins. Retreatment with penicillins in skin test-negative patients have reported virtually no reaction, even if clinical presentation was compatible; no catastrophic false-negative reactions have been reported in cases using penicillins.[23] Because more than 80% of history-positive patients will have negative penicillin skin tests, skin testing is a valuable tool that permits retreatment of many patients previously labelled as 'penicillin allergic'.

Patch tests and intradermal tests are useful in evaluating non-immediate reactions to penicillins, and both can reliably predict the results of re-challenge. More research is needed to confirm the consistency of these results and extrapolate the findings to other drug allergies.

SEROLOGICAL ASSAYS

Immunoassays like RAST and ELISA have been investigated as diagnostic modalities for a wide variety of drug allergies. These in vitro test results have been systematically compared with skin tests only in the case of penicillin allergy.[24] A diagnostic sensitivity of 65–85% compared with skin tests has been reported. Flow cytometry is rapidly gaining attention in the diagnosis of drug allergy.[25] Assessment of drug-induced basophil activation as detected by increase in surface markers such as CD63 may be helpful in the diagnosis of ADR to penicillin, aspirin/NSAIDs, and neuromuscular blocking agents. Determination of cysteinyl leukotrienes released from blood leukocytes after drug incubation has been suggested to increase the diagnostic value of flow cytometry. Mast cell tryptase or serum histamine levels may be helpful in retrospective diagnosis of an anaphylactic reaction if measured within 4 hours of the event. Detectable serum mast cell β tryptase (>1 ng/mL) or plasma histamine (>10 nmol/L) may be helpful.[26] Mild anaphylaxis without hemodynamic changes may still yield false negative results.

DRUG PROVOCATION TESTING

Definite diagnosis of drug allergy may be possible by a placebo controlled drug provocation testing (DPT).[27] Here, escalating doses of the offending drug are administered. Drug provocation tests should be contemplated only after evaluating the risk–benefit ratio for an individual patient and should be performed only by experienced centres. It may be necessary to accurately identify the responsible agent when multiple drugs have been given simultaneously prior to reaction. In clinical practice, only a small minority of history positive subjects have positive drug challenges. As previously mentioned, DPT is better avoided if the initial reaction was life threatening.

MANAGEMENT

The tasks involved in the management of drug allergy are[28]

1. To stabilise the patient experiencing drug reaction and ensure clinical safety

2. To confirm that the adverse event is related to a drug and pin point the culprit drug in case of polypharmacy

3. To elucidate the immune response to the drug and thereby confirm true drug allergy as opposed to pseudoallergy

4. To ensure that necessary therapy for the primary medical problem is instituted, if possible by a reasonable alternative with no cross reaction or structural similarity to the offending drug

5. To consider desensitization on a case to case basis if the clinical condition mandates that the offending drug needs to be mandatorily continued

In real-life practice, the first and fourth parameters assume paramount importance. Investigation into the adverse drug reaction, other than from prior records and history, is done at an interval of 4–6 weeks from the adverse event after stabilization. This is the optimal time to proceed with a skin test or drug provocation test, if these are deemed necessary. Drug-induced allergic syndromes are pharmacologically treated similar to non-drug-induced immunopathology except that the suspected culprit drug should be promptly withdrawn. Treatment of urticaria and angioedema, anaphylaxis, serum sickness, immune cytopenias, and contact sensitivity follows similar principles. In dramatic ADR like anaphylaxis, establishment and maintenance of airway has the utmost priority. Epinephrine 1 mg/mL (adults 0.3–0.5 mg; children 0.01 mg/kg) acts as a physiological antagonist to histamine. Supplemental oxygen to maintain saturation goals may be needed in hypoxic patients. Establishment of intravenous access is also a priority in the unstable patient. Beta-2 agonists administered via aerosolized route may be needed for bronchospasm. Systemic steroids and antihistamine agents ameliorate cutaneous reactions.

Withdrawal of the putative offending drug allergen is almost always the norm, and this may actually be therapeutic to attenuate the reaction. However, exceptions do exist. In case of mild type I reactions, it may be prudent to interrupt treatment because restarting treatment after a lapse may invoke more serious reactions like anaphylaxis. A classical example is a patient with serious enterococcal endocarditis who requires prolonged treatment with penicillin. Isolated episodes of urticaria and generalized pruritus in such patients may be self-limited and will resolve with continued therapy. Late-occurring maculopapular exanthems with minimal or no pruritus is another setting for continuing treatment, especially if the culprit drug is valuable with regard to clinical results. Spontaneous resolution of ampicillin rashes has been reported in many children despite continuation of therapy.

READMINISTRATION OF OFFENDING DRUG

Readministration should be reserved for patients where therapy with alternate drugs will have significantly inferior clinical outcomes, thereby rendering the drug indispensible. Readministration is to be avoided if the initial reaction was severe (Steven S-Johnson syndrome, toxic epidermal necrolysis, etc.). Readministration involves desensitization of causative drug.[29] The mechanism of achieving clinical tolerance by drug desensitization is complex. Antigen-specific basophil and mast cell desensitization is achieved by low level; sub-threshold antigen stimulation.[30] Low-dose therapy induces oligomer formation with generation of monovalent inhibitors, both of which may be involved in the desensitization process. Desensitization results in a reduced skin sensitivity to drug allergens in most patients. Desensitization is a reversible process and relies on the continuous presence of the drug. After drug discontinuation, the desensitized state dissipates over days to weeks, and repeat desensitization may be needed for later treatment courses. Desensitization is also drug-dose dependent; subsequent large dose exposure may result in recurrence of allergic symptoms.

Readministration of the drug is usually accomplished by graded challenge. Detailed protocols for desensitization have been previously charted out and reviewed.[3] If the reaction occurred within one hour of drug administration, then the starting challenge dose should be between 1:10000 and 1:10 of the therapeutic dose depending on the severity of the reaction. In case of severe reactions, 1:10000 to 1:1000 dilutions are initially preferred. Subsequent 3–10-fold incremental doses are administered in 30–60 min intervals in the absence of positive reaction. The test challenge can be completed in a day with usually 4–5 incremental doses for patients with a previous immediate-type reaction. For delayed or non-immediate types of reactions, the test may need days or sometimes weeks.

ADMINISTRATION OF POTENTIALLY CROSS-REACTING DRUGS

Administration of potentially cross-reacting drugs is of greater concern because if these options are also taken away, then the choices left for successful therapy is further compromised. In general, cross-reactivity is confined to the same drug class (e.g., within the quinolone or sulfa-antibiotics class); cross-reactivity occurring outside the class, although reported, is much less common. Clinical situation may compel the use of cephalosporins and carbapenems in penicillin-allergic subjects. Occurence of cross-allergic reactions is low (<25%) among beta lactam antibiotics like penicillins and cephalosporins.[31] Prior skin testing with the alternative agent and slow hiking to full dose will minimize the reaction severity. Potentially cross-reactive drugs should be avoided in case of severe ADR (SJS, TEN, etc.).

PREVENTION OF ADR

Although not always preventable, certain measures decrease the likelihood of ADR. Interrogation for previous drug allergy should be made by each doctor prior to prescribing, which is essential from both a medical and a medico-legal view-point. A list of drugs to be avoided with a list of reasonable alternatives should be given to patients with a DHR, who may be instructed to carry them. Lifelong avoidance of the agent and cross-reacting ones is advisable in cases of prior drug-induced anaphylaxis. Preventive approaches (slow injection, pre-treatment with glucocorticosteroids and H1-antihistamines, etc.) may be beneficial mainly for non-allergic DHRs. It may be noted that such attempts are not a safeguard against IgE-dependent anaphylaxis. Patients having high risk factors should be more carefully monitored.

PHARMACOVIGILANCE

Under reporting of ADR is a major stumbling block to the pharmacovigilance systems.[32] The Government of India's ministry of health and family welfare, supports and sustains the pharmacovigilance programme of India and encourages reporting of suspected ADR. Any healthcare professional can report a suspected ADR in a structured format designed by the Indian Pharmacopia commission. Designated ADR Monitoring Centres (AMC) conduct a causality assessment using the WHO-UMC scale. All reports from the country are periodically reviewed by the National Co-ordinating Centre, and interventions are suggested to clinicians. National reports are sent to the Global Pharmacovigilance database maintained by the WHO.

CONCLUSION

Adverse drug reactions constitute a serious hazard in clinical practice and account for substantial morbidity and health care costs. The reported rates of ADR vary. Distinguishing a true allergic drug reaction from its close mimics is challenging for the less experienced physician. The diagnosis of drug allergy is often challenging because of the wide variations in presentation, concurrent polypharmacy, limitations of available tests, and uncertainties in the natural history of drug allergy. Withdrawal of the offending drug is almost always the norm in the management and this may actually be therapeutic to attenuate the reaction. Readministration of the drug if indicated, is usually accomplished by graded challenge.

REFERENCES

1. Edwards IR, Aronson JK. Adverse drug reactions: definitions, diagnosis, and management. Lancet 2000; 356:1255–59.

2. Lazarou J, Pomeranz BH, Corey PN. Incidence of adverse drug reactions in hospitalized patients: a meta-analysis of prospective studies. JAMA 1998; 279:1200–05.

3. Çelik G, Pichler WJ, Adkinson NF Jr. Drug Allergy. In: Adkinson NF Jr., ed. Middleton's Allergy: Principles and Practice. 7th Ed. Philadelphia, Pa; Mosby Elsevier; 2008:1202–1226.

4. Ghandhi TK, Weingart SN, Borus J, et al. Adverse drug events in ambulatory care. N Engl J Med. 2003; 348:1556–64.

5. Gomes ER, Demoly P. Epidemiology of hypersensitivity drug reactions. Curr Opin Allergy Clin Immunol. 2005; 5:309–16.

6. Fiwszenson-Albala F, Auzerie V, Mahhe E, et al. A 6-month prospective survey of cutaneous drug reactions in a hospital setting. Br J Dermatol. 2003; 149:1018–22.

7. Adkinson NF Jr. Risk factors for drug allergy. J Allergy Clin Immunol. 1984;74:567–72.

8. Pirmohamed M, Park BK. Adverse drug reactions: back to the future. Br J Clin Pharmacol. 2003;55:486–92.

9. Mirakian R, Ewan PW, Durham SR, et al. BSACI guidelines for the management of drug allergy. Clin Exp Allergy. 2009;39:43–61.

10. Gordin FM, Simon GL, Wofsy CB, et al. Adverse reactions to trimethoprim-sulfamethoxazole in patients with the acquired immunodeficiency syndrome. Ann Intern Med. 1984; 100: 495–99.

11. Haddi E, Charpin D, Tafforeau M et al. Atopy and systemic reactions to drugs. Allergy 1990; 45:236–39.

12. Ebbesen J, Buajordet I, Erikssen J et al. Drug-related deaths in a department of internal medicine. Arch Intern Med. 2001; 161:2317–23.

13. Moore TJ, Cohen MR, Furberg CD. Serious adverse drug events reported to the Food and Drug Administration, 1998–2005. Arch Intern Med. 2007; 167:1752–59.

14. Dern RJ, Beutler E, Alving AS. The hemolytic effect of primaquine V. Primaquine sensitivity as a manifestation of a multiple drug sensitivity. J Lab Clin Med. 1955; 45:30–39.

15. P. Demoly, N. F. Adkinson, K. Brockow et al. International Consensus on drug allergy. Allergy 2014; 69: 420–37.

16. Johansson SG, Bieber T, Dahl R, et al. Revised nomenclature for allergy for global use: Report of the Nomenclature Review Committee of the World Allergy Organization, October 2003. J Allergy Clin Immunol. 2004;113:832–36.

17. Pichler WJ. Delayed drug hypersensitivity reactions. Ann Intern Med. 2003;139:683–93.

18. Ju C, Uetrecht JP. Mechanism of idiosyncratic drug reactions: reactive metabolites formation, protein binding and the regulation of the immune system. Curr Drug Metab. 2002; 3:367–77.

19. Pichler WJ. Pharmacological interaction of drugs with antigen-specific immune receptors: the p-i concept. Curr Opin Allergy ClinImmunol. 2002; 2:301–05.

20. Schnyder B. Approach to the patient with drug allergy. Immunol Allergy Clin N Am. 2009;29:405–18.

21. Gadde J, Spence M, Wheeler B, et al. Clinical experience with penicillin skin testing in a large inner-city STD clinic. JAMA 1993; 270:2456–63.

22. Antunez C, Blanca-Lopez N, Torres MJ, et al. Immediate allergic reactions to cephalosporins: evaluation of cross-reactivity with a panel of penicillins and cephalosporins. J Allergy ClinImmunol. 2006; 117:404–10.

23. Sogn DD, Evans R III, Shepherd GM, et al. Results of the National Institute of Allergy and Infectious Diseases Collaborative Clinical Trial to test the predictive value of skin testing with major and minor penicillin derivatives in hospitalized adults. Arch Intern Med. 1992; 152:1025–32.

24. Fontaine C, Mayorga C, Bousquet PJ, et al. Relevance of the determination of serum-specific IgE antibodies in the diagnosis of immediate beta-lactam allergy. Allergy 2007; 62:47–52.

25. Ebo DG, Laudy SJ, Bridts CH, et al. Flow-assisted allergy diagnosis: current applications and future perspectives. Allergy 2006; 61:1028–39.

26. Lin RY, Schwartz LB, Curry A, et al. Histamine and tryptase levels in patients with acute allergic reactions: an emergency department-based study. J Allergy Clin Immunol. 2000; 106:65–71.

27. Aberer W, Bircher A, Romano A, et al. European Network for Drug Allergy (ENDA); EAACI interest group on drug hypersensitivity. Drug provocation testing in the diagnosis of drug hypersensitivity reactions: general considerations. Allergy 2003; 58:854–63.

28. Sylvia LM. Drug allergy, pseudoallergy and cutaneous diseases. In: Tisdale JE, Miller DA, editors. Drug-induced diseases: prevention, detection, and management. 2nd ed. Bethesda: American Society of Health-System Pharmacists; 2010:71–122.

29. Sobotka AK, Dembo M, Goldstein B, et al. Antigen-specific desensitization of human basophils. J Immunol. 1979; 122:511–17.

30. Sullivan TJ. Antigen-specific desensitization of patients allergic to penicillin. J Allergy Clin Immunol. 1982; 69:500–08.

31. Kelkar PS, Li JT. Cephalosporin allergy. N Engl J Med. 2001; 345:804–9.

32. Mulchandani R, Kakkar AK. Reporting of adverse drug reactions in India: A review of the current scenario, obstacles and possible solutions. Int J Risk Saf Med 2019; 30(1):33–44.

8 Insect Allergy

Balachandran J

CONTENTS

INTRODUCTION

Insect allergies are very common in India because of the diversity of insects that live in the country, as well as the inadequate preventive measures in place.[1,2] Insects are the most diverse group of organisms within the animal kingdom. Insects can be stinging, biting, or non-stinging and non-biting. The wings, scales, saliva, dried faeces, and venom cause allergic diseases like allergic rhinitis, asthma, allergic conjunctivitis and urticaria. The allergens may be proteins, glycoproteins, or chemically complex substances of low molecular weight. There are three ways in which allergic reactions may develop in patients due to insects. It can be due to injection, in the form of bites or stings; ingestion, when it is orally taken either knowingly or unknowingly; or inhalation, due to non-stinging and non-biting insects like cockroaches and dust mites.

PREVALENCE

The worldwide prevalence of insect allergy ranges from 1–7%. There is a risk of allergy when insects or their parts are eaten. Worldwide, about two billion people consume insects as food and 1600 species of insects are consumed as food. It has been pointed out that insects may be an

DOI: 10.1201/9781003125785-8

alternative food source in the near future. As the number of insects is huge, body parts and faeces containing allergenic substances are carried to long distances and hence there is a high likelihood of various allergic diseases.

Insect allergies are classified according to the route of entry of allergens.

Insect Allergy Due to Stings— Stinging Insects

The 3 families of the Hymenoptera order are stinging insects. They are *Apidae* (for example, bees), *Vespidae* (for example, wasps), and *Formicidae* (for example, fireants). The honeybee is universally found. Yellow jackets (Vespula) are common in temperate regions.[1] Wasps (Polistes) and hornets (Vespa) are seen usually in the subtropical and tropical regions.

Pathophysiology

There are allergic as well as non-allergic components in the venom which may lead to various reactions.[3] The non-allergic components are the vasoactive amines like histamine, serotonin, dopamine, and norepinephrine. They cause local reactions lasting less than 24 hours. The reactions usually include redness, pain, and swelling. If a large quantity of these substances is injected, as happens when hundreds of insect stings occur together, anaphylactoid reactions may occur.

Another non-IgE mediated reaction to insect stings is serum sickness which is a Gell and Coombs type III hypersensitivity reaction.[4] Allergic reactions to insect stings occur due to type I hypersensitivity to insect venom, which is mainly peptides and enzymes. The enzymes phospholipase A and hyaluronidase are responsible for most allergic reactions.[3]

Clinical Features

Allergic manifestations caused by different species of insects differ from each other. Stings result almost exclusively from the Hymenoptera order.

Hymenoptera Venom Allergy (HVA)[5]

Sensitization may or may not be clinically relevant. If symptomatic, it is called hymenoptera venom allergy. Asymptomatic sensitization is common, especially in bee keepers.

1. Patients with HVA who are at high risk of severe allergic reaction are those with a history of previous severe allergic reaction

2. Cardiovascular comorbidities

3. Patients on beta-blockers and angiotensin converting enzyme inhibitors

4. Patients with elevated BST levels (Basal serum tryptase)

5. Mastocytosis

6. Elderly patients

Lepidoptera[6]

Lepidoptera includes moths, butterflies and their larvae. Only a few of 150,000 species of moths and butterflies have been noted to evoke reactions. Parlato reported in 1932, respiratory allergy caused by moths and butterflies. Wills and co-workers found in 2016 that allergic diseases are caused by the scales and toxic fluids of adult moths and butterflies. Localized reactions like pain, itchiness, or wheal may be caused by stinging caterpillars. Urticaria and dermatitis may be caused by hairs from caterpillars or moths. Haemorrhagic illness may also result from stings by some species of caterpillars. Ophthalmia nodosa (eye allergy resulting from caterpillar hairs) is another manifestation. Dendrolimiasis and pararamose are skin involvements, along with joint inflammation. Destruction and deformation of joints may occur.

Midges[7]

Midges differ from mosquitoes in that they do not have a proboscis. They also fly in swarms. Female midges bite birds and mammals for the maturation of their eggs. Midges can cause asthma by way of inhalation of allergenic particles. Freeze dried larvae of midges are used as fish food in Germany. This leads to allergic asthma among fish breeders. The prevalence of allergic rhinitis and asthma was found to be higher in midge-exposed villagers in Sudan. Both adult and larval body parts were found to contain allergenic substances.

Mosquitoes[8]

Mosquitoes belong to the family Culicidae. The females possess proboscis. Allergies due to mosquito bites are characterized by erythema, bulla, or even ulcer with or without fever. Hemo-phagocytic syndrome is a potential cause of death. Proteins within the saliva of mosquitoes can evoke an immunologic response, which is the basis of severe allergic reactions following their bites. The percentage of people who manifest clinically with significant allergic reactions following mosquito bites are, however, low. The most frequent type of allergic reactions seen following mosquito bites is a large local reaction (Skeeter syndrome).[9] Systemic reactions including anaphylaxis or asthma are rare following mosquito bites. It is to be noted that mosquitoes transmit numerous diseases, the details of which are beyond the scope of this book.

Type I Hypersensitivity to insect venom may present in three ways:

1. **Large local reactions (LLR)**

   The size is more than 10 cm, peaking in 1–3 days. LLR may start within a few minutes or several hours after injection. It may last days or even weeks. It may or may not be associated with lymphadenopathy or lymphangitis. LLR caused by a bite in the periorbital area may lead to swelling of the eyelids, and this may be confused with angioedema of systemic allergic reactions (SAR). The most frequent feature is skin reaction. Chronic urticaria can result from insect allergy without an immediate reaction.

2. **Generalized non-life-threatening systemic reactions**: Urticaria and angioedema are the usual manifestations of this type of SAR.

3. **Anaphylaxis**: Severe and life-threatening allergic reactions come under this category. It is characterized by either the presence of hypotension or the involvement of at least two organ systems of the following[10]:

   - Cutaneous (urticaria, angioedema, itching, flushing)
   - Pulmonary (bronchospasm)
   - Upper airway (swelling of the tongue or throat, laryngeal oedema)
   - Gastrointestinal (nausea, vomiting, diarrhoea and abdominal pain)
   - Neurological (seizures)
     - **Biphasic anaphylaxis**: It is the recurrence of anaphylactic reaction within 4–12 hours after resolution, which occurs without any further exposure to the insect.
     - **Beta-blockers and ACEIs**: If a patient is on beta-blockers or ACEIs, hymenoptera sting reaction can be very severe. In addition, beta-blockers may inhibit epinephrine, which is the life saving drug for anaphylaxis. ACEIs can increase the bradykinin levels and block the vasoconstrictor response by the renin-angiotensin mechanism. Thus ACEIs can aggravate hypotonia during anaphylaxis.
     - **Other**: Increased serum tryptase levels (as in mastocytosis, myelocytic

leukemia and myelodysplastic syndromes) can increase the severity of reactions.

Insect Allergy Due to Bites—Biting Insects

Insect bites are less likely to cause anaphylaxis than insect stings. Mosquitoes, bugs, fleas, ticks, and some types of flies that bite humans may evoke an allergic reaction. Formic acid is the chemical usually injected. It can cause blisters, redness, oedema, pain, and itching. Allergic reactions are usually large local reactions (LLR). However, they do not normally last as long as sting reactions.

SPECIAL MANIFESTATIONS
Kounis Syndrome[11]

It is an acute coronary syndrome resulting from an allergic or immunological reaction to an allergen. This was first reported by Kounis and Zavras in 1991. It is also termed "allergic angina" or "allergic myocardial infarction". Coronary artery vasospasm or atheromatous plaque rupture may result from inflammatory cytokines released by mast cell activation.

Takotsubo Cardiomyopathy[12]/ Stress Cardiomyopathy

It is characterised by acute coronary syndrome without angiographical evidence of coronary artery stenosis. The distinctive feature of it is reversible left ventricular apical ballooning.

Spontaneous Abortion

This may occur due to uterine contraction resulting from insect sting allergy.

Children[13]

Insect allergy is the second most common cause of severe reactions in children, the first being food allergy. Children with atopy tend to face a higher incidence of severe insect allergy than non-atopic children. Skin reactions are relatively more common in systemic reactions in children. In 60% of cases of systemic reactions in children, only the skin is involved; this is much higher in comparison to adults, in which 15% of cases fall into this category.

DIAGNOSIS
History[9]

Effort must be taken for the identification of the insect if possible. Place of the stinging or biting episode, location of the nest, whether the insect was aggressive or not, and presence or absence of a stinger in the wound are also to be noted. The duration between the stinging event and the development of symptoms is important. The details of symptoms also aid in the diagnosis.

Investigations

The following tests are used for the diagnosis of insect allergy.

Skin Test[14]

The skin test is the most common test employed, with an accuracy of 90–95%. This test, which is considered the gold standard, should be done at least 2 weeks after the insect sting. This is necessary because false negativity is possible during the refractory period. Prick tests are carried out first. If they are negative, intradermal tests are indicated.

Specific IgE[15]

If available, this is useful. Specific IgE in serum is ideally measured 1 to 4 weeks after the sting or bite. However, it can even be detected immediately after the sting or bite.

Total IgE

The utility of total IgE is in the correct interpretation of specific IgE levels, especially if they are low. Pollen sensitization can lead to high total IgE levels.

Basal Serum Tryptase (BST)[16]

It should be measured within 36 hours of the sting bite. It is indicated when there is a severe systemic reaction, lack of urticaria in a systemic reaction, or a systemic reaction with negative IgE result.

The Basophil Activation Test (BAT)[17]

It can identify about two-thirds of patients with a positive history and negative skin and negative IgE tests.

Component Resolved Diagnosis (CRD)[18,19]

Recombinant allergens are used to diagnose specific IgE antibodies.

CAP Inhibition Method[20,21]

This is time consuming and expensive. However, it has high accuracy in identifying sensitizations when cross-reactions exist.

Sting Challenge[22]

It is not widely practised because of the risk.

Insect Allergy Due to Ingestion[23,24]
Entomophagy

This is the term used to refer to the utilization of insects as a food source. There is a risk of allergy when insects or their parts are eaten.

There are three ways in which insects or their body parts enter the human body via ingestion.

1. Eating insects for taste and nutrition
2. Carmine dye from cochineal being used as a natural red pigment in food
3. Insects or its fragments, eggs, or larvae contaminating food or food products

Tropomyosin

This is a cross-reactive allergen among invertebrates and shellfish. Those who are allergic to shellfish can potentially develop an allergy to insect based foods. Carmine dye is extracted from crushed bodies of the female cochineal, *Dactylopiuscoccus*, which is native to South and Central America. About 17% of the female cochineal has cariminic acid.

The three orders of insects which can contaminate food or food products are:

1. Coleoptera (beetles)
2. Lepidoptera (butterflies and moths)
3. Psocoptera (booklice)

Diagnosis of orally ingested insect allergy:

- Clinical history
- Oral challenge (OFC)
- Skin prick test (SPT)
- Specific IgE (SIgE)

There is a risk of anaphylaxis during OFC. It is the first test tried when the clinical history is not suggestive of food allergy.

Insect Allergy by the Inhalational Route

It has been demonstrated that allergen sensitization is seen in the case of stinging insects like bees, even when the person had never been stung by an insect in their life. Skin reaction has been demonstrated equally among the non-stinging and the stinging insect extracts. This shows that sensitization is possible by any route of exposure to the insect antigens.

Adequate temperature, sufficient humidity, atmospheric pressure, and wind velocities determine the concentration of insects and thus the prevalence of insect allergy by the inhalant route. Allergic rhinitis and asthma can result from inhalation of insects or their parts or excreta. The cockroach is a common insect causing upper and lower respiratory allergy by this route. Though not insects, mites (belonging to Arachnida) are important causes for allergic rhinitis and asthma.

The prevalence of allergic diseases by inhalation of mosquito body parts is not frequent.

Allergic rhinitis and asthma may be caused by mayflies. Pellicles of mayflies are mainly responsible for allergic reactions. Caddis fly allergy can also cause similar reactions. Immunotherapy was found to be successful in the above two instances. Wings of caddis fly were found to be allergenic. Allergy due to inhalation of the house fly, fruit fly, bugs, honey bees, beetles, locusts, and crickets has been reported. The most potent allergen reported is locust faeces.

The clinical features, diagnosis, and management of asthma and allergic rhinitis have been described elsewhere in the book.

MANAGEMENT

Antihistamines with oral steroids are sufficient for the treatment of mild allergic reactions resulting from insects. Cold compresses may provide symptomatic relief. In an LLR in the oral cavity, treatment as in a systemic allergic reaction is needed.

Management of Anaphylaxis[25]

Management includes general and specific measures.

i. *General measures:* Monitoring of heart rare, arterial blood pressure and oxygen saturation is absolutely essential. Immediate intravenous isotonic saline solution is required the patient is positioned in the Trendelenburg position.

ii. *Specific measures*: Adrenaline must be administered intramuscularly in the lateral thigh. The dose is 0.01 mg/kg of a 1 in 1000 solution. The maximum recommended dose is 0.3 mg in children and 0.5 mg in adults.

Other medications which are useful in the treatment of anaphylaxis are dopamine, corticosteroids, bronchodilators, glucagon, and desmopressin. Anti-H1 antihistamines are useful only for the treatment of skin symptoms. The use of anti-H2 antihistamines are not recommended because there is no added benefit.

Self-Treatment

Those patients with a previous history of anaphylactic reaction should be advised to carry adrenaline auto injections with them. The patients, or parents in the case of small children, should be given adequate training of its use.

VENOM IMMUNOTHERAPY[26,27]

Venom Immunotherapy is the treatment of choice for systemic reaction after hymenoptera sting. The indications for venom immunotherapy include systemic reactions, patients with high risk of exposure, those with impaired quality of life and patients with a global mast cell disorder. It is the only causative treatment for HVA and reduces the risk of recurrent SAR. In addition, it improves quality of life. VIT is not recommended in patients with unusual, toxic and atypical reactions. Factors leading to the failure of VIT are older age, cardiovascular/pulmonary comorbidities, elevated BST levels, and mastocytosis. VIT protects almost all HVA patients from future allergic reactions.

PREVENTION[28]

It includes avoidance measures and prevention of anaphylaxis. Covering the body, especially the forearms and the legs are essential. Gloves may be needed in certain situations of outdoor activity. If possible, children with a history of anaphylaxis due to insects must wear identification tags showing the name of the insect to which they are allergic.

REFERENCES

1. Kausar MA. A review on respiratory allergy caused by insects. Bioinformation 2018; 14(9):540–53.

2. Shivpuri, DN, Shali, PL, Agarwal, MK, Prakash, D, Bhatnager PL. Insect allergy in India. Ann Allergy 1971;29(11):588–97.

3. Resiman RE. Allergy to stinging insects. In: Patterson R, Grammer LC, Greenberger PA eds. Allergic Diseases: Diagnosis and Management. 5th ed. Philadelphia: Lippincott Williams & Wilkins; 1997:253–64.

4. Yunginger JW. Insect allergy. In: Middleton E, Reed CE, Ellis EF, et al eds.: Allergy, Principle and Practice, 4th ed. St. Louis: Mosby-Year Book;1993:1511–20.

5. Alfaya Arias T, Gomis VS, Soto Mera T, Vega Castro A, Vega Gutierrez JM, Alonso Llamazares A, et al. (Hymenoptera Allergy Committee of the SEAIC) Key Issues in Hymenoptera Venom Allergy: An Update. J Investig Allergol Clin Immunol. 2017; 27(1): 19–31.

6. Osgood H. Comparison of reagins to separate species of caddis fly. Jour Allergy 1934; 5 (4): 367–72.

7. Baur X. Chironomid midge allergy. Arerugi 1992;41(2):81–85.

8. Crisp, HC, Johnson, KS. Mosquito allergy. Ann Allergy Asthma Immunol 2013;110(2):65–69.

9. Simons, FE, Peng Z. Skeeter syndrome. J Allergy ClinImmunol 1999;104(3):705–707.

10. Golden DBK, et al. Stinging insect hypersensitivity-A practice parameter update 2016. Ann Allergy Asthma Immunol. 2017; 118:28–54.

11. Kounis NG. Hymenoptera stings, anaphylactic shock and the Kounis syndrome. N Am J Med Sci 2013; 5: 159–60.

12. Mert GÖ, Biteker FS, Mert KU, et al. Takotsubo cardiomyopathy or Kounis syndrome or both? Int J Cardiol. 2015; 179: 16-21.

13. Tan, JW, Campbell, DE. Insect allergy in children. J Paediatr Child Health 2013; 49(9):E381–7.

14. Quirt JA, Wen X, Kim J, Herrero AJ, Kim HL. Venom allergy testing: is a graded approach necessary? Ann Allergy Asthma Immunol 2016; 116:49–51.

15. Goldberg A, Confino-Cohen R. Timing of venom skin tests and IgE determinations after insect sting anaphylaxis. J Allergy Clin Immunol 1997; 100:183–184.

16. Haeberli, G, Brönnimann, M, Hunziker, T, Müller U. Elevated basal serum tryptase and hymenoptera venom allergy: relation to severity of sting reactions and to safety and efficacy of venom immunotherapy. Clin Exp Allergy 2003; 33(9):1216–20.

17. Kucera P, Cvackova M, Hulikova K, Juzova O, Pachl J. Basophil activation can predict clinical sensitivity in patients after venom immunotherapy. J Investig Allergol Immunol 2010; 20:110–16.

18. Blank, S, Bilò, MB, Ollert M. Component-resolved diagnostics to direct in venom immunotherapy: Important steps towards precision medicine. Clin Exp Allergy 2018; 48(4):354–64.

19. Tomsitz, D, Brockow K. Component resolved diagnosis in hymenoptera anaphylaxis. Curr Allergy Asthma Rep 2017; 17(6):38. https://doi.org/10.1007/s11882-017-0707-0

20. Quercia O, et al. CAP-inhibition, molecular diagnostics, and total IgE in the evaluation of polistes and vespula double sensitization. Int Arch Allergy Immunol 2018; 177(4):365–69.

21. Savi, E, et al. Comparing the ability of molecular diagnosis and CAP-inhibition in identifying the really causative venom in patients with positive tests to Vespula and Polistes species. Clin Mol Allergy 2016; 14: 3. doi: 10.1186/s12948-016-0040-5.

22. Rueff F, Przybilla B, Muller U, Mosbech H. The sting challenge test in hymenoptera venom allergy. Allergy 1996; 51: 216–25.

23. Carlos Ribeiro J. Allergic risks of consuming edible insects: A systematic review. Mol Nutr Food Res 2018; 62(1). doi: 10.1002/mnfr.201700030.

24. de Gier, S, Verhoeckx, K. Insect (food) allergy and allergens. Mol Immunol 2018;100: 82–106.

25. Lieberman P, Nicklas RA, Randolph C, et al. Anaphylaxis: a practice parameter update 2015. Ann Allergy Asthma Immunol 2015; 115: 341–84.

26. Golden DB. Insect sting allergy and venom immunotherapy: a model and a mystery. J Allergy Clin Immunol 2005; 115: 439–47.

27. Reisman RE, Livingston A. Venom immunotherapy: 10 years of experience with administration of single venoms and 50 micrograms maintenance dose. J Allergy Clin Immunol. 1992; 89: 1189–95.

28. Bonifazi F, Jutel M, Bilo BM, Birnbaum J, Muller U. Prevention and treatment of hymenoptera venom allergy: guidelines for clinical practice. Allergy 2005; 60: 1459–70.

9 Life-Threatening Allergy

Benita Florence and Dodiy Herman

CONTENTS

INTRODUCTION

Allergy refers to the abnormal immune response to a certain substance in a susceptible host, causing life-threatening clinical syndromes to the latter. These reactions are reproducible each time the substance is introduced and, most of the time, are dose-independent. An acute, potentially life-threatening, generalised, hypersensitivity reaction that is characterised by a rapid onset of airway and/or breathing and/or circulatory problems usually associated with skin or mucosal changes, resulting from the sudden release of mediators derived from mast cells and basophils, is termed anaphylaxis. Human anaphylaxis is generally thought to be mediated by IgE, with mast cells and basophils as key players, although alternative mechanisms have been proposed. Neutrophils and macrophages have also been implicated in anaphylactic reactions, as have IgG-dependent, complement and contact system activation.

All allergic reactions are not anaphylactic, and the presence of co-factors may explain the reason why some conditions lead to anaphylaxis, while in other cases the allergen elicits a milder reaction. Co-factors that have reported to be relevant in up to 30% of anaphylactic episodes

are nonsteroidal anti-inflammatory drugs, exercise, estrogens, angiotensin-converting enzyme inhibitors, β-blockers, lipid-lowering drugs, and alcohol. Food allergens account for 33–56% of all cases and up to 81% of cases of anaphylaxis in children.

These reactions are associated with different mechanisms, triggers, clinical presentations, and varied severity. Hence the wide range of clinical manifestations, lack of laboratory confirmatory testing, and complex underlying mechanism leads to difficulty in establishing a standard definition and diagnostic criteria for anaphylaxis.

The rate of occurrence of anaphylaxis globally is unknown because of under-recognition by patients, caregivers and healthcare professionals, under-reporting, use of a variety of medical terms, under-coding and lack of disease-specific laboratory tests. Yet anaphylaxis is not rare, and the rate of occurrence appears to be increasing with geographic variations. Based on international studies, lifetime prevalence is estimated to be 0.05–2%.[1–5]

HYPERSENSITIVITY REACTIONS

Repeated exposure of the body to an allergen sensitizes and makes the individual susceptible to that allergen. At some time,

DOI: 10.1201/9781003125785-9

Table 9.1: The Types of Hypersensitivity Reactions, Their Mechanisms, Onset of Symptoms, and Examples[6-8]

Type	Reaction	Mechanism	Onset of Action	Examples
Type I immediate hypersensitivity	IgE mediated	Degranulation of mast cells and release of histamine	Minutes to hours	Urticaria, Food allergy, Allergic rhinitis
Type II antibody-mediated hypersensitivity	Non-IgE (IgG or IgM) mediated	Interaction of antibodies with cell surface antigens leads to complement activation and lysis or phagocytosis. Autoimmune reactions Antibody-mediated cytotoxicity	Hours to days	Hemolytic anaemia, Hashimoto's thyroiditis, Transfusion reaction
Type III immune complex-mediated hypersensitivity	Immune complex-mediated	Deposits of antigen - antibody complexes activate complement pathway and cause tissue injury.	10–21 days	Serum sickness Systemic lupus erythematosus
Type IV cell-mediated	Cell-mediated	Cytokines from CD4+ and CD8+ cells activate macrophages leading to inflammation and tissue damage Direct killing of affected cells by CD8+ T cells	2–4 days or more days	Tuberculin reaction, allergic contact dermatitis

the body may become hypersensitive to the exposed allergen and cause tissue injury and damage. Diseases resulting from this type of reaction are immunologic and known as hypersensitivity diseases. The types of hypersensitivity reactions, mechanisms, onset of action, and common causes are summarized in Table 9.1.[6-8]

PATHOPHYSIOLOGY

Anaphylaxis can be due to multiple triggers. The body undergoes widespread release of inflammatory mediators including histamine, leukotrienes and platelet-activating factor, primarily from mast cells, irrespective of the trigger. Mast cells are present in highest concentration in the skin followed by the respiratory tract, gastrointestinal tract, around the coronary vessels, and between the myocardial muscle fibres. This is the reason for the varied distribution of the clinical features. Bronchoconstriction, vasodilatation, increased vascular permeability, weakening of myocardial contractility, and coronary artery spasm are caused by the inflammatory mediators.

RISK FACTORS AND TRIGGERS FOR ANAPHYLAXIS

Cardiovascular disease, asthma, eczema, allergic rhinitis, increase in age, and coexisting comorbidities are risk factors. Medications which include beta-adrenergic blockers, angiotensin converting enzyme inhibitors, latex, horse-derived antitoxins (e.g. snake anti-venoms), helminthes, and insect stings are major triggers in adults, while foods including stinging insects are the triggers in children and adolescents. Contaminants in medications such as over-sulphated chondroitin sulphate in heparin and herbal formulations can also be triggers. Radiocontrast media are diagnostic substances, leading to anaphylaxis in patients with multiple coexisting diseases. Exercise, acute infection, such as fever, emotional stress, travel, which causes a change in the normal routine, and premenstrual status are co-factors that amplify anaphylaxis. Seminal fluid can be an allergen in atopic women.

Pregnant patients are vulnerable, and both the mother and baby are at increased risk of death or ischemic encephalopathy. Anaphylaxis in these patients is triggered by administration of oxytocin, or an antimicrobial, such as penicillin, or a cephalosporin for prophylaxis of group B hemolytic streptococcal infection in the neonate. Anaphylaxis can be difficult to recognize in the paediatric population, in patients with impaired vision or hearing, neurologic disease, psychiatric illness, such as depression, substance abuse, autism spectrum disorder, attention deficit hyperactivity disorder, or cognitive disorders, as they may not be able to describe their symptoms.[9-13]

CLINICAL PRESENTATION

A rapid assessment with prompt treatment should begin immediately upon arrival to the hospital.

Clinical assessment involving history and physical examination will then help in channelling the diagnosis and further investigations. A detailed history relevant enough to include exposures and events prior to the onset of symptoms should be recorded which may include exercise, ingestion of prescribed or non-prescribed medications, recreational drugs, ethanol, and food. History taking however should not delay treatment at any cost. Sudden onset of symptoms and signs within minutes to hours after exposure to a known or potential trigger, followed by rapid progression of symptoms and signs should help in diagnosis. Cutaneous involvement may not be seen in 20% of the cases making the diagnosis difficult. Various clinical presentations of anaphylaxis in different systems are given in Table 9.2.[4,6,10,13–16]

Based on the triggers identified anaphylaxis can be classified as drug-induced anaphylaxis, insect venom-induced anaphylaxis, food anaphylaxis, and so on.

CATAMENIAL ANAPHYLAXIS

Catamenial or cyclical anaphylactic reaction syndrome ranges from dermatitis, urticaria, angioedema, and asthma to anaphylactic shock, usually in the luteal phase of menstruation induced by endogenous progesterone secretion. Patients usually have a cyclical pattern of attacks during the premenstrual part of the cycle. The mechanism is most likely hypersensitivity to progesterone and probably the vasoactive component in menstrual fluid such as prostaglandin. This is more a diagnosis of exclusion and pattern study. Cessation of the menstrual cycle by means of medical or surgical menopause showed reduction in such anaphylactic reactions in these patients.[17,18]

IDIOPATHIC ANAPHYLAXIS

All symptoms suggestive of anaphylaxis can occur without any identifiable cause. Diagnosis is based primarily on the history and an exhaustive search for causative factors.[19]

DIFFERENTIAL DIAGNOSIS

Various differential diagnosis of acute anaphylaxis includes vaso-vagal syndrome, acute severe asthma, post-feeding generalized acute urticaria, and food-dependent exercise-induced anaphylaxis.

Other medical conditions like respiratory failure, globus hystericus, foreign body aspiration, pulmonary embolism, epiglottitis, myocardial infarction, hereditary angioedema, seizure, carcinoid syndrome, drug overdose, phaeochromocytoma, and the like should be considered if no clear cause suggestive of anaphylaxis is found by either history or physical examination.

Table 9.2: Clinical Features Seen as Part of Early Allergic Reactions or Anaphylaxis Based on the System Involved[4,6,10,13–16]

System	Features

Skin and Mucosal Involvement	Generalized urticaria
	Itching or flushing
	Swollen lips-tongue-uvula
	Angioedema
	Rash
	Periorbital swelling
	Conjunctival irritation
	  Tearing from eyes
	  Tingling of lips

Respiratory System	Nasal itching and congestion
	Rhinorrhea
	Sneezing
	  Throat itching and tightness
	Dysphonia
	Hoarseness
	Hypoxia
	Stridor
	Dry staccato cough
	Increased respiratory rate
	  Shortness of breath
	Chest tightness
	  Wheezing/bronchospasm
	Decreased peak expiratory flow
	  Cyanosis
	  Respiratory arrest

Cardiovascular System	Chest pain Tachycardia or bradycardia or other arrhythmias Palpitations Hypotension, syncope, shock Cardiac arrest

Gastrointestinal System	Crampy abdominal pain
	Nausea, vomiting
	  Diarrhoea
	  Dysphagia
	Urinary or faecal incontinence

Central Nervous System	Sense of impending doom Uneasiness (in infants and children, sudden behavioural change, e.g. irritability, cessation of play, clinging to parent) Throbbing headache (pre-epinephrine) Altered mental status Dizziness Confusion Tunnel vision Lipothymia
Others	Metallic taste in the mouth Cramps and bleeding due to uterine contractions in women

When anaphylaxis presents with generalised urticaria, it many mimic many cutaneous syndromes (Table 9.3).

MANAGEMENT

First attempt should be directed at eliminating the cause such as intravenous administration of drug, blood products, or anaesthetic agents.

Table 9.3: Conditions Mimicking Allergic Reactions with Urticaria[20]

Atopic Dermatitis

Bullous Pemphigoid

Contact Dermatitis

Erythema Multiforme

Fixed Drug Reactions

Mastocytoma

Urticaria Pigmentosa

Viral Exanthem

Vasculitis

Henoch Schonlein Purpura

Pityriasis Rosea

FIRST-LINE TREATMENT

Epinephrine (Adrenaline) is administered intramuscularly (in a dose of 0.01 mg/kg of a 1:1000 [1 mg/mL] solution to a maximum of 0.5 mg in adults and 0.3 mg in children) into the anterolateral thigh. Epinephrine being a nonselective adrenergic agonist increases peripheral vascular resistance through vasoconstriction, increases cardiac output, reverses bronchoconstriction, and reduces mucosal oedema, and helps in stabilizing mast cells and basophils.

In a state of circulatory insufficiency, subcutaneous administration may not be the best route for the drugs. The intramuscular route helps drugs reach their peak concentrations faster than the subcutaneous route. This will help in getting a quicker access till an intravenous cannula is secured in place. Rich vascularization of the muscle allows the medication to be readily absorbed with an immediate effect.[13]

SECOND-LINE TREATMENT

Agents of second-line treatments (see Table 9.4) should not be used in place of epinephrine. Antihistamines have slow onset of action and do not play a role in stabilizing or preventing mast cell degranulation. They also do not target additional mediators of anaphylaxis and will not help in immediate management of hypotension or bronchospasm. However, they are helpful in controlling the symptoms, especially generalized itching.

ADJUNCTIVE THERAPY

Glucocorticoids are used as an adjunctive therapy for anaphylaxis, even though there is lack of evidence in supporting clinical benefits. They may help in preventing a relapse.[13–15,21]

REFRACTORY ANAPHYLAXIS[13,22]

In cases of refractory anaphylaxis, the following treatments may be considered:

1. Glucagon 1–2 mg intramuscular or intravenous every 5 minutes, if there is no response to epinephrine (especially may be beneficial in patients on beta-blockers).

2. In patients requiring more than one dose of adrenaline, a half dose of adrenaline may be safe in patients on amitriptyline, imipramine, or beta-blockers.

3. Vasopressors may be beneficial in persistent hypotension. Anticholinergic agents may help in those with persistent bradycardia (Atropine) or ipratropium, in those with epinephrine-resistant bronchospasm.

4. Think of other causes like cardiac tamponade, acute coronary syndrome, etc., if no positive response to treatment is seen.

5. Anaphylaxis caused due to C1 esterase inhibitor deficiency will be resistant to adrenaline, steroids, and antihistamines and will need treatment with C1 esterase inhibitor concentrate or fresh frozen plasma.

Epinephrine should be administered in life-threatening anaphylactic reactions, even when there is relative contraindications like coronary artery disease, uncontrolled hypertension, serious ventricular arrhythmia, or if the candidate is in the second stage of labour.

The ABCs of treating anaphylaxis are addressed in Table 9.5.

Do not make these patients suddenly sit, stand, or stay in the upright position. If they experience respiratory distress or vomiting, place them in a position of comfort with their

Table 9.4: Classes of Second-Line Agents, Their Dosage and Route of Administration

Class of Drugs	Medication	Adult	Children	Route
H1-antihistamine	Chlorpheniramine Or Diphenydramine	10 mg 25-50 mg	2.5-5 mg 1 mg/kg (max 50 mg)	Intravenous
ß2-adrenergic agonist	Salbutamol	5 mg	2.5 mg	Nebuliser/Face mask
Glucocorticoids	Hydrocortisone Or Methylprednisolone	200 mg 50-100 mg	2.5 mg/kg (max 100 mg) 1 mg/kg (max 50 mg)	Intravenous
H2-antihistamine	Ranitidine	50 mg	1 mg/kg (max 50 mg)	Intravenous

Table 9.5: The ABCs of Treating Anaphylaxis

Airway	Maintain patent airway/Keep difficult airway trolley at hand in the event of swollen tongue or other features causing obstruction.
Breathing	Oxygen via nasal cannula/mask. Maintain SpO_2 <=94%.
Circulation	Epinephrine 1:1000 (1 mg/mL). Children: 0.01 mg/kg up to a maximum of 0.3 mg intramuscular, in the anterolateral thigh. Adults: 0.5 mg intramuscular, in the anterolateral thigh. Repeat if necessary, every 5–15 min. Monitor – heart rate, blood pressure. Epinephrine at dilutions of 1:10,000 intravenous only in cases of cardiorespiratory arrest or profound hypotension not responding to volume expansion or multiple intramuscular injections of epinephrine.
Volume expansion 0.9% Saline solution or Ringer's lactate	Children: 5–10 mL/kg IV in the first 5 min and 30 mL/kg in the first hour. Adolescents: 1–2 litres at 500 ml boluses. Regulated by pulse rate and blood pressure. Establish IV access with the highest calibre of cannula possible. Monitor for volume overload.
Position	Maintain adequate position preferably supine with elevated lower limb. Getting up or sitting down suddenly is associated with fatal outcomes ("empty ventricle syndrome").

lower limbs elevated. This helps in achieving the therapeutic goals:

1. Preservation of fluid in the central vascular compartment—helps in managing distributive shock.

2. Prevention of the empty vena cava/empty ventricle syndrome—occurs immediately when patients with anaphylaxis suddenly are placed in an upright position. These patients are at high risk for sudden death. Epinephrine does not act as required because it does not reach the heart and hence cannot be circulated throughout the body.[23]

LABORATORY INVESTIGATIONS AND THEIR ROLE IN DIAGNOSIS

Tryptase levels may help in diagnosis when there is a doubt. Blood sample for measurement of tryptase level is best obtained from 15 minutes to 3 hours after symptom onset. Histamine levels in blood are obtained 15–60 minutes after symptom onset. It is important to note that these tests are not available in all institutions, need not be performed on an emergency basis, and are not specific for anaphylaxis. Anaphylaxis cannot be ruled out with normal levels of either tryptase or histamine. The measurement of the IgE specific for the food allergen components may be helpful as well.[13,24]

FOOD PROTEIN–INDUCED ENTEROCOLITIS SYNDROME[25,26]

Food protein–induced enterocolitis syndrome (FPIES) also known as delayed food allergy is a non–IgE mediated food allergy. This is characterized by repetitive, projectile vomiting associated with pallor and generalised weakness within 1–4 hours. This condition is treated with:

1. Fluid resuscitation: 10–20 mL/kg body weight in bolus.

2. Methylprednisolone: 1 mg/kg body weight IV, maximum of 60–80 mg.

3. Ondansetron IV or IM: 0.15 mg/kg body weight.

Resuscitation is started in the Emergency Department, and the patient should be admitted for hydration and further evaluation. Replacement of electrolytes is necessary with monitoring of pulse rate, temperature, capillary filling time, blood pressure, and input output charting.

BIPHASIC ANAPHYLAXIS

Biphasic anaphylaxis is recurrent anaphylaxis occurring 1–72 hours after resolution of an initial anaphylactic episode.

Risk factors for biphasic anaphylaxis are:

1. Severe anaphylaxis

2. Patients who required more than 1 dose of epinephrine

3. Wide pulse pressure

4. Unknown anaphylaxis trigger

5. Cutaneous signs and symptoms

6. Drug trigger in children

DISPOSITION

Patients should be observed and monitored for a minimum of 6 hours after the resolution of symptoms. This may need to be longer for patients in the vulnerable or high risk groups:[14]

- Extremes of age
- Multiple comorbidities
- Severe asthma
- Continued absorption of the substance
- History of previous biphasic reaction
- Out of hours presentation
- Difficulty accessing emergency care

ANTIBIOTIC ALLERGY LABELS

The initial allergy reaction documented for a drug might not have been an allergy, it could have been an intolerance, a viral rash, or a drug infection interaction. Even if the original reaction was immunological, it may not recur with re-challenge. If T-cell mediated mild delayed reactions do not occur with re-challenge, it could be possible that the immune responses were lost in the absence of ongoing drug exposure. In a study conducted among admitted patients with a documented penicillin allergy who were skin tested and re-challenged, 95% were not allergic and were de-labelled. More than 98% of out-patients with previous documented penicillin allergies have also been tolerant to penicillin. Global variation in the frequency of confirmed IgE-mediated penicillin allergy exists. These variations might be due to differential antibiotic prescribing patterns, differences in patient selection, or demographic and genetic differences.[27–31]

PREVENTION

A detailed understanding of predisposing and augmenting factors could lead to the development of prophylactic and therapeutic approaches on individual patient to patient basis.

Patients should be instructed on identifying triggers and how to avoid being exposed to them.

Patients must understand the need to carry an epinephrine autoinjector syringe at all times and learn how to use it at the earliest onset of symptoms. Unused syringes should be replaced when they reach their expiry date.

Other important patient instructions include:

a. An anaphylaxis emergency action plan should be explained verbally and a written copy given to patient

b. The use of EpiPen (autoinjector) should be taught

c. Follow-up investigations by an allergy/ immunology specialist should be arranged

CONCLUSION

Life-threatening allergy or anaphylaxis is an acute hypersensitivity reaction presenting with respiratory and/or haemodynamic compromise. Other manifestations of hypersensitivity reactions, such as urticarial or angioedema, may coexist. Common causes for anaphylaxis are food and drugs. At the same time any allergen can cause this in susceptible individuals. Identification of the offending antigen is the most important measure to be taken to avoid further reaction if exposed to the same allergen. Management strategies include early detection, restoration of respiratory and haemodynamic function, administration of epinephrine and systemic corticosteroids, and other supportive measures.

REFERENCES

1. Sampson HA, Muñoz-Furlong A, Campbell RL, Adkinson NF Jr, Bock SA, Branum A, et al. Second symposium on the definition and management of anaphylaxis: summary report—Second National Institute of Allergy and Infectious Disease/Food Allergy and Anaphylaxis Network Symposium. J Allergy Clin Immunol. 2006;117:391–7.

2. Ben-Shoshan M, Clarke AE. Anaphylaxis: past, present and future. Allergy. 2011;66:1–14.

3. Wang J, Sampson HA. Food anaphylaxis. Clin Exp Allergy. 2007;37:651–60.

4. Metcalfe DD, Peavy RD, Gilfillan AM. Mechanisms of mast cell signaling in anaphylaxis. J Allergy Clin Immunol. 2009;124:639–46.

5. Lieberman P, Camargo CA Jr, Bohlke K, Jick H, Miller RL, Sheikh A, et al. Epidemiology of anaphylaxis: findings of the American College of Allergy, Asthma and Immunology Epidemiology of Anaphylaxis Working Group. Ann Allergy Asthma Immunol. 2006;97:596–602.

6. Mahmoudi M. ed. Allergy and Asthma: Practical Diagnosis and Management. Second edition Springer International Publishing AG; Switzerland 2016. ProQuest E book Central, http://ebookcentral. proquest.com/lib/sthl/detail.action?docID=4537989. Created from sthl on 2020-10-31 13:38:09.

7. Abbas AK, Lichtman AH. Cellular and Molecular Immunology. 5th ed. Philadelphia: Elsevier Saunders; 2005.

8. Sell S. Immunology, Immunopathology, and Immunity. 6th ed. Washington, DC: ASM Press; 2001.

9. Chaudhuri K, Gonzales J, Jesurun CA, Ambat MT, Mandal-Chaudhuri S. Anaphylactic shock in pregnancy: a case study and review of the literature. Int J Obstet Anesth. 2008;17:350–7.

10. Simons FE, Ardusso LR, Dimov V, Ebisawa M, El-Gamal YM, Lockey RF, Sanchez-Borges M, Senna GE, Sheikh A, Thong BY, Worm M, World Allergy

Organization anaphylaxis guidelines: 2013 update of the evidence base. Int Arch Allergy Immunol. 2013;162:193–204.

11. Kishimoto TK, Viswanathan K, Ganguly T, Elankumaran S, Smith S, Pelzer K, et al. Contaminated heparin associated with adverse clinical events and activation of the contact system. N Engl J Med. 2008;358: 2457–67.

12. Ji K, Chen J, Li M, Liu Z, Xia L, Wang C, et al. Comments on serious anaphylaxis caused by nine Chinese herbal injections used to treat common colds and upper respiratory tract infections. Regul Toxicol Pharmacol. 2009;55:134–8.

13. Simons FER, Ardusso LRF, Bilò MB, El-Gamal YM, Ledford DK, Ring J, et al. World Allergy Organization guidelines for the assessment and management of anaphylaxis, WAO Journal. 2011; 4:13–37.

14. Soar J, Pumphrey R, Cant A, Clarke S, Corbett A, Dawson P, et al. Emergency treatment of anaphylactic reactions: guidelines for healthcare providers. Resuscitation. 2008;77:157–69.

15. Lieberman P, Nicklas RA, Oppenheimer J, Kemp SF, Lang DM, Bernstein DI, et al. The diagnosis and management of anaphylaxis practice parameter: 2010 update. J Allergy Clin Immunol. 2010;126:477–480.

16. Sampson HA, Munoz-Furlong A, Campbell RL, Adkinson NF Jr, Bock SA, Branum A, et al. Second symposium on the definition and management of anaphylaxis: summary report: Second National Institute of Allergy and Infectious Disease/Food Allergy and Anaphylaxis Network Symposium. J. Allergy Clin. Immunol. 2006;117:391–97.

17. Lin K, Rasheed A, Lin S, Gerolemou L. Catamenial anaphylaxis: a woman under monthly progesterone curse BMJ Case Rep. 2018; Jan 4

18. Burstein M, Rubinow A, Shalit M. Cyclic anaphylaxis associated with menstruation. Ann Allergy. 1991;66:36–8.

19. Nwaru BI, Dhami S, Sheikh A. Idiopathic Anaphylaxis. Curr Treat Options Allergy. 2017; 4(3):312-19.

20. Schaefer P. Acute and chronic urticaria: evaluation and treatment. Am Fam Physician. 2017; 95(11):717–724.

21. Endo T, Shinozawa Y. Practice guidelines 2005: management of anaphylaxis. Nippon Naika Gakkai Zasshi. 2006;95:2463–8.

22. Wyatt, JP, Taylor, RG, de Wit, K, Jotton, EJ. Life threatening emergencies. Oxford Handbook of Emergency Medicine. 5th ed. Oxford: University of Oxford Press; 2020; 45.

23. Pumphrey RSH. Fatal posture in anaphylactic shock. J. Allergy Clin. Immunol. 2003;112:451–2.

24. Schwartz LB. Diagnostic value of tryptase in anaphylaxis and mastocytosis. Immunol Allergy Clin North Am. 2006;26:451–463.

25. Holbrook T, Keet CA, Frischmeyer-Guerrerio PA, Wood RA. Use of ondansetron for food protein-induced enterocolitis syndrome. J Allergy Clin Immunol. 2013;132:1219–20.

26. Fernandes BN, Boyle RJ, Gore C, Simpson A, Custovic A. Food protein-induced enterocolitis syndrome can occur in adults. J Allergy Clin Immunol. 2012;130:1199–200.

27. Romano A, Gaeta F, Valluzzi RL, Zaffiro A, Caruso C, Quaratino D. Natural evolution of skin-test sensitivity in patients with IgE-mediated hypersensitivity to cephalosporins. Allergy. 2014; 69: 806–9. [PubMed: 24673580]

28. Blanca M, Romano A, Torres MJ, Férnandez J, Mayorga C, Rodriguez J, et al. Update on the evaluation of hypersensitivity reactions to betalactams. Allergy. 2009; 64: 183–93. [PubMed: 19133923]

29. Sacco KA, Bates A, Brigham TJ, Imam JS, Burton MC. Clinical outcomes following inpatient penicillin allergy testing: a systematic review and meta-analysis. Allergy. 2017; 72: 1288–96. [PubMed: 28370003]

30. Macy E, Ngor EW. Safely diagnosing clinically significant penicillin allergy using only penicilloyl-poly-lysine, penicillin, and oral amoxicillin. J Allergy Clin Immunol Pract. 2013; 1: 258–63. [PubMed: 24565482]

31. Tucker MH, Lomas CM, Ramchandar N, Waldram JD. Amoxicillin challenge without penicillin skin testing in evaluation of penicillin allergy in a cohort of Marine recruits. J Allergy Clin Immunol. Pract. 2017; 5: 813–15. [PubMed: 28341170]

10 Allergy Testing

Devasahayam J Christopher and Jefferson Daniel

CONTENTS

INTRODUCTION AND OVERVIEW

History

Allergy skin testing was first introduced in 1865 by Charles H. Blackley of Lancashire, England. He demonstrated the very first skin test on himself by applying grass pollen in denuded skin. Later, Helmtraud Ebruster described the skin prick test in medical literature for the first time in 1959. The test had since been further refined and standardized. Skin tests can confirm the presence of sensitization to specific allergens and aid in the diagnosis of various allergic diseases—Allergic rhinitis, Asthma, Atopic dermatitis, Urticaria, Anaphylaxis, Eczema, and Food and Drug allergy.

Biological Mechanism

An allergy develops to certain substances when they are exposed for the first time. Allergens come in contact with the immune system when the innate barrier of skin or mucosa is breached. Antigen-presenting cells process the allergens and present them to T cells. After interaction with T cells, allergen-specific IgE is produced by B cells. This T cell-mediated class switching of the B cell is mediated by IL-4 and IL-13. Allergen-specific IgE will get bound to the surface of mast cells and basophils. An individual is known to be sensitized if there are mast cells with allergen-specific IgE. Allergy skin testing can demonstrate sensitization.

DOI: 10.1201/9781003125785-10

Table 10.1: Differences between the Skin Prick Test and Intradermal Test

	Skin Prick Test (SPT)	Intradermal Test (IDT)
1	The SPT has a simple technique and is easy to teach.	The technique needs to be mastered as the depth at which allergens are injected. Dilution and amount of allergen injected can all affect the interpretation of the study.
2	It is very safe and no fatalities have been reported.	Few cases of anaphylaxis have been reported (0.02 to 1.4%) and few fatalities have occurred.
3	It results in significantly less pain in the hands of a trained person.	Painful
4	The sensitivity of the test is lower than IDT, but the specificity is higher.	Higher sensitivity
5	The SPT can be done quickly and results will be available within 20 minutes.	Requires more time

Sensitization or presence of allergen-specific IgE bound mast cells does not always progress to clinical allergy. In patients who develop an allergic disorder, upon exposure to an offending allergen, the mast cells with specific IgE bind to the allergens, and trigger intracellular signalling. This results in the degranulation of the inflammatory secretory granules, such as histamine, tryptase, chymase, and carboxypeptidase, resulting in local inflammation and allergic symptoms. Histamine is the primary mediator of the wheal and flare response which has an area of skin oedema enclosed by erythema. This wheal and flare represent immediate reaction. Late-phase reactions may occur after 2 hours of testing. Patient may develop swelling, tenderness, pruritus, and redness that may take 1–2 days to resolve (1).

Atopy, Sensitization, and Clinical Allergy

'Atopy' is defined as a genetic predisposition to produce allergen-specific IgE to offending allergens. 'Sensitization' is understood as the presence of allergen-specific IgE bound mast cells to the offending allergens. Sensitization does not always result in an allergic disorder. When sensitization and allergic clinical symptoms are both present, we can diagnose allergy.

Role of Skin Testing in Diagnosis

In order to diagnose an allergic disease, the offending allergen needs to be identified, and sensitization to that allergen needs to be confirmed with the help of a skin prick test. Alternatively, an in vitro test to detect a specific IgE could also be done. A positive allergen skin test is not diagnostic of the disease but means that the subject is sensitized to a particular antigen which tested positive. A clinical history which correlates well with the allergen skin test is essential to diagnose an allergic disorder. Sensitization precedes clinical allergy. Sensitization without a clinical history of an allergic disorder does not warrant treatment.

Three methods of skin testing are widely practised (Table 10.1):

1. *Skin prick testing (SPT)*

2. *Intradermal testing (IDT) – This method has a higher risk of adverse reactions, including anaphylaxis. Because of their high sensitivity, they are useful if prick/puncture tests are negative*

3. *Patch testing – Useful in the evaluation of contact hypersensitivity and delayed-type hypersensitivity*

Advantages over In Vitro Tests

Allergy skin testing has several advantages over in vitro tests:

1. It is cost-effective, and results are available rapidly.

2. Patients can understand sensitization better as they can see the swelling and erythema corresponding to the allergen.

3. A negative test is reassuring to patients.

4. Skin tests can be performed for a vast number of antigens compared to in vitro tests.

5. Skin test solutions of certain allergens can be self made, making it easier to use in cases of food allergy.

6. Sensitivity is greater in comparison to in vitro tests.

To their advantage, in vitro test results are not affected by any drug intake, and there is no risk for patient safety.

INDICATIONS

1. In screening patients for atopy and planning preventive measures from the development of allergic disease

1. In allergic asthma, rhinitis, and conjunctivitis, the establishment of sensitization to aeroallergens is needed along, with a strong history for diagnosis

2. In food allergy, it is the initial test of choice before the food challenge

3. In IgE-mediated drug allergies, especially antibiotics, chemotherapeutic agents, anaesthetic agents, etc., it is used to as an initial test to decide on a drug challenge

4. In venom allergies, especially of the Hymenoptera species, it is the investigation of choice

5. In the evaluation of latex allergy

6. In epidemiologic studies to identify sensitization pattern in different geographical locations

7. In the process of allergen extract standardization

8. In eosinophilic esophagitis and eosinophilic gastroenteritis

CONTRAINDICATIONS

1. Poorly controlled asthma

2. Poor baseline lung function

3. Past history of a severe reaction

4. Recent anaphylactic event (within 1 month)

5. Use of beta-blockers (they may interfere with the treatment of anaphylaxis since it interferes with adrenaline action)

6. Dermographism, urticaria, and cutaneous mastocytosis, it may lead to erroneous interpretation of the skin test

Relative Contraindications

1. Active angina and cardiac arrhythmias

2. Frail health of older adults

3. Pregnancy

4. Atopic dermatitis (since test needs to be done in unaffected skin)

Medications That Should Be Withheld

The following classes of drugs interfere with the response to skin prick tests and should be withheld:

1. *Antihistamines:* H1 antihistamines will inhibit the allergic reaction mediated by histamine and the typical wheal and flare will not be seen, resulting in a false-negative test. First-generation H1 antihistamines such as ketotifen can have inhibitory effects up to 5 days. Second-generation H1 antihistamines such as cetirizine, levocetirizine, desloratadine, fexofenadine, etc., can have inhibitory effects up to 7 days. Multiple doses of inhaled antihistaminics will also interfere with the test results.

2. *Tricyclic antidepressants* such as imipramine can have negative effects on the test for up to 2 weeks.

3. *Phenothiazines* have an H1 antihistamine property.

4. *Corticosteroids:* Short-term oral steroids do not have an effect; however, long-term steroids can alter the nature of the skin and cutaneous mast cell reactivity, potentially altering the interpretation of the results. Topical steroids also affect skin reactivity.

5. *ACE inhibitors* increase the reactivity of the skin to allergens and histamine.

6. *Clonidine* decreases skin test reactivity.

Risk of Anaphylaxis

Vasovagal syncope is a common systemic side effect that may mimic anaphylaxis. Systemic introduction of the allergen may happen if the skin prick is too deep, and the intradermal test becomes a subdermal test. Patients may develop urticaria, angioedema, bronchospasm, or hypotension. In most cases, the reactions are usually mild and are easily managed. Studies report a 0.03 to 0.04% prevalence of anaphylaxis; however, most of them are likely to be syncope. Delayed systemic reactions due to late-phase responses such as wheezing in asthmatics may occur and can be managed with inhalers (2).

Based on case series and individual reports, some of the risk factors for anaphylaxis with skin prick testing are (3):

- Children less than 6 months of age

- Previous history of anaphylaxis, especially with food panel antigens

- Self-made food antigens rather than standardized commercial kits

- Latex allergens

- Unstable asthma

WHO SHOULD TEST?

Allergy skin testing should be performed only by health care professionals who are trained appropriately to perform the test. Interpreting the test requires a thorough history, and a good understanding about sensitization and clinical allergy. Physicians and allied health care personnel trained in allergy are best suited to request and interpret the test. Albeit in extremely rare cases, there is a possibility of severe allergic reactions and rarely anaphylaxis. Therefore, it is essential to perform the test in a well-equipped lab. Personnel who perform the skin test should periodically be assessed for repeatable skin test results with the same prick device and control, to ensure standard practice and consistency.

HOW MANY ANTIGENS TO TEST?

1. A focused approach is to be deployed when the clinical history is clear about the offending agent, like a peanut allergy or penicillin allergy.

2. In diseases like asthma and allergic rhinitis where sensitization needs to be established, and the possible offending allergens are not known, a broad panel of allergens need to be tested. A typical panel of allergens would cover the following:

   • Pollens of common tree, grass, and other aeroallergens based on the 'patient's locality

   • Fungal antigens such as *Alternaria alternata, Aspergillus fumigatus*, and *Cladosporium*

   • House dust mites: *Dermatophagoides pteronyssinus/farina*

   • Cockroaches

   • Animal danders of cats and dogs

In general, even the presence of sensitization to one allergen is sufficient to label atopy. The choice of the allergens in the panel should be clinically relevant.

TECHNICAL FACTORS THAT INFLUENCE ALLERGY SKIN TESTS
Allergen Preparation

Allergens that cause sensitization are usually glycoproteins and lipoproteins that are foreign to the human body. Several allergens that cause allergy in humans have been identified, and commercial standardized antigens are available for testing. Allergen obtained from natural sources are superior to those that are manufactured by other techniques such as recombinant technology. Since multiple proteins of an offending substance can be allergic, recombinant

allergens may not be as sensitive compared to natural allergens. Commercial extracts use proteins extracted from the allergens and are preserved in 50% glycerol. Certain food and moulds can have naturally occurring histamine and need chemical processing to remove it. *Examples:* Cheese, tomatoes, eggplant, spinach. In such cases, commercial preparation chemically removes histamine and is preferred for testing.

Quality and Standardization of Allergens

Allergen solutions should contain all allergenic proteins from a particular allergen and should not be cross-contaminated with other allergens. The results of the AST may vary if unstandardized allergens are used. Standardization is a process that ensures the same quantity of allergen proteins with the same potency is manufactured with each batch. Each allergen contains major and minor allergenic determinants, and patients can be allergic to different antigens within an individual extract. Composition of different commercial solutions vary. Some manufacturers standardize a fixed weight of proteins per mL, whereas others standardize based on the potency of the antigen (4).

SPT results are comparable across different centres only if the allergen extract utilized was from the same manufacturer or if the protocol for standardization protocols used were the same. Preservatives that can cause false-positive reactions should be avoided in the allergen solution; e.g., Sodium Merthiolate. Allergen solutions should be stored at +2°C to +8°C to maintain stability.

Generally, food allergy testing solutions are made by the allergist in the lab and are not standardized (5).

Choice of Test Device

AST involves a prick through the applied allergen drop into the epidermis of the skin using a sharp-pointed lancet. Another method of doing the test is dipping the device into the allergen extract and then performing the prick. Metal lancets and intravenous needles are widely used and are more sensitive than plastic lancets. Similarly, multi-headed devices are available but produce more false negatives than single-headed devices. Hypodermic needles are not recommended as a uniformly deep skin prick cannot be achieved.

In the interest of keeping the costs low, the same lancet device is used for several pricks, wiping with an alcohol swab between each prick. However, the risk of cross-contamination and needle stick injury is likely.

Cross-Reactivity of Antigens

Cross-reactivity is defined as the reaction of IgE to more than one similar allergen at the same time, despite a lack of exposure to the other allergen. This occurs due to the preservation of the protein structure of particular antigen across species. When designing the allergy skin test panel, cross-reacting allergens can be excluded. Example: Grass pollen belonging to three families (Pooideae, Chloridoideae and Panicoideae) cross react. Hence, testing for one of them is sufficient (6).

Skin Testing Food Allergens

Positive tests may be present without clinical allergy, and a negative test does not rule out allergy. Hence generalized testing with a panel of food allergens is not advised. A detailed history of the allergenic food is obtained first. A cause-effect relationship is established before proceeding to SPT for historically confirmed food allergens only. Fresh food are preferable, and the prick-by-prick method (explained below) should be used for better results.

Positive and Negative Controls (Table 10.2)

Patients may have a hyper- or hypo-sensitive reaction to allergens. In dermatographism, a small prick can cause a large wheal. Drugs such as ACE inhibitors can cause increased sensitivity to histamine, leading to large wheals, causing a false positive test. Similarly, drugs such as antihistamines can cause reduced wheal size, leading to a false negative test.

A positive control should produce a wheal of at least 4 mm. If the size of the wheal is smaller, the test should not be performed, and the drug history should be revisited. Histamine is usually used as a positive control.

Table 10.2: Requirements before Performing Allergy Skin Testing

1. Allergen extract solutions that need to be tested.
2. Fresh food in cases of food allergy and appropriate dilutions of drugs in case of drug allergy.
3. Histamine for positive control and saline for negative control.
4. Sterile lancets for skin pricking; or an alcohol swan to wipe the lancet, if a single device is used.
5. Sharps container for disposal of lancets.
6. Marker pen for marking the controls and allergen on the skin.
7. Measuring tape to read the wheals.
8. Documentation sheets that can be custom made for AST (as shown in Figure 10.1).
9. Personal protective equipment.
10. A bed and emergency trolley with adrenaline, hydrocortisone, and other essential drugs.

The negative control is the same commercial solution in which the allergens are constituted without any allergen in it. It is usually a saline buffer with 50% glycerol. A negative control should ideally be 0 mm. Nevertheless, if the negative control shows a wheal, the test should be interpreted as positive only if the allergen-induced wheal is 3 mm more significant in size than the negative control. Negative control of >3 mm maybe because of dermatographism and AST should thus be avoided.

When using drugs for skin testing, a third person should be used as a control to look for the irritating property of the drug that can mimic a wheal.

Site of Study

The anterior surface of the forearm and the back are usually the preferred sites for testing. The size of wheals tend to vary in the same patient at different sites in the following order: (1) lower back; (2) upper back; (3) upper forearm; (4) near the wrist. However, the positive and negative controls will aid in the correct interpretation of the tests. The test site should be 5 cm proximal to and 3 cm distal to the antecubital fossa. Usually, the back is preferred in children. Young children, babies, and older people have low skin reactivity compared to adolescents and middle-aged people.

TECHNIQUE (SEE TABLE 10.3)
Skin Prick/Puncture Test (Figure 10.1)

- Clean the skin site with alcohol.

- Mark the spot for positive and negative control.

- Number and label areas where allergy solution drops will be placed in a prefixed order, according to the allergen panel available.

- Skin prick tests should be at least 2 cm apart to avoid overlapping reactions and false-positive results.

- A single drop of the allergen solution is laid on the pre-labelled area using the dropper onto the skin before pricking the skin.

Table 10.3: Pre-Procedure Patient Preparation

1. Explain to the patient information regarding the test, including the possible risks.
2. Assess for risk factors of anaphylaxis (as explained earlier).
3. Check and document vitals.
4. Check the patient's prescriptions for drugs that need to be avoided.
5. Expose the area to be tested and remove clothes to prevent friction with the test site.

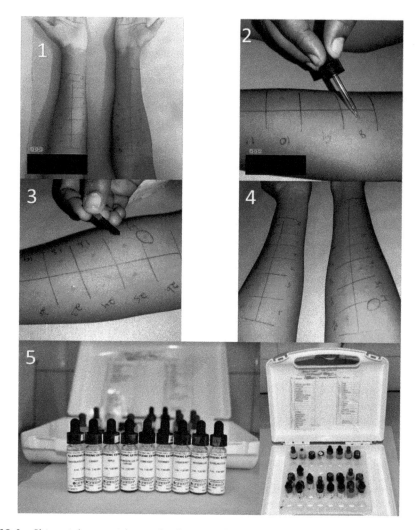

Figure 10.1 Skin prick test with standard antigen kit. (Photo Credit: Andrew, Institutional Photographer.) (1 – Skin markings as per allergen panel number; 2 – Placing the allergen solution in the appropriate place; 3 – Prick using lancet; 4 – Measuring the induration; 5 – A standard set of allergen solutions.)

- If a hypodermic needle is used, the bevel should face upward while nibbling the skin.
- The epithelial layer of the skin should be penetrated without inducing bleeding.
- Care should be taken to avoid insufficient penetration of the skin as well.
- The solution dropper must not touch the skin.
- One allergen drop should not run onto the next prick site.
- The time at which the skin prick was made should be documented. In case there was a delay in skin prick due to the patient or child not cooperating, different pricks may have been done at different times, and the interpretation should be made accordingly. Histamine and negative control test results should be read 10 minutes after application.
- The allergen extract drop should be blotted after completing the prick.
- Allergy pricks should be read 15–20 minutes after the skin prick was made.

Intradermal Tests

- Clean the skin site with alcohol.
- Mark the spot for positive and negative control.

- Number and label areas where allergy solution drops will be placed in a prefixed order according to the allergen panel available.

- The quantity of allergen solution used is 0.02 to 0.05 mL of a 1:500 to 1:1000 weight/volume ratio.

- A 26/27 F needle, inserted at a 45° angle with the bevel facing downward is used, and the solution is inserted to create a small bleb of 2 to 3 mm intradermally, similar to a Mantoux test.

- Before administration of the injection, bubbles must be expelled to avoid a splash reaction.

- Saline is used as intradermal-negative control.

- A positive control is a histamine injected intradermally at a concentration of 0.001 mg/mL.

- Time to read the intradermal test is similar to the prick test, at 15–20 minutes.

- Since skin test reactions disappear after 30 minutes, a visual record of the results can be obtained. Mark the edges of the wheals with a marker, apply cellophane tape on the test site and transfer the markings to a paper.

MEASUREMENT

- Before measuring the size of wheals, the leftover allergen solution should be carefully blotted out from each prick site.

- Measure the mean diameter of the wheal, using a transparent ruler on the longest and shortest perpendicular axis. An average of these 2 diameters is obtained.

- Similarly, the average diameter of the flare is obtained. If there is an overlapping of the flares, then only the width is considered.

- A single figure measurement is obtained for wheal and flares separately in mm.

- Pseudopods are not measured but are mentioned separately in the report.

- Some centres describe the wheals in mm^2; however, mean diameter is universally accepted and is considered as standard practice.

- Qualitative marking (e.g. +, ++) as the primary method of reporting is not recommended (7).

POST-PROCEDURE CARE AND MONITORING

- Clean the test area with an alcohol solution.

- Itching subsides within 15 minutes.

- An ice pack could be applied at the test site to alleviate pain.

- Possibility of a late-phase reaction with an increase in swelling/pain and wheezing, etc., must be clearly explained to the patient. An action plan should also be provided.

- If the test is negative, patients can leave the centre after completion.

- A more extended holding period for monitoring is needed for intradermal skin tests.

- Patients with a history of asthma or anaphylaxis should be monitored for 30 minutes after the test.

REPORTING

SPT result should contain the following information (Table 10.4):

- Name of the centre performing the test

- Name, Age, Sex, Hospital identification number of the patient

- Date and time of the test

- Name of the physician who requested the test

- Name of the technician/physician who performed the test

- Region tested (forearm/back)

Table 10.4: A Sample Reporting Form

ALLERGY PRICK SKIN TESTING

NAME:	HOSPITAL ID:	REFERED BY:
AGE:	DATE:	TESTED BY:
SEX:	TIME IN:	

INHALANTS ADULT SCREEN

S. No.	Allergens	Wheal Diameter (in mm)
1	Dust mite mix (D and F)	
2	Cockroach	
3	Prosopis	
4	Parthenium	
5	*Amaranthus spinosus*	
6	*Sorghum halipase*	
7	*Morus alba/rubra*	
8	*Alternaria tenius*	
9	Penicillium	
10	*Aspergillus niger*	
11	Dog dander	
12	Cat dander	

SALINE CONTROL

HISTAMINE CONTROL

- Name of each allergen tested
- Negative control and positive control with concentration
- Size of the resultant wheal for each allergen
- Standardised quantitative reporting should be done with the mean diameter method or mm^2 method
- Qualitative reporting such as. 0, +, ++, etc., alone is not recommended to avoid misinterpretation of the report. However, qualitative reporting may facilitate patients' understanding (8)

INTERPRETATION

A positive reaction appears as a raised wheal with surrounding erythema. A wheal diameter larger than 3 mm or if the wheal is equal or larger compared to the normal-sized histamine control, is a positive reaction. AST has a high negative predictive value (>95%). A wheal which is smaller than histamine control or absent wheal is a negative reaction. A positive-intradermal result is a wheal of 5 mm or larger or 3 mm greater than the negative control.

A positive allergy test only indicates sesnsitization. Allergy is diagnosed only if the patient develops symptoms upon exposure to the allergen. A positive skin test that does not correlate with history could either represent (1) currently developing allergy; or (2) reduced exposure to allergens to trigger a disease; or (3) a genuinely false positive.

Wheal size usually does not correlate with the severity of the clinical allergy (Table 10.5). If the wheal size is equivocal or does not correlate with clinical history, a controlled challenge with the suspected allergen is indicated.

VARIATIONS IN ALLERGY SKIN TESTING
Endpoint Dilution Testing

This is a variant of intradermal testing used to establish a relation between the concentration of administered allergen and the size of the wheal produced. The concentration required to create a wheal of a specific size is lesser in more sensitive patients. The same allergen is injected at different sites in increasing doses from minimum to maximum, to identify the dose at which a predefined sized wheal is obtained. This technique is used to standardize the strength of allergen extract, to measure the response of immunotherapy treatment and to determine the initial concentration of allergen to be used in nasal or bronchial challenge testing (12).

Prick-by-Prick Testing

This is a variation of skin prick testing mainly used in food allergy. Since fresh food in its raw form is usually associated with a food allergy, it is directly used instead of commercial food allergens. A crushed extract of fresh food should be made and used as a test solution. Third-party control is also needed before labelling a test positive to account for skin irritation and local non-allergic reactions (13).

CONCLUSION

AST is a useful tool to recognize sensitization to allergens; a useful aid in diagnosing a clinical allergy. It is easy to perform, cheap, reliable, and a safe investigation.

It is the initial tool of investigation in allergy evaluation. Specifically designed allergen panels that are locally and clinically relevant should be used. Limiting the choice of allergens to those that are clinically meaningful is the best practice compared to testing large numbers of allergens without clear direction.

Table 10.5: Performance of Different Classes of Allergens (9–11)

Allergen	Sensitivity	Specificity
Aero-allergens	70–95%	80–97%
Food allergens	30–90%	20–60%
	PPV	NPV
Cows milk	76%	—
Hens egg	89%	—
Penicillin	—	98.5%

REFERENCES

1. Subcommittee on skin tests of the European Academy of Allergology and Clinical Immunology. Pathophysiology of skin tests. Allergy. 1989;44(s10): 13–21.

2. Liccardi G, Salzillo A, Spadaro G, Senna G, Canonica WG, D'Amato G, et al. Anaphylaxis caused by skin prick testing with aeroallergens: Case report and evaluation of the risk in Italian allergy services. J Allergy Clin Immunol. 2003 Jun 1;111(6):1410–2.

3. Devenney I, Fälth-Magnusson K. Skin prick tests may give generalized allergic reactions in infants. Ann Allergy Asthma Immunol Off Publ Am Coll Allergy Asthma Immunol. 2000 Dec;85(6 Pt 1):457–60.

4. Dreborg SKG. Skin Testing in Allergen Standardization and Research. Immunol Allergy Clin. 2001 May 1;21(2):329–54.

5. Henzgen M, Ballmer-Weber BK, Erdmann S, Fuchs T, Kleine-Tebbe J, Lepp U, et al. Skin testing with food allergens. Guideline of the German Society of Allergology and Clinical Immunology (DGAKI), the Physicians' Association of German Allergologists (ADA) and the Society of Pediatric Allergology (GPA)

together with the Swiss Society of Allergology. J Dtsch Dermatol Ges J Ger Soc Dermatol JDDG. 2008 Nov;6(11):983–8.

6. Esch RE. Allergen immunotherapy: what can and cannot be mixed? J Allergy Clin Immunol. 2008 Sep;122(3):659–60.

7. Frati F, Incorvaia C, Cavaliere C, Di Cara G, Marcucci F, Esposito S, et al. The skin prick test. J Biol Regul Homeost Agents. 2018 Feb;32(1 Suppl. 1):19–24.

8. Antunes J, Borrego L, Romeira A, Pinto P. Skin prick tests and allergy diagnosis. Allergol Immunopathol (Madr). 2009 Jun;37(3):155–64.

9. Wood RA, Phipatanakul W, Hamilton RG, Eggleston PA. A comparison of skin prick tests, intradermal skin tests, and RASTs in the diagnosis of cat allergy. J Allergy Clin Immunol. 1999 May;103(5 Pt 1):773–9.

10. Mostafa HS, Qotb M, Hussein MA, Hussein A. Allergic rhinitis diagnosis: skin-prick test versus laboratory diagnostic methods. Egypt J Otolaryngol. 2019 Jul 1;35(3):262–8.

11. Heinzerling L, Mari A, Bergmann K-C, Bresciani M, Burbach G, Darsow U, et al. The skin prick test - European standards. Clin Transl Allergy. 2013 Feb 1;3(1):3.

12. Nadarajah R, Rechtweg JS, Corey JP. Introduction to serial endpoint titration. Immunol Allergy Clin. 2001 May 1;21(2):369–81.

13. Cantani A, Micera M. The prick by prick test is safe and reliable in 58 children with atopic dermatitis and food allergy. Eur Rev Med Pharmacol Sci. 2006 Jun;10(3):115–20.

PART II
ASTHMA IN ADOLESCENTS AND YOUNG ADULTS

11 Epidemiology of Asthma in Children and Young Adults

Anitha Kumari and Sanjeev Nair

CONTENTS

INTRODUCTION

Asthma is a common disease, causing severe morbidity and mortality in India and around the world. The Global Initiative for Asthma (GINA) defines Asthma as "a heterogeneous disease, usually characterized by chronic airway inflammation. It is defined by the history of respiratory symptoms such as wheeze, shortness of breath, chest tightness and cough that vary over time and in intensity, together with variable expiratory airflow limitation. Airflow limitation may later become persistent" (1).

EPIDEMIOLOGY

Asthma is one of the most common chronic diseases worldwide with an estimated 300 million affected individuals. Prevalence is increasing in many countries, especially in children and it is a major cause of school/ work absence. The current global estimates for asthma, as for other diseases, is available as part of the Global Burden of Diseases (GBD) estimates. These have been summarized in Table 11.1a (2). As per GBD 2019 estimates, asthma caused an estimated 461,069 deaths (95% CI: 366,579, 559,006) globally and 198,799 (95% CI: 129,622, 271,916) deaths in India (3).

Earlier estimates of asthma prevalence in India are available from the INSEARCH study data. This study estimated a prevalence of 2.05% and an age adjusted prevalence of 1.97%; it estimated the number of asthma for all ages in India to be 21 million. As per this study, the lowest proportions of asthma were in the 15–24 years age group.

There has been a paradigm shift in the causes of death in India from 1990 to 2019. The leading causes of death in India in 1990 were diarrheal diseases, neonatal disorders, and lower respiratory tract infections. However, by 2019 these dropped down the list, occurring behind ischemic heart disease, COPD, and stroke. Asthma, which was the 12th leading cause of death in 1990, is currently (2019 GBD estimated) the 13th leading cause of death, with an 18% decline in mortality. Overall, mortality from asthma in India in 2019 is estimated by GBD to be 14.29 deaths/100,000 population. The age-wise mortality due to asthma for children and young adults can be seen in Table 11.1b. Among the 5 years and under age group and the 5 to 15 years age group, asthma does not figure in the top 20 causes of death. Death due to asthma in the below 5 years age group is estimated to have declined by 84% and in the 5 to 15 years age group by 60%. Therefore, overall, there is a decline in death due to asthma in the younger age groups. However, the decline in disability-adjusted life years (DALYs) between 1990 and 2019, while being significant in the under 5 years age group at 71%, is less so in the 5 to 5 years age group, where the decline in number of DALYs is at only 7.62%. Overall, the prevalence of asthma in the under 25 years age group in India, as per the GBD estimates for 2019 is 9,845,406, and mortality in this age group is estimated to be 2322. Asthma accounts for 0.12% of the total deaths in the under 20 years age group, as per the GBD 2019 estimates.

The International Study of Asthma and Allergies in Childhood (ISAAC), a unique worldwide epidemiological research program, was established in 1991 to investigate asthma, rhinitis, and eczema in children due to considerable concern that these conditions were increasing in western and developing countries (4). The results of the ISAAC study showed that there is consistently more variation between countries than within countries. India, which had 14 centres, had a low prevalence of childhood asthma as compared with countries like Italy, which were in the middle prevalence group, and countries like the United Kingdom, which were in the high prevalence group. The limitation was that the countries and centres within the countries were self-selected and might not be representative. Overall, the

DOI: 10.1201/9781003125785-11

Table 11.1a: Global Estimates for Asthma, as per GBD 2019

Age Group	Prevalence			DALYs			Deaths		
	Number	Percentage[a]	Rate[b]	Number	Percentage[a]	Rate[b]	Number	Percentage[a]	Rate[b]
Under 5	21,809,765	3.81%	3290.3	1,404,783	1.06%	264.6	6102	0.12%	1.20
5–9	33,602,368	4.63%	5132.5	1,494,273	2.48%	228.2	6102	0.53%	0.31
10–14	26,308,484	4.46%	4096.7	1,217,854	2.10%	189.6	2109	0.81%	0.39
15–19	18,591,623	4.48%	3000.9	954,563	1.23%	154.1	2970	0.68%	0.55
20–24	13,805,155	3.31%	2300.3	825,914	0.88%	137.6	4178	0.68%	0.80

Abbreviation: DALYs, disability-adjusted life years.
[a] Percentage of overall death/DALYs/prevalence in that age group.
[b] Rate per 100,000 population.

prevalence was lower in developing countries as compared to developed countries (5).

RISK FACTORS FOR ASTHMA IN CHILDREN AND ADOLESCENTS

Asthma is a heterogeneous disease whose development and persistence is influenced by gene–environment interactions (1).

Genetic factors: Maternal asthma was most strongly associated with asthma in children of all ages in both univariate (OR 5 3.2, 95% CI 5 1.5 to 6.7) and multivariate (OR 5 4.1, 95% CI 5 1.7 to 10.1) models. In the univariate model, paternal asthma was weakly associated with childhood asthma (OR 5 1.4, 95% CI 5 0.6 to 3.2). This association increased in magnitude in the multivariable model (OR 5 2.7, 95% CI 5 1.0 to 7.2). Among children below 5 years of age, the risk for childhood asthma associated with maternal asthma (OR 5 5.0, 95% CI 5 1.7 to 14.9) was greater than the risk associated with paternal asthma (OR 5 1.6, 95% CI 5 0.5 to 5.9). Both maternal asthma and paternal asthma were associated with similar risks among children greater than 5 years of age (OR 5 4.6, 95% CI 5 1.1 to 19.0 and OR 5 4.1, 95% CI 5 1.0 to 16.0,

respectively). The probability of having a child with asthma were three times greater in families with one asthmatic parent and six times greater in families with two asthmatic parents than in families where only one parent had inhalant allergy without asthma (6).

Studies conducted on twins have shown that concordance rates for asthma are significantly higher in monozygotic twins than in dizygotic twins. Broad-sense heritability estimates derived from twin studies range from 36 to 75% (7). Twin studies have revealed a 0.74 concordance between monozygotic twins and a 0.35 concordance between dizygotic twins. These studies implicate a genetic contribution to asthma development (8).

Maternal obesity: A meta-analysis showed that maternal obesity in pregnancy was associated with higher odds of asthma. Each 1 kg/m^2 increase in maternal BMI was associated with a 2–3% increase in the odds of childhood asthma.

Childhood obesity: A meta-analysis of 18 studies found that being either overweight or obese was a risk factor for childhood asthma and wheeze. This is seen mainly in girls.

Childhood exposure to antigens: Dampness, visible mould, and mould odor in the home

Table 11.1b: Estimates for India for Asthma, as per GBD 2019

Age Group	Prevalence			DALYs			Deaths		
	Number	Percentage[a]	Rate[b]	Number	Percentage[a]	Rate#	Number	Percentage[a]	Rate[b]
Under 5	1,172,973	1.07%	1001.9	78,181	0.10%	66.8	362	0.04%	0.31
5–9	2,961,784	2.49%	2358.4	132,636	1.01%	105.6	170	0.22%	0.14
10–14	2,529,045	1.99%	1894.5	119,855	0.89%	89.8	244	0.34%	0.18
15–19	1,780,964	1.37%	1325.6	113,137	0.65%	84.2	587	0.52%	0.44
20–24	1,400,640	1.11%	1081.7	119,498	0.55%	92.3	959	0.57%	0.74

Abbreviation: DALYs, disability-adjusted life years.
[a] Percentage of overall death/DALYs/Prevalence in that age group.
[b] Rate per 100,000 population.

environment are associated with increased risk of developing asthma in at-risk children. Sensitization to indoor, inhaled aero-allergens is more important than sensitization to outdoor allergens for the development of asthma. A linear relationship exists between exposure and sensitization to house dust mites.

Breastfeeding: Breastfeeding decreases wheezing episodes in early life, but it may not prevent development of persistent asthma.

Maternal smoking: A meta-analysis concluded that pre-natal smoking had its strongest effect on young children. Post-natal maternal smoking seemed relevant to asthma development only in older children.

Microbial effects: The 'hygiene hypothesis', and the more recently coined 'microflora hypothesis' and 'biodiversity hypothesis', suggest that human interaction with microbiota may have a benefit in preventing asthma. This is being discussed in detail in a subsequent chapter.

Viral infections and asthma: The link between viral respiratory infections and asthma has been well established. Respiratory syncytial virus (RSV) infection is associated with wheezing in infants. Rhinovirus is more common in children. Other viruses associated with wheezing include para-influenza virus, influenza virus, adenovirus, corona virus, and picorna virus. Rhinovirus is more commonly associated with hospital admissions for asthma in children. Bronchiolitis in children can cause reduced FEV_1 and FEF 25–75% in childhood. There is elevated eosinophillic cationic protein (ECP) and leukotriene C_4 in the nasal lavage fluid of infants with RSV bronchiolitis. Continued follow-up of patients with RSV bronchiolitis in infancy revealed a persistent increase in allergic asthma in early adulthood (9).

Environmental pollution: Exposure to outdoor pollutants is associated with increased risk of asthma. A recent study suggests that up to 4 million new pediatric asthma cases (13% of the global incidence) may be attributable to exposure to traffic-related air pollution (TRAP).

Allergic March: The term 'Allergic March' is also called 'Atopic March'. It refers to the natural history of atopic manifestations, which is characterized by a typical sequence of immunoglobulin E (IgE) antibody responses and clinical symptoms which may appear early in life, persist over years or decades and often remit spontaneously with age (10). The atopic march begins with atopic dermatitis, and progresses to IgE-mediated food allergy, asthma, and allergic rhinitis (11).

Drugs: Antibiotic use during pregnancy and in infants and toddlers has been associated with the development of asthma later in life (12,13). However, all studies have not shown this association (14). Intake of the analgesic, paracetamol may be associated with asthma in both children and adults (15). Frequent use of paracetamol by pregnant women has been associated with asthma in their children (16).

PREVENTION OF ASTHMA IN CHILDREN

Prevention of asthma is discussed in the GINA guidelines based on the results of cohort and observational studies and the ARIA guidelines (1,17). The risk of child developing asthma can be reduced by avoiding exposure to environmental tobacco smoke during pregnancy and after birth, encouraging vaginal delivery, advising breastfeeding, and discouraging use of broad-spectrum antibiotics during the first year of life.

CONCLUSION

Asthma is a common disease causing morbidity and mortality. It still remains the 13th leading cause of death in India. The GBD estimates for India for 2019 show the prevalence of asthma in the below 25-year age group to be 9,845,406 and mortality to be 2322. The major risk factors for asthma include genetic factors, maternal and childhood obesity, maternal smoking, not breastfeeding, allergen exposure, antibiotic use in early childhood, viral infections in childhood and other allergies. Major preventive measures include avoiding exposure to environmental tobacco smoke during pregnancy and after birth, encouraging vaginal delivery, advising breastfeeding, and discouraging use of broad-spectrum antibiotics during the first year of life.

REFERENCES

1. GINA-2020-full-report_-final-_wms.pdf [Internet]. [cited 2020 Oct 23]. Available from: https://ginasthma.org/wp-content/uploads/2020/04/GINA-2020-full-report_-final-_wms.pdf

2. GBD Results Tool | GHDx [Internet]. [cited 2020 Oct 23]. Available from: http://ghdx.healthdata.org/gbd-results-tool

3. GBD India Compare | IHME Viz Hub [Internet]. [cited 2020 Oct 23]. Available from: http://vizhub.healthdata.org/gbd-compare/india

4. Asher MI, Keil U, Anderson HR, Beasley R, Crane J, Martinez F, et al. International Study of Asthma and Allergies in Childhood (ISAAC): rationale and methods. Eur Respir J 1995 Mar 1; 8(3):483–91.

5. Worldwide variations in the prevalence of asthma symptoms: the International Study of Asthma and Allergies in Childhood (ISAAC). Eur Respir J 1998 Aug 1; 12(2):315–35.

6. Litonjua AA, Carey VJ, Burge HA, Weiss ST, Gold DR. Parental history and the risk for childhood asthma. Am J Respir Crit Care Med 1998 Jul 1; 158(1):176–81.

7. Masoli M, Fabian D, Holt S, Beasley R, Global Initiative for Asthma (GINA) Program. The global burden of asthma: executive summary of the GINA Dissemination Committee report. Allergy 2004 May; 59(5):469–78.

8. Bijanzadeh M, Mahesh PA, Ramachandra NB. An understanding of the genetic basis of asthma. Indian J Med Res 2011 Aug; 134(2):149–61.

9. Chang C. Asthma in children and adolescents: a comprehensive approach to diagnosis and management. Clin Rev Allergy Immunol 2012; Aug; 43(1–2):98–137.

10. The Allergic March | World Allergy Organization [Internet]. [cited 2020 Nov 27]. Available from: https://www.worldallergy. org/education-and-programs/education/ allergic-disease-resource-center/professionals/ the-allergic-march

11. The epidemiologic characteristics of healthcare provider-diagnosed eczema, asthma, allergic rhinitis, and food allergy in children: a retrospective cohort study [Internet]. [cited 2020 Nov 27]. Available from: https://www.ncbi.nlm.nih.gov/pmc/articles/ PMC4992234/

12. Marra F, Marra CA, Richardson K, Lynd LD, Kozyrskyj A, Patrick DM, et al. Antibiotic use in children is associated with increased risk of asthma. Pediatrics 2009 Mar; 123(3):1003–10.

13. Stensballe LG, Simonsen J, Jensen SM, Bønnelykke K, Bisgaard H. Use of antibiotics during pregnancy increases the risk of asthma in early childhood. J Pediatr 2013 Apr; 162(4):832–838.e3.

14. Celedón JC, Fuhlbrigge A, Rifas-Shiman S, Weiss ST, Finkelstein JA. Antibiotic use in the first year of life and asthma in early childhood. Clin Exp Allergy J Br Soc Allergy Clin Immunol 2004 Jul; 34(7):1011–6.

15. Cheelo M, Lodge CJ, Dharmage SC, Simpson JA, Matheson M, Heinrich J, et al. Paracetamol exposure in pregnancy and early childhood and development of childhood asthma: a systematic review and meta-analysis. Arch Dis Child 2015 Jan; 100(1):81–9.

16. Eyers S, Weatherall M, Jefferies S, Beasley R. Paracetamol in pregnancy and the risk of wheezing in offspring: a systematic review and meta-analysis. Clin Exp Allergy 2011 Apr; 41(4):482–9.

17. Brozek JL, Bousquet J, Baena-Cagnani CE, Bonini S, Canonica GW, Casale TB, et al. Allergic Rhinitis and its Impact on Asthma (ARIA) guidelines: 2010 revision. J Allergy Clin Immunol 2010 Sep; 126(3):466–76.

12 Hygiene Hypothesis and Global Increase in the Incidence of Asthma

Surinder K Jindal and Aditya Jindal

CONTENTS

INTRODUCTION

There is a global increase in both the incidence and prevalence of respiratory allergies and bronchial asthma. Asthma is a chronic respiratory disease which constitutes one of the major non-communicable diseases (NCD). It is a more common disease among children, teenagers and young adults than among older populations. As per global estimates in 2016, there were more than 339 million people of asthma world wide (1). It has been also estimated that the number is likely to exceed 400 million by the year 2025. Asthma is ranked 28th in the list of causes of disease burden measured by disability-adjusted life years (DALY) and ranked 16th among the leading causes of years lived with disability (2). According to World Health Organization (WHO) estimates, asthma was responsible for about 25 million DALYs in 2016 (3). Over 400,000 deaths were attributed to asthma at the global level (4). Notably, asthma prevalence is generally higher in high-income countries, even though asthma-related deaths are more common in low- and middle-income countries (4).

Globally, there have been major changes in lifestyle with more people, particularly children, moving indoors. This trend has resulted in increased sensitization to indoor allergens, diet, and decreased physical activity. Urbanization and increased industrialization have added to an increase in ambient and household air pollution from vehicular and industrial exhausts. There is greater consumption of foods with synthetic and chemical additives. The sequential changes in lifestyle in the last few decades have led to increases in different forms of allergic diseases almost parallel to the adoption of hygienic conditions, indoor entertainment, changes in diet, or physical activity which were never predicted (5). Some of these observations have given birth to the idea that there existed a protective environment and personal microbiome which bore a paradoxical relationship with allergic and other hypersensitivity disorders.

RISK FACTORS OF ASTHMA

Asthma is present all over the world, but there are large variations in its prevalence, severity, and mortality. The exact aetiology of asthma is not known, but both genetic and environment exposures are responsible for causing asthma (Table 12.1). Exposure to inhaled substances and particles in the air provokes allergic reactions and asthma episodes in a genetically predisposed individual. Some of the common environmental risk factors which can cause and/or trigger asthma include exposure to aeroallergens, house-dust mites, dander and hair of pet animals such as cats and dogs, insect proteins (urine, faeces and body parts scattered in the air), tobacco smoke and environmental tobacco smoke exposure (passive smoking), and industrial and occupational dusts. Microbial infections by viruses and bacteria constitute another important risk factor that precipitate or trigger acute asthma episodes.

Living in an urbanized and polluted atmosphere is an important risk factor because of heightened exposures to environmental and occupational pollution, tobacco smoking, and viral and bacterial infections (6). On the other hand, a high prevalence of asthma is reported from some of the least polluted Western countries with a minimum level of infectious diseases. There is thus a great dichotomy between the type of risk factors and prevalence of asthma among different populations. The

DOI: 10.1201/9781003125785-12

Table 12.1: Etiological Risk Factors and/or Important Triggers of Asthma

1. Non-modifiable: Genetic predisposition— Family history of asthma and allergies
2. Pre-natal exposures:
   • Maternal tobacco smoking or mother's exposure to smoking from others at home
     • Pre-natal maternal diet, nutrition and level of stress
     • Maternal use of antibiotics
     • Emergency cesarean section—2 to 3 times more likely among infants
3. Risk factors during early childhood:
   • Lower rates of asthma in babies exclusively breastfed for at least 3 months
   • Protective effect of large and joint family structure
   • Living a farm and dairy life in rural/farm homes—exposure to microbial endotoxins
   • Living in inner-city homes—exposure to pets, pests and indoor endotoxins
   • Repeated antibiotic use for respiratory and other infections
4. Risk factors during teenage years and adulthood:
   • Aeroborne allergens
   • Viral and bacterial infections
   • Tobacco smoking and environmental tobacco smoke exposure
   • Exposure to pets at home
   • Occupational exposures
   • Obesity
   • Miscellaneous (cold exposure, exercise, psychological stress, certain foods, drugs and chemicals)

'hygiene hypothesis' seems to address and explain this dichotomy with reference to infections.

HYGIENE HYPOTHESIS

The term 'hygiene' owes its origin to *'Hygeia'* the goddess of good health in Greek and Roman mythology, who was a daughter and attendant of Asclepius, the god of medicine. In today's context, the WHO describes hygiene as "conditions and practices that help to maintain health and prevent the spread of diseases." Humans have always attempted to prevent diseases that threatened human life. The need for sanitation and water quality improvements was recognized, and cleanliness practices were introduced in Europe and North America largely during the 19th century. Adoption of measures such as toilets and sewer systems, hand-washing, cleanup of city streets, and cleaner food resulted in a significant decline in the incidence of infectious diseases during the early 20th century. Infections accounted for a clear division between the developed versus the developing and under-developed countries.

Later observations suggested that the incidence of allergies had increased almost in parallel to the decrease in infections. In Britain, allergic problems of hay fever and eczema were more commonly reported in larger families with greater chances of unhygienic practices and increased transmission of infections from siblings within a household (7). It was presumed that there were lesser chances of inter-personal contact, better household amenities and standards of cleanliness in small families, indirectly suggesting that these hygienic conditions promoted the occurrence of allergies among children. This view was somewhat antagonistic to the previously held view that an increase in the incidence of allergies was attributable to an increase in pollution. Soon thereafter, there were other reports that supported the observations that overcrowding and unhygienic conditions accounted for a higher prevalence of atopic conditions including asthma and hay fever (8,9). Hygiene hypothesis was also known as the 'old friends/microbiota hypothesis', which implied a mutually beneficial relationship with the commensal non-pathogenic microorganisms, which provided immuno-modulatory signals against immune-mediated allergic disorders.

It was therefore implied that an 'unhygienic contact' was protective against allergic disorders and asthma. The various types of unhygienic contacts included fecal-oral contact through repeated mouth-touching with unclean hands, and environmental inhalational exposure to dusts on farms with domesticated animals and in the 'inner-city' houses infested with pests and insects (Table 12.2).

There is contradictory evidence in the reported literature in support of and against the hygiene hypothesis.

1. *Epidemiological evidence:* The incidence of asthma is significantly less in the developing low- and middle-income countries (LMIC) than in the industrialized and developed countries (10). People in LMIC more

Table 12.2: Types of 'Unhygienic Contact' during Early Life Considered to Be Protective of Asthma

1. Fecal-oral contact
   • Viral infections—Hepatitis A
   • Parasitic infections—helminths, *Toxoplasma gondii*
   • Bacterial infections—*Helicobacter pylori*
   • Commensal microorganisms
2. Inhalational exposures in farms
   • Endotoxins emitted by farm animals—cows, pigs
   • Inhalational exposures in crowded, unclean homes—pets (cats, dogs) and pests (mice, cockroach, mites)

commonly live in rural or semi-urban areas with farming surroundings. There is greater exposure to domestic animals and dairy farming. There is less exposure to air pollution and consumption of artificial foods and synthetic agents. Urban residence and urbanization are important factors for an increased prevalence of asthma in LMIC. The hypothesis gets strong support from the case study on Amish farmers who had emigrated to America from Sweden and lived a simple dairy farming life. The prevalence of asthma in Amish children in America (5.2%) was significantly lower compared to Swedish farm children (6.8%) and Swedish non-farm children (11.2%), whose lifestyles had evolved in keeping with modern times (11,12). Similar trends were seen in the case of hay fever, atopic eczema, and aero-allergen sensitization (11,12).

The urbanization process is likely to be responsible for an increase in risk factors for asthma. Some of these risk factors include changes in diet, lack of physical activity, reductions in childhood infections, smaller family size, more frequent use of antibiotics, and environmental pollution (13). These factors were considered antagonistic to human microbiomes and the development of requisite immunological responses. This has been also supported by the observation of a higher incidence of asthma in homes with low levels of the bacterial protein lipopolysaccharide (LPS) in a multi-centre, follow-up study from Germany where newborns were followed up for about 7 years for the development of childhood asthma (14). Early childhood infections and LPS-exposure are considered important protective factors against asthma.

Exposure to allergens from pests, mice, cockroaches, and pets such as cats and dogs during early life is also shown to protect against asthma. In the United States, the Urban Environment and Childhood Asthma (URECA) Inner City, Birth-Cohort study demonstrated a negative association of these exposures with recurrent wheezing at 3 years of age. In addition, the exposure to house-dust microbiomes with bacterial forms such as Firmicutes and Bacteriodes phyla was additive to this negative association (11,15).

2. *Antibiotic use:* Asthma has been linked with antibiotic use during childhood. This has been attributed to the alterations of gut microbiomes due to excessive use of antibiotics that play an important role in maintaining the essential immunological balance. Others, however, believe that asthmatic children are likely to be administered antibiotics more frequently than the non-asthmatic children and that excessive use has no causative relationship.

3. *Childhood vaccination:* Childhood vaccination—in particular with Bacillus Calmette-Guerin (BCG) against tuberculosis—is believed to demonstrate a protective effect against asthma (16). This is possibly mediated through a modulation of the immune maturation process. A similar effect has been attributed to pertussis vaccination (17). There are other studies and meta-analyses that support the hypothesis. This effect is however inconsistent, as demonstrated in several other epidemiological studies. The Manchester Community Asthma Study cohort clearly showed that the protective effect of BCG vaccination on childhood asthma lasted only for a short period (18).

SCIENTIFIC BASIS

Different mechanisms have been proposed to explain the hygiene hypothesis, even though there are conflicting opinions and evidences. The two commonly believed explanations are discussed as follows:

1. *Immunological imbalance:* There is a balance between the two subtypes of T helper cells (TH1 and TH2) involved in immunological responses to various allergens and other challenges (Figure 12.1). Various inhalational and other allergens activate TH2 cells which produce interleukin (IL)-4, IL-5, IL-6, IL-13 and immunoglobulin (Ig)-E (19). On the other hand, several viruses, bacteria, and other microbes activate TH1 cells. TH1 type immune response produces pro-inflammatory mediators such as IL-2, IFN γ and TNF α. TH1 activation also down-regulates TH2 cells. Normally, there exists a 'see-saw'-like reciprocal relationship—stimulation of one arm suppresses the other, and vice-versa (20,21). An increase in TH1 immune response due to an infection is likely to cause suppression of TH2—type response responsible for allergic reactions.

2. *Immaturity of regulatory T-cell response:* The immune system is meant to defend invasion by microbial and other harmful particles that enter the body. It matures with time for this fight when repeatedly challenged

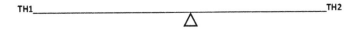

A dominant TH1 response weakens TH2 type responses.

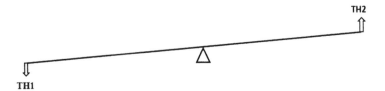

Figure 12.1 Balance of regulatory TH1 response to microbial infections and TH2 types of immune responses predominantly for allergic immune responses.

by stimuli (infections and endotoxins) that are therefore 'essential' to educate the regulatory T-cells of the immune system during early childhood in its developing stage (21). The period of exposure to microbes may in fact begin 'in-utero' and is likely to end by school age. An absence of this challenge when the environment is 'too clean' does not allow the immune system to get appropriately trained. This inadequate education allows the development of allergic problems, asthma, and autoimmune diseases whenever there is an environment challenge.

MICROBIAL ASSOCIATION

There is a significant association of some viral, bacterial, and helminthic infections with lower prevalence of asthma and other allergic disorders. This association however is not consistent since asthma is also known to be more likely in children with other infections (Table 12.3). Measles, mumps, hepatitis A, Schistosoma mansonii, and croup are shown to be protective and bear inverse relationships with asthma, while several other worm infestations may have a positive relationship (22,23). Bronchiolitis and infection with respiratory syncytial virus (RSV) causing pneumonia during childhood also increases the possibility of childhood asthma. Hypopharyngeal colonization of 1 month-old infants by *Streptococcus penumoniae*, *Haemophilus influenzae* or *Moraxella catarrhalis* was significantly associated with persistent wheeze, acute exacerbation of wheeze, and hospitalization. This was, however, not seen with *Staphylococcus aureus*. An inverse relationship of asthma has also been shown with household levels of pro inflammatory agents, such as bacterial endotoxins and

microbial components (peptidoglycans, extracellular polysaccharides and fungal glucans etc.).

ASSOCIATION WITH INTESTINAL MICROBIOTA

There is epidemiologic evidence to suggest that microbial colonization of the gut—for example with lactobacilli due to the consumption of raw milk—and the gut microbiota may play a key role in development of allergic disorders such as asthma (23–25). Commensal microbes and intestinal helminths have developed along with the immune system and are therefore vital to promote normal immune maturity. Human GI microbiome during the first year of life is important for the maturation of immune function and development of allergic

Table 12.3: Factors Which Differentially Favour TH1 or TH2 Types of Phenotypes

1. Favouring TH1 phenotypes—protective of asthma:
   - Large family size
   - Older sibling
   - Daycare attendance
   - Tuberculosis and BCG vaccination
   - Other infections—Measles, mumps, rubella, chicken pox, hepatitis,
   - Schistosoma mansonii and croup
   - Living on farms and having contact with animals
   - Unpasteurised milk consumption
2. Favouring TH2 phenotypes—promoting asthma:
   - Urban environment
   - Western lifestyle
   - High antibiotic use
   - Sensitivity to house-dust mites and cockroaches
   - Bronchiolitis and some other early life respiratory infections—respiratory syncytial virus (RSV) causing pneumonia

disease. An inverse relationship has been shown between the number of microorganisms in the drinking water and the prevalence of childhood atopy assessed by prick skin tests. There are also reports that unpasteurized cow milk during the first year of life reduces the incidence of allergic disease and asthma in children.

Manipulation of bacterial microbiota with use of pro- and pre-biotics has been suggested for management of atopic disorders and some other diseases (26). Treatment with live helminths and/or their secretory or excretory products is also an option for treatment and prevention of these diseases (27).

ASSOCIATION WITH FARM AND DOMESTIC ANIMALS

Exposure to domestic animals is reported to offer protection against asthma (28,29). Asthma is less common in rural homes and in farming communities among children as well as adults. It is likely that living in a home or a farm with domestic animals like cattle and pigs provides a surrounding akin to the early 20th century environment; this may create a microbiome with more bacterial but fewer fungal species and lead to a lower risk of allergic disease. It is unclear whether it is the consumption of raw, unpasteurized milk or the inhalation of endotoxins that is actually preventive. Keeping pets like cats and dogs is also reported to prevent the development of atopy in childhood. This relationship is however dubious since exposure to pets is frequently reported to trigger acute asthma attacks.

It is also relevant to mention that the exposure to farms and animals as well as the consumption of cow's raw milk is protective earlier, rather than later in life. Consumption of raw milk in early childhood has been also shown to reduce the incidence of rhinitis, otitis, respiratory tract infections, and fever (30). Ingestion of raw, unpasteurized milk, however, was fraught with risk of infections. It was frequently associated with an increased occurrence of gastrointestinal tuberculosis due to bovine tuberculous bacilli. The incidence of bovine tuberculosis in humans is believed to disappear with the introduction of pasteurization.

Work on a modern farm is not necessarily protective. It may involve exposure to a number of irritants and allergens, which include organic and inorganic dusts, particulate matter, microbial agents, and gases. There are higher concentrations of volatile organic compounds, cleaning agents, fertilizers, and other chemical agents that are commonly used in the farms for different purposes. Some of these exposures can precipitate asthma and other respiratory problems.

PROBLEMS WITH THE HYGIENE HYPOTHESIS

There are several limitations to the foregoing discussion in favour of evidence in support of the protective effect of exposure to microbes and microbial products during early childhood.

1. *Asthma in less affluent countries:* Most epidemiological studies on global prevalence of asthma suggest widely variable figures. Nonetheless, the resource-poor and developing nations have a significantly high burden (31,32). A very high incidence in fact has been reported from countries with low income in a secondary analysis of the WHO's world health survey data among adults in 70 countries (10). The analysis reported that symptoms of asthma were more frequent in the extremes: low-income and high-income countries. There are also reports on an increasing prevalence of asthma in both children and adults in LMIC. This is particularly so in the urban areas. Infection rates as well as asthma prevalence are high in many Latin American countries (33,34). Some of the Indian reports have also reported similar high trends of asthma prevalence (35,36). It is also likely that the low prevalence frequently reported in some studies may actually be due to under-diagnosis and under-reporting.

   Less affluent countries in fact suffer from a number of environmental factors that have been frequently listed as asthma triggers. Air pollution, largely attributed to the ever-ongoing process of urbanization is an important factor. Frequent respiratory infections during childhood and early infancy may also trigger asthmatic attacks and impairment of lung function.

2. *Decline in asthma:* Asthma in the last decade, particularly in the developed Western countries has either declined or reached a plateau (37–39). A plateau of prevalence has been reached in several parts of Europe and the United States, while the severity and rate of mortality have declined. This has happened in spite of the continued standards of hygiene and cleanliness. A cohort study from Israel has shown a significant decrease in both the prevalence and severity of asthma in teenage boys (40). A systematic review, however, showed that asthma prevalence continued to increase

or remain stable in most parts of the world (39). Nonetheless, there is no linear correlation of either an increase or decline in prevalence of asthma with standards of hygiene or exposure to a farming life.

3. *Atopic versus non-atopic asthma:* Atopic asthma constitutes only about half the cases of asthma, which should have increased as per 'hygiene hypothesis'. There is, however, evidence to suggest that there is a greater increase in non-atopic asthma (41). It has been also seen in repeated surveys among pre-school children that besides the increase in classic asthma wheezing, there has been an increase in all different kinds of wheezing, including the 'virus-induced' wheezing, that do not involve the atopic immune responses.

4. *Contradictory influences of exposures:* Early exposures to many of the so-called protective exposures can also aggravate asthma and precipitate acute attacks. Exposures to pets and animal dander, house-dust mites, and insects such as cockroaches are important triggers for asthma and frequently responsible for an uncontrolled disease. Similarly, all kinds of respiratory infections are known to precede asthma attacks. For example, RSV infection may cause rather than prevent asthma. Moreover, a number of infections that might help prevent asthma can cause other health problems. Intestinal worm infestations are considered important causes of asthma in childhood. It is quite a routine clinical practice in several tropical countries to administer anti-helminthic treatment in patients with asthma. Apparently, the protective effects are limited to early life exposures only, notably during the first year of life (42,43).

5. *Inconsistency of relationship:* The relationship of atopy and asthma with intestinal worms and helminths is not consistent. Exposures to fungi or fungal products can also cause an increased risk of allergic disease. Infestation with helminth and other parasites is a known cause of asthma and other allergic diseases (44). Anti-helminthic treatment given for chronic helminthic infection or atopies in schoolchildren resulted in an increased prevalence of eczema and skin allergies, while asthma or allergic rhinitis remained unchanged. Infestations with Trichuris and Ascaris are also unrelated to asthma prevalence. The relationship between parasites, anti-helminth immunity, and allergic disorder is fairly complex but it is quite important to study the pathomechanisms of asthma (45).

All this evidence suggests that the 'hygiene hypothesis' does not satisfy the essential criteria needed to explain the rising incidence of asthma and should therefore be abandoned. Moreover, it tends to suggest that 'unhygienic' practices' such as not washing hands before eating may prevent asthma and other allergies. This is obviously an incorrect statement—good hygiene is a way of life which cannot be discarded. Personal hygienic practices have an immensely significant relationship with infection control and prevention. Most of all, it is not practical to adopt lifestyle measures considered protective according to the 'hygiene hypothesis'—such as having a large family or living on farms—for the prevention of asthma.

CONCLUSION

The current evidence seems to suggest that the 'hygiene hypothesis' should not be considered in a narrow sense linking asthma or other immune diseases with personal hygienic habits. The hygiene hypothesis and the role of microbiomes appears to be relevant in a broader sense, which signifies a more general version of relationships of diverse exposures to various microbes in early life with the development of immune mechanisms involved in the aetiology of asthma. The terminology seems to require rephrasing to suit a broader concept of an aetiological relationship.

REFERENCES

1. GBD 2016 Disease and Injury Incidence and Prevalence Collaborators. Global, regional, and national incidence, prevalence, and years lived with disability for 328 diseases and injuries for 195 countries, 1990–2016: a systematic analysis for the Global Burden of Disease Study 2016. Lancet 2017; 390: 1211–59.

2. Dharmage SC, Perret JL, Custovic A. Epidemiology of asthma in children and adults. Front Pediatr 2019; 7: 246–256 (published online).

3. Global Health Estimates 2016: Disease burden by Cause, Age, Sex, by Country and by Region, 2000–2016. Geneva, World Health Organization; 2018.

4. Global Health Estimates 2016: Deaths by Cause, Age, Sex, by Country and by Region, 2000–2016. Geneva, World Health Organization; 2018.

5. Platts-Mills TAE. The allergy epidemics: 1870–2010. J Allergy Clin Immunol 2015;136(1):3–13.

6. Elina Toskala E, Kennedy DW. Asthma risk factors. Int Forum Allergy Rhinol 2015;5:S11–S16.

7. Strachen DP. Hay fever, hygiene, and household size. BMJ. 299 (6710): 1259–60.

8. Ball TM, Castro-Rodriguez JA, Griffith KA, et al. Siblings, day-care attendance, and the risk of asthma and wheezing during childhood. N Engl J Med 2000; 343:538–43.

9. Ring J, Krämer U, Schäfer T, Abeck D, Vieluf D, Behrendt H. Environmental risk factors for respiratory and skin atopy: results from epidemiological studies in former East and West Germany. Int Arch Allergy Immunol 1999; 118(2–4):403–7.

10. Cruz ÁA, Stelmach R, Ponte EV. Asthma prevalence and severity in low-resource communities. Curr Opin Allergy Clin Immunol 2017; 17(3):188–93.

11. Liu AH. Revisiting the hygiene hypothesis for allergy and asthma. J Allergy Clin Immunol 2015; 136:860–5.

12. Holbreich M, Genuneit J, Weber J, Braun-Fahrlander C, Waser M, von Mutius E. Amish children living in northern Indiana have a very low prevalence of allergic sensitization. J Allergy Clin Immunol 2012; 129:1671–3.

13. Rodriguez A, Brickley E, Rodrigues L, Normansell RA, Barreto M, Cooper PJ. Urbanisation and asthma in low-income and middle-income countries: a systematic review of the urban-rural differences in asthma prevalence. Thorax 2019 Nov; 74(11):1020–30.

14. Lau S, Nickel R, Niggemann B, Grüber C, Sommerfeld C, Illi S, Kulig M, Forster J, Wahn U, Groeger M, Zepp F, Kamin W, Bieber I, Tacke U, Wahn V, Bauer CP, Bergmann R, von Mutius E; MAS Group. The development of childhood asthma: lessons from the German Multicentre Allergy Study (MAS). Paediatr Respir Rev 2002;3(3):265–72.

15. Lynch SV, Wood RA, Boushey H, Bacharier LB, Bloomberg GR, Kattan M, et al. Effects of early-life exposure to allergens and bacteria on recurrent wheeze and atopy in urban children. J Allergy Clin Immunol 2014; 134:593–601.e12.

16. Park SS, Heo EY, Kim DK, Chung HS, Lee CH. The Association of BCG Vaccination with Atopy and Asthma in Adults. Int J Med Sci 2015; 12(8):668–73.

17. Vogt H, Bråbäck L, Kling AM, Grünewald M, Nilsson L. Pertussis immunization in infancy and adolescent asthma medication. Pediatrics 2014; 134(4):721–8.

18. Linehan MF, Nurmatov U, Frank TL, Niven RM, Baxter DN, Sheikh A. Does BCG vaccination protect against childhood asthma? Final results from the Manchester Community Asthma Study retrospective cohort study and updated systematic review and meta-analysis. J Allergy Clin Immunol. 2014; 133(3):688–95.e14.

19. Okada H, Kuhn C, Feillet H, Bach J-F. The 'hygiene hypothesis' for autoimmune and allergic diseases: an update. Clin Exp Immunol 2010 Apr; 160 (1): 1–9.

20. Weinberg EG. Urbanization and childhood asthma: An African perspective. JAllergy Cinical Immunol. 2000 Feb; 105(2): 224–31.

21. Bufford JD, Gern JE. The hygiene hypothesis revisited. Immunol Allergy Clin North Am. 2005, 25(2): 247–62.

22. Matricardi PM, Rosmini F, Riondino S, et al. Exposure to foodborne and orofecal microbes versus airborne viruses in relation to atopy and allergic asthma: epidemiological study. BMJ 2000; 320:412–17.

23. Brooks C, Pearce N, Douwes J. The hygiene hypothesis in allergy and asthma: an update. Curr Opin Allergy Clin Immunol 2013; 13:70–7.

24. Kalliomaki M, Kirjavainen P, Eerola E, et al. Distinct patterns of neonatal gut microflora in infants in whom atopy was and was not developing. J Allergy Clin Immunol 2001; 107:129–34.

25. Bisgaard H, Li N, Bonnelykke K, et al. Reduced diversity of the intestinal microbiota during infancy is associated with increased risk of allergic disease at school age. J Allergy Clin Immunol 2011; 128:646–52.

26. Stiemsma L, Reynolds L, Turvey S, Finlay B. The hygiene hypothesis: current perspectives and future therapies. ImmunoTargets Ther 2015; 4:143–57.

27. Nutman TB, Santiago HC. Human helminths and allergic disease: The hygiene hypothesis and beyond. Am J Trop Med Hyg. 2016; 95(4):746–53.

28. Downs SH, Marks GB, Mitakakis TZ, et al. Having lived on a farm and protection against allergic diseases in Australia. Clin Exp Allergy 2001; 31:570–5.

29. Douwes J, Travier N, Huang K, et al. Lifelong farm exposure may strongly reduce the risk of asthma in adults. Allergy 2007; 62:1158–65.

30. Waser M, Michels KB, Bieli C, et al. Inverse association of farm milk consumption with asthma and allergy in rural and suburban populations across Europe. Clin Exp Allergy 2007; 37:661–70.

31. To T, Stanojevic, S, Moores G, Gershon, AS, Bateman ED, Cruz AA, Boulet L-P. Global asthma prevalence in adults: findings from the cross-sectional world health survey. BMC Public Health 2012;12:204–210.

32. van Tilburg Bernardes E,Arrieta, M-C. Hygiene hypothesis in asthma development: is hygiene to blame? Arch Med Res 2017; 48(8):717–26.

33. Mallol J, Solé D, Baeza-Bacab M, Aguirre-Camposano V, Soto-Quiros M, Baena-Cagnani C; Latin American ISAAC Group. Regional variation in asthma symptom prevalence in Latin American children. J Asthma 2010; 47(6):644–50.

34. Forno E, Gogna M, Cepeda A, Yañez A, Solé D, Cooper P, Avila L, Soto-Quiros M, Castro-Rodriguez JA, Celedón JC. Asthma in Latin America. Thorax. 2015; 70(9):898–905.

35. Jindal SK, Aggarwal AN, Gupta D, Agarwal R, Kumar R, Kaur T, Chaudhry K, Shah B. Indian study on epidemiology of asthma, respiratory symptoms and chronic bronchitis in adults (INSEARCH). Int J Tuberc Lung Dis 2012; 16(9):1270–7.

36. Paramesh H. Air pollution and allergic airway diseases: social determinants and sustainability in the control and prevention. Indian J Pediatr 2018 Apr; 85(4):284–94.

37. Ponsonby AL, Glasgow N, Pezic A, Dwyer T, Ciszek K, Kljakovic M. A temporal decline in asthma but not eczema prevalence from 2000 to 2005 at school entry in the Australian capital territory with further consideration of country of birth. Int J Epidemiol 2008; 37:559–69.

38. van Schayck CP, Smit HA. The prevalence of asthma in children: a reversing trend. Eur Respir J 2005; 26:647–50.

39. Anandan C, Nurmatov U, van Schayck OCP, Sheikh A. Is the prevalence of asthma declining? systematic review of epidemiological studies. Allergy 2010; 65:152–67.

40. Cohen S, Berkman N, Avital A, Springer C, Kordoba L, Haklai Z, Eshel A, Goldberg S, Picard E. Decline in asthma prevalence and severity in Israel over a 10-year period. Respiration 2015; 89(1):27–32.

41. Thomsen SF, Ulrik CS, Larsen K, Backer V. Change in prevalence of asthma in Danish children and adolescents. Ann Allergy Asthma Immunol 2004; 92:506–11.

42. Kramer U, Heinrich J, Wjst M, Wichmann HE. Age of entry to day nursery and allergy in later childhood. Lancet 1999; 353:450–4.

43. Johnson CC, Ownby DR. The infant gut bacterial microbiota and risk of pediatric asthma and allergic diseases. Transl Res 2017; 179: 60–70.

44. Alexandre-Silva GM, Brito-Souza PA, Oliveira ACS, Cerni FA, Zottich U, Pucca MB. The hygiene hypothesis at a glance: early exposures, immune mechanism and novel therapies. Acta Tropica. 2018;188:16–26.

45. Bohnacker S, Troisi F, Jiménez MdeLR, von Bieren JE. What can parasites tell us about the pathogenesis and treatment of asthma and allergic diseases. Front Immunol 2020 Sep; 11:2106.

13 Pathophysiology of Asthma

Ajith Kumar and Tisekar Owais Rafique Ahmed

CONTENTS

INTRODUCTION

Asthma is a heterogeneous disorder characterized by airway hyperresponsiveness and variable airflow limitation during expiration. The classical symptoms of asthma are cough, breathlessness, wheeze, and chest tightness that vary over time (1). Genetic predisposition plays a major role in the etiology of asthma with 50–70% of cases found to be inherited (2,3). The involved genes however follow a non-Mendelian pattern of inheritance. Besides, there is complex genetic heterogeneity with different combinations of genetic variants predisposing to specific phenotypes (4). The pathogenesis of asthma involves bronchoconstriction, airway hyperresponsiveness, and remodelling in response to a variety of stimuli (5).

This chapter focuses on the complex interplay between genetic and environmental factors in the pathogenesis of asthma, along with the phenotypes for individualized treatment in severe cases.

GENETICS OF ASTHMA

Multiple genes are involved in the transmission of asthma. The syndrome of asthma is characterized by locus heterogeneity, polygenic inheritance, and pleiotropy. Locus heterogeneity is defined as multiple genes leading to the same phenotype, whereas multiple genes acting together in one individual are termed as polygenic inheritance. Pleiotropy describes the association of genes involved in asthma with autoimmune and inflammatory disorders (6).

Using whole-genome linkage studies and case-control studies, at least five asthma genes were identified, i.e. disintegrin and metalloprotease 33 (ADAM33), dipeptidyl peptidase 10 (DPP10), plant homeodomain (PHD) zinc finger protein 11, G protein-coupled receptor for asthma susceptibility (GPRA), and prostaglandin D2 receptor (PGD2) (7). However, the application of the analyses to a complex disease like asthma has not been successful. This paved the way for association studies and next-generation sequencing (NGS).

Candidate or genome-wide association studies (GWAS) have revolutionized the understanding of asthma genetics. GWAS arrays are designed on the principle of linkage disequilibrium i.e. non-random association of alleles (specific forms) at different loci of genes. GWAS uses microarrays of single nucleotide polymorphism (SNP) chips to test the association between alleles (8). The EVE consortium studied more than 30,000 asthma cases and controls in groups of European Americans, African Americans, and U.S. Hispanics. The consortium found a strong association at the ORMDL3/GSDMB locus on chromosome 17q21, and near the IL1RL1, IL-13, TSLP, IL-33, SMAD3, and PYHIN1 genes. The PYHIN1 (interferon-inducible protein X) gene is unique for African descent individuals whereas

DOI: 10.1201/9781003125785-13

the interleukin 33 (IL 33) and interleukin 1 receptor-like 1 (IL1RL1) are strongly associated with atopic asthma (9,10).

NGS is a much faster sequencing platform compared with conventional sequencing that can be used to sequence a part or the whole genome (11). A few examples of NGS include the exome sequencing and targeted deep resequencing. The exome sequencing involves sequencing the protein-coding region of the gene. Exome sequencing has a limited role in complex traits like asthma, in which the genes are predominantly affected in the non-coding regions, but are useful in Mendelian traits in which alleles disrupt the protein-coding loci (12). The targeted deep resequencing has identified variants in the ARDB2 (beta-2 adrenergic receptor), *NCAM1* (neural cell adhesion molecule-1), *NOS1* (nitric oxide synthase-1), and *FLG* (filaggrin) genes. The findings helped us to understand that rare variants are also implied in asthma pathophysiology for some individuals. Further research is needed to understand their functional significance (13,14).

Part of the genetic risk for asthma is thought to result from genotype-specific responses to environmental factors during infancy and childhood. GWAS found an association between the *CDHR3* (cadherin-related family member-3) gene and rhinovirus C. The *CDHR3* gene mediates rhinovirus C binding and replication, and increases the frequency of hospitalization in asthmatics (15). Studies have demonstrated that a polymorphism in the promoter region of the CD14 gene was protective against asthma among children with high exposure to bacterial products like lipopolysaccharide (LPS) and its endotoxin moiety. In contrast, the same polymorphism conferred a risk for asthma in children with low endotoxin exposure (16).

GWAS have identified thousands of alleles involved in asthma, but the interpretation remains challenging. Multi-omics studies involve the use of genomics, transcriptomics (the study of RNA transcripts), proteomics (the study of proteins), metabolomics (the study of small molecules or metabolites), and epigenomics (the study of the modification of genetic material) (17,18). These studies together with GWAS have been incorporated in asthma research. The role of multi-omics studies is poorly understood at present and needs further research.

Environmental Risk Factors (19)

1. *Ethnicity:* In the United States, prevalence is higher in African American children compared with the white population (10.1% vs 8.1%) (20).

2. *Prematurity:* Low birth weight (LBW) increases the risk of asthma. Premature babies carry a risk for bronchopulmonary dysplasia and heightened airway responsiveness.

3. *Vitamin D levels:* Low vitamin D levels are associated with a high risk of exacerbation, more severe disease, and lower lung functions.

4. *Indoor and outdoor allergens:* Exposure to allergens like animals (cats, dogs, rodents), insects (mites, cockroaches), plants (grass, weed, pollen), and the workplace dampness (fungi) can trigger an acute exacerbation of asthma.

5. *Tobacco exposure:* Smoking and environmental tobacco smoke (ETS) exposure contribute to increased airway hyperreactivity. Maternal smoke exposure in utero increases the risk of asthma in the first few years of life.

6. *Respiratory viruses:* Respiratory syncytial virus (RSV) is associated with an increase in IgE levels. Rhinovirus can cause bronchiolitis in early childhood and can lead to asthma later in life. The viruses like influenza, parainfluenza, and human metapneumovirus (HMPV) trigger exacerbations.

7. *Obesity:* It is associated with a sixfold risk of hospitalization. The cytokines produced by adipose tissue including IL-6, IL-8, plasminogen activator inhibitor-1 (PAI-1), monocyte chemotactic factor-1 (MCP-1), and TNF-α are implicated in the pathogenesis of asthma (21).

ACUTE INFLAMMATORY RESPONSE

The acute inflammatory response in asthma is categorized into an early- and late-phase response (Figure 13.1).

EARLY ALLERGIC RESPONSE (EAR)

Asthma is an inflammatory response that begins with an exposure to a foreign antigen. When a novel antigen enters the airway, it is trapped in the mucosal lining. The antigen is then taken up by the dendritic cells. The dendritic cells, which are the antigen-presenting cells, transport the antigen to the pulmonary lymph nodes to naive T cells (Th0). GM-CSF stimulates the naive T cells and transforms them into Th2 cells. Upon re-challenge with the same antigen, the Th2 cells are recruited to the airways by the chemokines CCL 17 and CCL 22 secreted by dendritic cells. This is followed by the expression of interleukins IL-4, IL-5, IL-9, and IL-13 at the site of inflammation. B cells produce antigen-specific IgE that binds to the mast cells

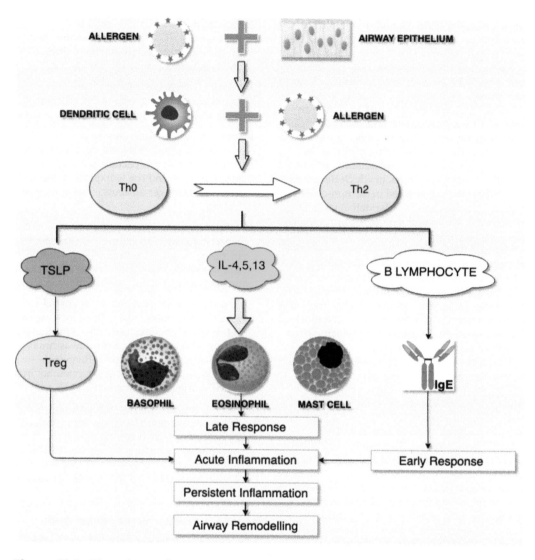

Figure 13.1 The asthma inflammatory response.

and basophils via the F_c receptor. The cross-linking between IgE and mast cell leads to mast cell degranulation and release of preformed mediators, and the activation of eicosanoid pathways replenish the used mediators. The release of inflammatory mediators leads to local tissue damage, bronchoconstriction, and airway edema (eosinophil mediated). The early response reaches a maximum by 15–30 minutes and resolves within 1–3 hours (22).

LATE ALLERGIC RESPONSE

The late phase response occurs several hours after the immediate hypersensitivity response. It is driven by Th2 mediated allergic response and airway hyperresponsiveness. There is an influx of inflammatory cells of both innate and adaptive immune responses like the mast cells, eosinophils, neutrophils, lymphocytes, and dendritic cells. The recruitment of inflammatory cells leads to airway smooth muscle contraction and bronchoconstriction. The onset occurs usually between 3–7 or more hours after allergen exposure and reaches a peak between 8–12 hours of exposure (23). The allergen-induced airway hyperresponsiveness can last up to 3 weeks (24). The late allergic response (LAR) is characterized by a decrease in the airway Tregs (regulatory T cells), which is not seen in the early phase response (25).

Role of Inflammatory Mediators and Cellular Elements

The role of various inflammatory cells in asthma is described below:

Mast Cells

The mast cells are commonly found in blood vessels, nerves, and surfaces. They are subdivided into two types (26).

a. MC_T: They contain only neutrophil protease tryptase and lack chymase. These are most commonly located in the subepithelium of bronchi, bronchioles, and the alveoli.

b. MC_{TC}: These mast cells contain chymase, carboxypeptidase A, tryptase, and cathepsin G like protease. They dominate the pleura and the pulmonary vasculature.

In severe asthma, there is a class switch of mast cells from MC_T to MC_{TC} type, especially in the smaller airways. These infiltrate airway smooth muscles and release both preformed and newly synthesized mediators (Table 13.1). These are as follows (27):

1. Preformed mediators:

    i. Histamine

    ii. Serotonin

    iii. Proteases (tryptase, chymotryptase, carboxypeptidase)

2. Newly synthesized mediators:

    i. Platelet-activating factor (PAF)

    ii. Growth factors like GM-CSF (granulocyte-macrophage colony-stimulating factor), VEGF (vascular

Table 13.1: Role of Inflammatory Mediators Released by Mast Cells in Asthma

Mediators	Role in Asthma
PREFORMED MEDIATORS	
Histamine	• Bronchoconstriction • Vasodilatation • Chemotaxis
Serotonin	• Modulates airway hyperresponsiveness
Proteases	• Regulates Th2 response
NEWLY SYNTHESIZED MEDIATORS	
Cysteinyl-LTs (LTC4, LTD4)	• Capillary leak • Bronchoconstriction
LTB_4	• Chemotaxis
PGD_2	• Bronchoconstriction • Chemotaxis.
.PAF (28)	• Chemotaxis • Bronchoconstriction
Growth Factors (VEGF, FGF-2) (29)	• Angiogenesis • Proinflammatory

endothelial growth factor), FGF-2 (fibroblast growth factor 2)

iii. Cytokines like IL-4, IL-5, IL-8, IL-13

iv. Arachidonic acid metabolites including LTB4 (leukotriene B4), cysteinyl leukotriene like LTC4 (leukotriene C4) and LTD4 (leukotriene D4), TXA2 (thromboxane A2), and prostaglandins (PGD2). The cysteinyl leukotrienes are the most potent bronchoconstrictors

Basophils

Basophils are present in the peripheral circulation, and they act as antigen-presenting cells (APCs). Basophils are involved in asthma in two different pathways. The IL-3 elicited basophils act through the IgE mediated pathway and cause inflammation. These basophils synthesize and release histamine, LTC4, IL-4, and IL-13. The basophils elicited by thymic stromal lymphopoietin (TSLP) do not respond to IgE-antigen complexes and secrete IL-18 and IL-33 for inflammation (30).

Eosinophils

These are one of the predominant inflammatory cells in the airways. The Th2 cells cause the release of eosinophils from the bone marrow in response to a foreign antigen. Their production is dependent upon stimulation by GM-CSF and IL-13 (31). The eosinophils are then recruited to the airways via several cytokines like IL-5, RANTES (Regulated upon Activation, Normal T Cell Expressed and Presumably Secreted), MIP-1α (macrophage inflammatory protein), MCP (monocyte chemo-attractant protein), and eotaxin. These recruited eosinophils then secrete primary and secondary granule proteins. Primary granules contain Charcot Leyden crystals, whereas secondary granules contain eosinophilic cationic protein (ECP), major basic protein (MBP), eosinophil-derived neurotoxin (EDN), and eosinophil peroxidase (EPO) (32).

The role of different eosinophil-derived products is described below.

a. *Granule proteins:*

They cause local tissue damage. The granule proteins cause mast cell induction, basophil degranulation, increased airway mucus production, and the generation of reactive oxygen species.

• ECP: Stimulation of mast cells and lymphocytes (33)

• MBP: Stimulation of mast cells, basophils, and neutrophils; bronchoconstriction (34)

- EDN: Causes neuronal damage along with antiviral property (35)
- EPO: Generation of reactive oxygen species (36)

b. *Cytokines:*

The cytokines up-regulate the expression of adhesion markers with the activation of other inflammatory cells. They are involved in airway remodelling.

- GM-CSF contributes to the growth, maturation, and survival of eosinophils (37).
- IL-3 is indicated in airway hyperresponsiveness, mucus production, and survival of eosinophils (38).
- IL-4 helps in the differentiation of Th0 cells into the Th2 subtype and upregulates IgE and vascular cell adhesion molecule-1 (39).
- IL-5 is essential for eosinophil production, growth and survival; and also airway remodelling (40).
- IL-13 stimulates eosinophil recruitment to airways, induces glandular hyperplasia, and cause airway remodelling (41).
- IL-25 has a role in trafficking of eosinophil progenitors to the airway and local differentiation of eosinophils (42).
- IL-33 is a potent activator of eosinophils, degranulation, and release of superoxides (43).
- TSLP suppresses Treg cells and enhances pro-inflammatory response (44).

c. *Chemokines:*

The chemokines are small cytokines produced by the eosinophils that promote the localization of immune cells to the site of inflammation and local cellular activation. A few examples include RANTES, MIP-1α, MCP, Eotaxin, CXCR4, CCR8, CCL11, and CCL22 (45).

d. *Lipid mediators:*

The function of lipid mediators like PGD2, PAF, TXA2, and cysteinyl leukotrienes (LTB4, LTC4) is to increase airway smooth muscle contraction, mucus production, vascular permeability, and the recruitment of inflammatory cells (46).

Neutrophils

The neutrophils are normally present in the bloodstream and body tissues, including lung. The neutrophils contain primary azurophilic and secondary specific granules. The cytokines recruit neutrophils to the airways. They in turn secrete cytokines like IL-1, IL-8, IL-18, and TNF-α. This leads to heightened airway inflammation with increased mucus production and bronchial hyperresponsiveness. They are not only important as chemoattractants, but they also play a major role in the release of reactive oxygen species. Such patients with neutrophil predominance are less responsive to steroids (47).

Lymphocytes

The cytokines and the APCs recruit the Th2 lymphocytes to the airway leading to increased production of GM-CSF, IL-3, IL-4, IL-5, and IL-13 cytokines. Th2 lymphocytes express the chemokine receptors (CCR4 and CCR8) and the chemoattractant receptor-like molecule (CRTH2). CRTH2 plays an important role in the activation of mast-cell dependent and mast cell-independent activation of Th2 cells (48).

Invariant Natural Killer T Cells

The invariant natural killer T (iNKT) expresses a conserved T-cell receptor that rapidly produces IL-4 and IL-13. The iNKT cells constitute less than 2% of the T cells in the airway lumen and the lung parenchyma (49). They recognze glycolipid antigens like the plant pollens (50).

Nitric Oxide (NO)

Nitric oxide can have both beneficial and deleterious effects in asthma pathophysiology. The protective effects by the production of NO through constitutive forms include smooth muscle relaxation, leading to bronchodilation and vasodilation. Nitric oxide synthesis by inducible forms leads to capillary leak, mucus hypersecretion, oxidative stress, and chemotaxis of inflammatory cells (51).

Immunoglobulin E (IgE)

Serum IgE is the hallmark of the immediate type of hypersensitivity reaction in asthma (early allergic response), but it is also indicated in the late phase of the allergen response. IgE is indicated in the initiation and propagation of the inflammatory cascade and the allergic response (52).

PATHOLOGICAL CHANGES IN AIRWAYS

The airway bronchial hyperresponsiveness describes an acute but temporary drop in maximal flow in expiration in response to inhaling bronchial provocation agents like histamine or methacholine (53). Children with airway hyperresponsiveness have twice the risk for the development of asthma (54). The baseline bronchomotor tone contributes to increased airway responsiveness (55). The probable mechanism for airway hyperreactivity includes the release of inflammatory mediators, airway epithelial changes, alteration in airway smooth muscle, and abnormalities in the neural pathway (5).

Forced expiratory volume 1 (FEV_1) depends on the balance between the resistance of airways that limits the expiratory flow and the elastic recoil that promotes the flow during the respiratory cycle. The inflammatory response leads to decreased flow rates in larger airways, while small airway obstruction (diameter <2 mm) leads to an increase in residual volume (RV) and air trapping. This leads to an increase in total lung capacity (TLC), functional residual capacity (FRC), and an increase in RV/TLC ratio (56).

Airway remodelling involves structural changes in the epithelium and the mesenchyme. There is an irreversible limitation in airflow due to structural changes in the airways. There is an increase in the proliferative growth factors like insulin-like growth factor (IGF-1), platelet-derived growth factor (PDGF), endothelin (ET-1), and transforming growth factor beta-2 (TGF β2). These factors act on smooth muscle and fibroblast to increase matrix deposition in the airways (57,58). There is an increase in the subepithelial basement membrane thickness via enhanced expression of matrix metalloproteinase-9 (MMP-9) and epidermal growth factor receptor (EGFR) (59,60). Histologically, there is damage to the pseudostratified ciliated epithelial lining with an increase in mucus-producing goblet cells and fibrosis in the subepithelial basement membrane. The vascularity is increased, along with an increase in smooth muscles, myofibroblasts, and extracellular matrix. All these changes contribute to the progressive loss of lung function (61).

ASTHMA PHENOTYPES

Patients with severe asthma present with variable clinical features, more progressive disease, and a non-uniform response to anti-inflammatory medicines, including glucocorticoids. The patients are typed into clinically discrete phenotypes based on demographic, clinical, and physiological variables (62). The variables include patient characteristics (age of onset, obesity), severity, atopic or non-atopic etiology, inflammatory biomarkers, glucocorticoid responsiveness, etc. Although this phenotypic approach may not have a clinical advantage, it helps to improve the understanding of the disease process.

Asthma is commonly classified into the following six subgroups (62–64):

1. *Early-onset atopic (classical)*: Childhood-onset asthma (before the age of 12 years) often has a strong family and allergic history. It is characterized by eosinophilic inflammation of airways and responds well to corticosteroids.

2. *Late-onset atopic*: This subgroup comprises a minority of individuals. They often have a history of allergic rhinitis in childhood.

3. *Late-onset non-atopic*: Adult-onset non-atopic asthma is seen mainly in women. The onset of symptoms is seen following a viral illness, aspirin ingestion, or occupational exposure. Such patients show partial response to steroids.

4. *Non-allergic*: This cluster is characterized by neutrophilic or pauci-granular inflammation.

5. *Asthma with persistent airflow obstruction*: Airway remodelling leads to persistent airflow limitation with partial or no reversibility on spirometry.

6. *Asthma with obesity*: Obese patients with asthma tend to have non-atopic inflammation.

The Severe Asthma Research Programme (SARP) cohort classified severe asthmatics into five clusters using three variables (baseline FEV_1, maximal FEV_1 after six to eight puffs of albuterol, and age of onset of asthma) with clusters ranging from milder asthma (Cluster 1) to more severe disease (Clusters 4 and 5) (Figure 13.2) (62).

There are a few other phenotypic classifications attempted by several authors, which have been categorized below (Table 13.2).

CONCLUSION

Asthma is a complex heterogeneous disorder characterized by reversible airflow limitation and airway inflammation. The inflammatory response not only leads to flow limitation and smooth muscle contraction but also airway remodelling. Airway remodelling contributes to irreversible airflow limitation and functional limitation. The pathophysiology of asthma can be approached as genotypic as well as phenotypic variants causing variable inflammatory response. About 50–70% of asthmatics exhibit a genetic predisposition in a complex non-Mendelian pattern. There is genetic heterogeneity with different combinations of genetic variants predisposing to a specific phenotype. The genetic studies on asthma help not only in understanding the biological effects of cytokines in the pathophysiology but also in

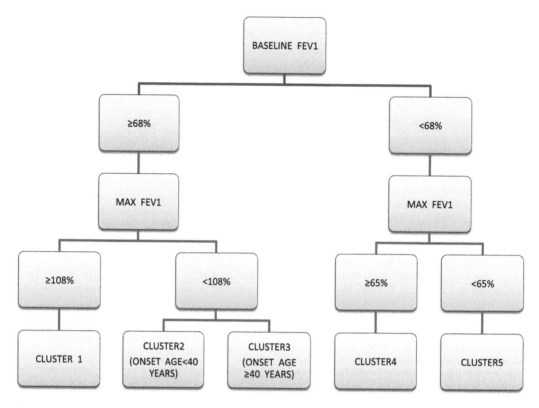

Figure 13.2 Cluster analysis as per the Severe Asthma Research Programme Cohort.

Table 13.2: Other Phenotyping Studies besides the Severe Asthma Research Programme

Study	Population	N	Phenotypes
Haldar et al. (2008) (65)	Adults	187	1. Early-onset, atopic 2. Obese, non-eosinophilic 3. Early symptom predominant(atopic) 4. Inflammation predominant (late-onset)
Kim et al. (2013) (66)	Adults	2567	1. Severe obstructive asthma 2. Smoking-induced asthma 3. Early-onset atopic 4. Late-onset mild asthma
Amelink et al. (2013) (67)	Adults	200	1. Severe eosinophilic inflammation 2. Frequent symptoms, high healthcare utilization, and low sputum eosinophils 3. Mild to moderate, well-controlled asthma
Schatz et al. (2014) (68)	Children	518	1. Atopic white males with no smoke exposure 2. Female sex 3. Non-atopic status 4. Passive smoke exposure 5. Non-white race
Schatz et al. (2014) (68)	Adolescents and adults	3,612	1. White female with adult-onset asthma and lower total IgE levels 2. Highest atopy 3. Male sex 4. Non-white race 5. Aspirin sensitivity
Newby et al. (2014) (69)	Adults	349	1. Atopic with early-onset 2. Obese with late-onset 3. Least severe asthma 4. Eosinophilic with late-onset disease 5. Significant fixed airflow obstruction

Table 13.2: (*Continued*)

Study	Population	N	Phenotypes
Zaihra et al. (2016) (70)	Adults	125	1. Severe asthma with late-onset disease 2. Obese females with severe asthma 3. Early-onset atopic disease with severe asthma 4. Moderate asthmatics with good lung functions
Lefaudeux et al. (2017) (71)	Adults	418	1. Moderate to severe well-controlled asthma 2. Obese late-onset severe asthma with airflow obstruction 3. Late-onset atopic asthma with severe airflow obstruction 4. Obese females with 5. Severe asthma
Ortega et al. (2014) (72)	Adults	616	1. Severe asthma with low blood eosinophil count 2. Severe asthma with low airflow reversibility 3. Severe asthma with high airflow reversibility 4. Obesity with high airflow reversibility

formulating targeted therapies. The role of cytokines in Th2 response has been a target for various anti-cytokine therapies. The phenotypic classification has been used in severe asthma to identify sub-group specific therapies for the difficult-to-treat cases. The future looks forward to the correlation of asthma pathophysiology to genotyping, as well as phenotyping in order to aid in the early identification of at risk individuals, implementation of preventive strategies, and, finally, in the delivery of an effective customized therapy to each patient.

REFERENCES

1. Expert Panel Report 3: Guidelines for the Diagnosis and Management of Asthma. 2007;440.

2. Thomsen SF, Sluis SVD, Kyvik KO, Skytthe A, Backer V. Estimates of asthma heritability in a large twin sample. Clin Exp Allergy. 2010;40(7):1054–61.

3. Duffy DL, Martin NG, Battistutta D, Hopper JL, Mathews JD. Genetics of Asthma and Hay Fever in Australian Twins. Am Rev Respir Dis. 1990 Dec 1;142(6_pt_1):1351–8.

4. Thomsen SF. Genetics of asthma: an introduction for the clinician. Eur Clin Respir J. 2015 Jan 1; 2(1):24643.

5. Kudo M, Ishigatsubo Y, Aoki I. Pathology of asthma. Front Microbiol. [Internet]. 2013 [cited 2020 Oct 16]; 4. Available from: https://www.frontiersin.org/articles/10.3389/fmicb.2013.00263/full

6. Meyers DA. Approaches to genetic studies of asthma. Am J Respir Crit Care Med. 1994 Nov 1;150(5_pt_2):S91–3.

7. Lee S-H, Park J-S, Park C-S. The search for genetic variants and epigenetics related to asthma. Allergy Asthma Immunol Res. 2011 Oct 1;3(4):236–44.

8. Weiss ST, Silverman EK. Pro: Genome-Wide Association Studies (GWAS) in asthma. Am J Respir Crit Care Med. 2011 Sep 15;184(6):631–3.

9. Myers RA, Himes BE, Gignoux CR, Yang JJ, Gauderman WJ, Rebordosa C, et al. Further replication studies of the EVE Consortium meta-analysis identifies 2 asthma risk loci in European Americans. J Allergy Clin Immunol. 2012 Dec 1;130(6):1294–301.

10. Torgerson DG, Ampleford EJ, Chiu GY, Gauderman WJ, Gignoux CR, Graves PE, et al. Meta-analysis of genome-wide association studies of asthma in ethnically diverse North American populations. Nat Genet. 2011 Jul 31;43(9):887–92.

11. Shendure J, Ji H. Next-generation DNA sequencing. Nat Biotechnol. 2008 Oct;26(10):1135–45.

12. DeWan AT, Egan KB, Hellenbrand K, Sorrentino K, Pizzoferrato N, Walsh KM, et al. Whole-exome sequencing of a pedigree segregating asthma. BMC Med Genet. 2012 Oct 9;13(1):95.

13. Torgerson DG, Giri T, Druley TE, Zheng J, Huntsman S, Seibold MA, et al. Pooled sequencing of candidate genes implicates rare variants in the development of asthma following severe RSV bronchiolitis in infancy. PLOS ONE. 2015 Nov 20;10(11):e0142649.

14. Torgerson DG, Capurso D, Mathias RA, Graves PE, Hernandez RD, Beaty TH, et al. Resequencing candidate genes implicates rare variants in asthma susceptibility. Am J Hum Genet. 2012 Feb 10; 90(2):273–81.

15. Bochkov YA, Watters K, Ashraf S, Griggs TF, Devries MK, Jackson DJ, et al. Cadherin-related family member 3, a childhood asthma susceptibility gene product, mediates rhinovirus C binding and replication. Proc Natl Acad Sci. 2015 Apr 28;112(17):5485–90.

16. Eder W, Klimecki W, Yu L, Mutius E von, Riedler J, Braun-Fahrländer C, et al. Opposite effects of CD14/-260 on serum IgE levels in children raised in different environments. J Allergy Clin Immunol. 2005 Sep 1;116(3):601–7.

17. Forno E, Wang T, Yan Q, Brehm J, Acosta-Perez E, Colon-Semidey A, et al. A multiomics approach to identify genes associated with childhood asthma risk and morbidity. Am J Respir Cell Mol Biol. 2017 Jun 2;57(4):439–47.

18. Hasin Y, Seldin M, Lusis A. Multi-omics approaches to disease. Genome Biol. 2017 May 5;18(1):83.

19. Miraglia del Giudice M, Allegorico A, Parisi G, Galdo F, Alterio E, Coronella A, et al. Risk factors for asthma. Ital J Pediatr. 2014 Aug 11;40(Suppl 1):A77.

20. Most Recent National Asthma Data | CDC [Internet]. 2020 [cited 2020 Oct 16]. Available from: https://www.cdc.gov/asthma/most_recent_national_asthma_data.htm

21. Mohanan S, Tapp H, McWilliams A, Dulin M. Obesity and asthma: pathophysiology and implications for diagnosis and management in primary care. Exp Biol Med Maywood NJ. 2014 Nov;239(11):1531–40.

22. Gauvreau GM, El-Gammal AI, O'Byrne PM. Allergen-induced airway responses. Eur Respir J. 2015 Sep;46(3):819–31.

23. Diamant Z, Gauvreau GM, Cockcroft DW, Boulet L-P, Sterk PJ, de Jongh FHC, et al. Inhaled allergen bronchoprovocation tests. J Allergy Clin Immunol. 2013 Nov;132(5):1045–1055.e6.

24. Durham SR, Craddock CF, Cookson WO, Benson MK. Increases in airway responsiveness to histamine precede allergen-induced late asthmatic responses. J Allergy Clin Immunol. 1988 Nov;82(5 Pt 1):764–70.

25. Kinoshita T, Baatjes A, Smith SG, Dua B, Watson R, Kawayama T, et al. Natural regulatory T cells in isolated early responders compared with dual responders with allergic asthma. J Allergy Clin Immunol. 2014 Mar 1;133(3):696–703.

26. Méndez-Enríquez E, Hallgren J. Mast Cells and Their Progenitors in Allergic Asthma. Front Immunol [Internet]. 2019 [cited 2020 Oct 16];10. Available from: https://www.frontiersin.org/articles/10.3389/fimmu.2019.00821/full

27. Holgate ST. The role of mast cells and basophils in inflammation. Clin Exp Allergy J Br Soc Allergy Clin Immunol. 2000 Jun;30 (Suppl 1):28–32.

28. Kasperska-Zajac A, Brzoza Z, Rogala B. Platelet-activating factor (PAF): a review of its role in asthma and clinical efficacy of PAF antagonists in the disease therapy. Recent Pat Inflamm Allergy Drug Discov. 2008 Jan 1;2(1):72–6.

29. Laddha AP, Kulkarni YA. VEGF and FGF-2: Promising targets for the treatment of respiratory disorders. Respir Med. 2019 Sep 1;156:33–46.

30. Siracusa MC, Kim BS, Spergel JM, Artis D. Basophils and allergic inflammation. J Allergy Clin Immunol. 2013 Oct;132(4):789–801.

31. Possa SS, Leick EA, Prado CM, Martins MA, Tibério IFLC. Eosinophilic Inflammation in Allergic Asthma. Front Pharmacol [Internet]. 2013 [cited 2020 Oct 16];4. Available from: https://www.frontiersin.org/articles/10.3389/fphar.2013.00046/full

32. Trivedi SG, Lloyd CM. Eosinophils in the pathogenesis of allergic airways disease. Cell Mol Life Sci. 2007 Mar 15;64(10):1269.

33. Zheutlin LM, Ackerman SJ, Gleich GJ, Thomas LL. Stimulation of basophil and rat mast cell histamine release by eosinophil granule-derived cationic proteins. J Immunol. 1984 Oct 1;133(4):2180–5.

34. Frigas E, Loegering DA, Solley GO, Farrow GM, Gleich GJ. Elevated levels of the eosinophil granule major basic protein in the sputum of patients with bronchial asthma. Mayo Clin Proc. 1981 Jun;56(6):345–53.

35. Durack DT, Ackerman SJ, Loegering DA, Gleich GJ. Purification of human eosinophil-derived neurotoxin. Proc Natl Acad Sci U S A. 1981 Aug 1;78(8):5165–9.

36. Wu W, Chen Y, Hazen SL. Eosinophil peroxidase nitrates protein tyrosyl residues implications for oxidative damage by nitrating intermediates in eosinophilic inflammatory disorders. J Biol Chem. 1999 Sep 3;274(36):25933–44.

37. Su Y-C, Rolph MS, Hansbro NG, Mackay CR, Sewell WA. Granulocyte-macrophage colony-stimulating factor is required for bronchial eosinophilia in a murine model of allergic airway inflammation. J Immunol. 2008 Feb 15;180(4):2600–7.

38. Pope SM, Brandt EB, Mishra A, Hogan SP, Zimmermann N, Matthaei KI, et al. IL-13 induces eosinophil recruitment into the lung by an IL-5– and eotaxin-dependent mechanism. J Allergy Clin Immunol. 2001 Oct 1;108(4):594–601.

39. Steinke JW, Borish L. Th2 cytokines and asthma. Interleukin-4: its role in the pathogenesis of asthma, and targeting it for asthma treatment with interleukin-4 receptor antagonists. Respir Res. 2001;2(2):66–70.

40. Pelaia C, Paoletti G, Puggioni F, Racca F, Pelaia G, Canonica GW, et al. Interleukin-5 in the Pathophysiology of Severe Asthma. Front Physiol [Internet]. 2019 [cited 2020 Oct 16];10. Available from: https://www.frontiersin.org/articles/10.3389/fphys.2019.01514/full

41. Nair P, O'Byrne PM. The interleukin-13 paradox in asthma: effective biology, ineffective biologicals. Eur Respir J. 2019;53(2).

42. Tang W, Smith SG, Du W, Gugilla A, Du J, Oliveria JP, et al. Interleukin-25 and eosinophils progenitor cell mobilization in allergic asthma. Clin Transl Allergy. 2018 Feb 13;8(1):5.

43. Johnston LK, Bryce PJ. Understanding interleukin 33 and its roles in eosinophil development. Front Med. [Internet]. 2017 [cited 2020 Oct 16];4. Available from: https://www.frontiersin.org/articles/10.3389/fmed.2017.00051/full

44. West EE, Kashyap M, Leonard WJ. TSLP: A key regulator of asthma pathogenesis. Drug Discov Today Dis Mech. 2012 Dec 1;9(3–4).

45. Lukacs NW. Role of chemokines in the pathogenesis of asthma. Nat Rev Immunol. 2001 Nov;1(2):108–16.

46. Monga N, Sethi GS, Kondepudi KK, Naura AS. Lipid mediators and asthma: scope of therapeutics. Biochem Pharmacol. 2020 Sep;179:113925.

47. Ciepiela O, Ostafin M, Demkow U. Neutrophils in asthma—A review. Respir Physiol Neurobiol. 2015 Apr 1;209:13–6.

48. Vinall SL, Townsend ER, Pettipher R. A paracrine role for chemoattractant receptor-homologous molecule expressed on T helper type 2 cells (CRTH2) in mediating chemotactic activation of CRTH2+ CD4+ T helper type 2 lymphocytes. Immunology. 2007;121(4):577–84.

49. Vijayanand P, Seumois G, Pickard C, Powell RM, Angco G, Sammut D, et al. Invariant natural killer T cells in asthma and chronic obstructive pulmonary disease. N Engl J Med. 2007 Apr 5;356(14):1410–22.

50. Oki S, Miyake S. Invariant natural killer T (iNKT) cells in asthma: a novel insight into the pathogenesis of asthma and the therapeutic implication of glycolipid ligands for allergic diseases. Allergol Int. 2007 Jan 1;56(1):7–14.

51. Prado CM, Martins MA, Tibério IFLC. Nitric oxide in asthma physiopathology. ISRN Allergy. 2011;2011:832560.

52. Sandeep T, Roopakala MS, Silvia CRWD, Chandrashekara S, Rao M. Evaluation of serum immunoglobulin E levels in bronchial asthma. Lung India Off Organ Indian Chest Soc. 2010;27(3):138–40.

53. Schoor JV, Joos GF, Pauwels RA. Indirect bronchial hyperresponsiveness in asthma: mechanisms, pharmacology and implications for clinical research. Eur Respir J. 2000 Sep 1;16(3):514–33.

54. Valerio MA, Andreski PM, Schoeni RF, McGonagle KA. Examining the association between childhood asthma and parent and grandparent asthma status: implications for practice: Clin Pediatr. (Phila) [Internet]. 2010 May 27 [cited 2020 Oct 17]; Available from: https://journals.sagepub.com/doi/10.1177/0009922809356465

55. Bossé Y, Rousseau É, Amrani Y, Grunstein MM. Smooth muscle hypercontractility in airway hyperresponsiveness: innate, scquired, or nonexistent? J Allergy [Internet]. 2013 [cited 2020 Oct 17];2013. Available from: https://www.ncbi.nlm.nih.gov/pmc/articles/PMC3703427/

56. Mitchell HW, Sparrow MP. Increased responsiveness to cholinergic stimulation of small compared to large diameter cartilaginous bronchi. Eur Respir J. 1994 Feb 1;7(2):298–305.

57. Hough KP, Curtiss ML, Blain TJ, Liu R-M, Trevor J, Deshane JS, et al. Airway remodeling in asthma. Front Med. [Internet]. 2020 [cited 2020 Oct 17];7. Available from: https://www.frontiersin.org/articles/10.3389/fmed.2020.00191/full

58. Zhang S, Smartt H, Holgate ST, Roche WR. Growth factors secreted by bronchial epithelial cells control myofibroblast proliferation: an in vitro co-culture model of airway remodeling in asthma. Lab Invest J Tech Methods Pathol. 1999 Apr;79(4):395–405.

59. Le Cras TD, Acciani TH, Mushaben EM, Kramer EL, Pastura PA, Hardie WD, et al. Epithelial EGF receptor signaling mediates airway hyperreactivity and remodeling in a mouse model of chronic asthma. Am J Physiol-Lung Cell Mol Physiol. 2010 Dec 17;300(3):L414–21.

60. Ohbayashi H, Shimokata K. Matrix metalloproteinase-9 and airway remodeling in asthma. Curr Drug Targets Inflamm Allergy. 2005 Apr;4(2):177–81.

61. Bergeron C, Tulic MK, Hamid Q. Airway remodelling in asthma: from benchside to clinical practice. Can Respir J. 2010 Aug;17(4):e85–93.

62. Moore WC, Meyers DA, Wenzel SE, Teague WG, Li H, Li X, et al. Identification of Asthma Phenotypes Using Cluster Analysis in the Severe Asthma Research Program. Am J Respir Crit Care Med. 2010 Feb 15;181(4):315–23.

63. Wenzel SE. Asthma phenotypes: the evolution from clinical to molecular approaches. Nat Med. 2012 May 4;18(5):716–25.

64. Bel EH. Clinical phenotypes of asthma. Curr Opin Pulm Med. 2004 Jan;10(1):44–50.

65. Haldar P, Pavord ID, Shaw DE, Berry MA, Thomas M, Brightling CE, et al. Cluster analysis and clinical asthma phenotypes. Am J Respir Crit Care Med. 2008 Aug 1;178(3):218–24.

66. Kim T-B, Jang A-S, Kwon H-S, Park J-S, Chang Y-S, Cho S-H, et al. Identification of asthma clusters in two independent Korean adult asthma cohorts. Eur Respir J. 2013 Jun;41(6):1308–14.

67. Amelink M, de Nijs SB, de Groot JC, van Tilburg PMB, van Spiegel PI, Krouwels FH, et al. Three phenotypes of adult-onset asthma. Allergy. 2013;68(5):674–80.

68. Schatz M, Hsu J-WY, Zeiger RS, Chen W, Dorenbaum A, Chipps BE, et al. Phenotypes determined by cluster analysis in severe or difficult-to-treat asthma. J Allergy Clin Immunol. 2014 Jun;133(6):1549–56.

69. Newby C, Heaney LG, Menzies-Gow A, Niven RM, Mansur A, Bucknall C, et al. Statistical cluster analysis of the British Thoracic Society Severe Refractory Asthma Registry: clinical outcomes and phenotype stability. PLOS ONE [Internet]. 2014 Jul 24 [cited 2020 Oct 17];9(7). Available from: https://www.ncbi.nlm.nih.gov/pmc/articles/PMC4109965/

70. Zaihra T, Walsh CJ, Ahmed S, Fugère C, Hamid QA, Olivenstein R, et al. Phenotyping of difficult asthma using longitudinal physiological and biomarker measurements reveals significant differences in stability between clusters. BMC Pulm Med. 2016 May 10;16(1):74.

71. Lefaudeux D, De Meulder B, Loza MJ, Peffer N, Rowe A, Baribaud F, et al. U-BIOPRED clinical adult asthma clusters linked to a subset of sputum omics. J Allergy Clin Immunol. 2017 Jun;139(6):1797–1807.

72. Ortega H, Li H, Suruki R, Albers F, Gordon D, Yancey S. Cluster analysis and characterization of response to mepolizumab. A step closer to personalized medicine for patients with severe asthma. Ann Am Thorac Soc. 2014 Sep;11(7):1011–7.

14 Smoking and Vaping in Young Adults and Their Influence on Asthma

Sujeet Rajan

CONTENTS

INTRODUCTION

Smoking has long had devastating effects on human health. A growing awareness of its impact has resulted in recent decades, in the reduction of cigarette consumption and stricter government regulations. In response, tobacco companies began promoting new tobacco products, such as flavoured electronic cigarettes (e-cigs).

E-cigs are battery-operated devices that deliver nicotine, flavourings and other constituents to the user by heating flavoured e-cig liquid (e-liquid) solutions to temperatures sufficient to form an aerosol. Despite a variety of names for these products, they all basically contain the same components, which include a battery, an atomiser, and a tank or cartridge to hold the e-liquid. This e-liquid is composed of propylene glycol (PG) and vegetable glycerine (VG).

Over the past few years, many researchers have suggested that asthmatics who smoke should shift to e-cigarettes. Recent data also suggests that with a decrease in cigarette smoking (15.8% in 2011 to 8% in 2016), e-cigarette use has increased (1.5% in 2011 to 11.3% in 2016) (1).

Michigan in the United States is the first state to ban flavoured e-cigarettes, a product closely associated with youth vaping. US federal regulators are now pursuing a nation wide ban of most flavoured e-cigarettes.

The FDA implemented a rule in 2016 to bring regulation of e-cigarettes within its tobacco division, stating it did so "to prevent youths from initiating tobacco use, inform consumers about the risks, prevent false and misleading claims, encourage cessation, and decrease the harms from tobacco use."

Tobacco use, of any type, is the leading cause of preventable death all over the world. Nearly all adult smokers started using tobacco products before they turned 18 years of age. Data about youth smoking rates isn't perfect. The rapid change in tobacco technology, coupled with young people likely not wanting to get in trouble for breaking the law and changing survey approaches trying to keep up with new cultural practices, make teen smoking rates difficult to measure. Nevertheless, the data is clear about the rising trend: more youth are using tobacco products and more youth are vaping.

THE COMPONENTS OF E-LIQUIDS AND THEIR PULMONARY EFFECTS

Propylene glycol (PG) and vegetable glycerine (VG) form a major portion of the e-liquid volume. They also have an ability to retain moisture and give the user a feeling of 'throat hit' similar to cigarette smoking. Propylene glycol can activate irritant receptors in sensory nerves in airways. These receptors can provoke airway inflammation and bronchial hyper reactivity as well (2). Another concern is that PG and VG can form toxic compounds on thermal decomposition. Newer e-cigarette devices allow the user to increase the voltage applied to the atomiser, thereby increasing the heating coil temperature. Therefore more aerosols are generated at higher temperatures. Significant amounts of

DOI: 10.1201/9781003125785-14

formaldehyde, acetaldehyde, and even acrolein are being generated and these are all known to exacerbate asthma (3).

Nicotine

Unlike PG and VG, Nicotine can increase arterial stiffness and affect microcirculation, thereby being a possible risk factor for cardiovascular disease. Physiological effects of nicotine by virtue of its ability to affect the release and metabolism of neurotransmitters include increased blood pressure and pulse rate, mobilisation of blood sugar, increased free fatty acids in the plasma, and increased concentrations of catecholamines in the bladder (4–9).

Most manufactured cigarettes contain 10–15 mg of nicotine per cigarette (10). However, the e-cigarette refill liquids are available with varying concentrations of nicotine ranging from 0–36 mg per ml. Because of this variation, it is still unclear whether vaping will result in significantly greater exposure to nicotine than smoking. Even though nicotine induces an anti-inflammatory response in the lung, it has also been associated with increased susceptibility to viral infections, which are major triggers of asthma exacerbations (11).

Flavouring Agents

E-liquids use many flavours. However, its safety to the lung at levels inhaled by the user is uncertain. Flavours are the major difference between cigarettes and e-cigarettes. In 2009, the United States banned the use of flavour for cigarettes to prevent smoking amongst children and adolescents. This significantly enhanced the use of e-cigarettes in the United States. The emphasis was on flavour variety and consumer choice (11).

The concern has been that flavouring agents will promote e-cigarette use among youth, increase nicotine dependence, and thwart the steady decline of smoking in this demographic. Additionally, the use of flavouring agents pose some immediate health concerns—for example, di acetyl (2, 3-butanedione) is a common food flavouring agent which has been shown to cause acute onset bronchiolitis obliterans, an irreversible obstructive lung disease when inhaled by workers exposed to flavouring agents containing diacetyl (12–15).

Airway Irritants and Chemical Sensitizers

Low-molecular-weight chemicals with highly reactive side chains pose an even greater risk, and are frequently identified as chemical sensitizers and airway irritants. A few examples on this list include di acetyl and acetoin (buttery flavour, camphor (minty flavour), benzaldehyde (cherry or almond flavour), cresol (leathery or medicinal flavour), and isoamyl acetate (banana flavour) (11).

Mint Flavouring Agents

Although these are the most popular among the e-cig and e-liquid users, there are reports of these causing or exacerbating respiratory conditions. Menthol is an example, though there is limited evidence on its harmful effects. However, mixed with other products, we still don't know whether menthol-based products will have harmful effects on the lungs or not (16).

DEGRADATION PRODUCTS (ALDEHYDES)

Multiple reports have suggested that aldehydes have a harmful effect. These are formed by the degradation of PG and VG by high temperatures. It is for this reason that many new e-cig devices limit the temperature to minimise formation of these harmful degradation products, which include glycidol, acetol, and acrloein. Glycidol is not only an irritant but also a tightly controlled carcinogen. Acrolein is a potent irritant and the major non-cancer hazard in tobacco smoke.

THE HUMAN HARM

There is inconsistent data about the long-term health effects of e-cigarettes, their effectiveness as smoking cessation agents, and the effect on children. This could be due to the rapid release of new devices, lack of a standard device, and the dual use of combustible cigarettes with other tobacco products including e-cigarettes, hookah, and marijuana. Many of the important outcomes related to chronic toxicity (for example, COPD) take many years to develop, so the exact effects may not be known for decades. Finally, the effect on patients with chronic lung disease may differ from those seen in young healthy people.

It is clear that e-cigarette use among young adults is a clear risk factor for future use of regular combustible cigarettes (10). Data is scant that e-cigarette use can really help in smoking cessation or that it is superior to pharmacotherapy for smoking cessation.

MATERNAL AND FETAL EFFECTS

Smoking during pregnancy is a large modifiable risk factor for pregnancy-related morbidity and mortality and is easily the most important modifiable risk factor for asthma. In fact, reports have even found lower efficacy of inhaled corticosteroids in asthmatic children of mothers exposed to smoking in pregnancy, irrespective of the current environmental tobacco exposure (17).

Smoking in pregnancy is further associated with increased risk of intrauterine growth retardation (IUGR) and this IUGR can also be a risk factor for poor lung function. It is also a risk for pre-term birth and birth complications like premature rupture of membranes. Smoking is also associated with an increased risk for viral respiratory illnesses in pregnancy.

In general, maternal smoking in pregnancy can have persistent effects on lung development, lung function, and respiratory health later in life. Reduction of environmental tobacco exposure in pregnant women has shown good success and can be associated with substantial reductions in preterm birth and reductions in hospital attendance for asthma. Caregivers of all infants and children and, in particular, those with a high risk of asthma, should be counselled on avoidance of tobacco smoke as an asthma prevention strategy. It is evident that avoiding maternal smoking during pregnancy will reduce the risk of development of asthma (17).

VAPING PRODUCT USE ASSOCIATED ACUTE LUNG INJURY (EVALI)

E-cigarette or vaping, product use associated lung injury (EVALI) was reported and detailed guidelines were released in the United States. The first case of EVALI was reported from India (18). Initial symptoms include cough, dyspnoea, pleuritic chest pain, gastrointestinal symptoms like vomiting and diarrhoea, headache, fatigue, and weight loss. Patients are often hypoxic, with fever and tachypnoea. There is often a history of use of e-cigarette (vaping) or dabbing (inhaled concentrated liquid) within the past 30 days. The CDC case definition includes vaping use within the past 90 days.

Imaging reveals diffuse bilateral infiltrates on chest X-ray, and the chest CT shows nonspecific bilateral ground-glass opacities with or without subpleural sparing. Organising pneumonia and diffuse lung nodules can also be seen. Laboratory tests should include CBC, ESR, CRP, LDH, renal and liver profiles, urinalysis and an ECG. It is essential to rule out other aetiologies by blood cultures, atypical pneumonia profiles, and HIV testing. If EVALI is suspected, urine screening for tetrahydrocannabinol (THC) is also recommended. Oxygen and respiratory support may be required. Empiric antibiotics should be administered for at least 48 hours if the history is unclear. During an influenza season, antivirals should also be considered until influenza is excluded. If the patient does not improve, systemic steroids may be considered on an individual basis. The duration of steroid use should be completely based on

the patient's course of recovery. It would be ideal to report such cases to a local poison control centre for case surveillance (19).

It is still not clear whether a specific toxin or a clear pathological mechanism explains the disease process of EVALI. While most case reports revealed the combined use of nicotine and cannabinoid containing products, there are some cases that report exclusive use of nicotine containing products alone.

Almost 90% of patients in a study with EVALI had a urine toxicology screen that was positive for THC. Interestingly, this study noted that the THC cartridges were loaded with a less viscous material than usual and did not produce the same concentration as the previous THC containing cartridges. Therefore, one hypothesis is that counterfeit, low cost, THC-containing cartridges might be contributing to the epidemic of EVALI. Often, the well-described presentations of typical exogenous lipoid pneumonia are not always seen in EVALI.

Whenever counselling patients, families, and/or the public in general, the appropriate guidance is that the use of any vaping product should be stopped. It is also very important to counsel anyone who is vaping to help quit combustible cigarette use to wean off vaping as soon as possible and avoid converting back to combustible cigarette use. It is important to remember that nicotine-based e-cigarettes are not an approved US FDA cessation approach, unlike transdermal nicotine patches that are approved and have proven benefits (19).

MANAGEMENT OF VAPING AND SMOKING IN CHILDREN

Surveys in the United States have shown that the majority of middle and high school students who use e-cigarettes report using e-liquids that contained only flavouring. However, 99% of e-liquids actually do contain nicotine. It is in this context that there is now a growing consensus that e-cigarettes increase the risk of subsequent use of cigarettes, marijuana, alcohol, and other substances. Almost one-third of adolescents who have used e-cigarettes in the past have used an e-cigarette to vape marijuana, often including high potency cannabis oils and concentrates (20).

Exposure to nicotine during adolescence can harm the developing brain, which may affect brain function and cognition, attention, and mood (21–24). Approximately 15% of patients hospitalised with EVALI were younger than 18 years of age. Interestingly, nearly 90% of adult daily smokers smoked their first cigarette by the age of 18 years (25). Another area of concern is the self-promotion of e-cigarette products through applications on social media.

Since e-cigarettes have become the primary source of nicotine exposure among youth in the span of a few years, it is important to have some kind of management algorithm to manage these children and adolescents (20).

PREVENTION AND MANAGEMENT

There is unfortunately a lack of adequately powered studies on behavioural counselling interventions and a lack of studies on medications as primary care interventions for tobacco cessation among school aged children and adolescents who already smoke. This brings up a significant challenge in the management of these children.

Behavioural counselling interventions should be considered to prevent tobacco use. This should be enclosed face-to-face counselling, telephone counselling, and computer-based and print-based interventions. The evidence here is not sufficient to recommend *for or against* providing interventions for cessation of tobacco use. This is because existing studies on behavioural interventions have been too heterogeneous and too small to detect benefits. Additionally, no medications are currently approved by the US FDA for tobacco cessation in children and adolescents. Therefore, it is best to use clinical judgement to decide how best to help these children and adolescents who use tobacco (25).

Interventions to Prevent Tobacco Use

Aged 7–10: Print-based materials predominantly

Age > 10 years: Face-to-face counselling, or telephone- and computer-based interventions

Interventions targeting parents: Largely print or telephone-based (25)

No medications are approved for preventive use so far. Varenicline is not indicated in children and adolescents below 16 years of age as efficacy has not been demonstrated. The Nicotine Replacement Therapy (NRT) trial found a greater incidence of headaches, cough, abnormal dreams, muscle pain, and related adverse events (6). Two clinical trials with bupropion sustained-release preparations did not find any significant difference in quit rates at the end of treatment. Bupropion also carries a box warning for increased risk of suicidality in children, adolescents, and young adults with other concerns for increased risk of seizure, hypertension, mania, visual problems, and unusual thoughts and behaviours (25).

Most studies reported that fewer youth initiated smoking when they received a behavioural counselling intervention (follow-up was usually at 12 months but ranged from 7 to 36 months). None of the trials reported adverse events or harms associated with behavioural counselling interventions (25).

FUTURE DIRECTIONS

Larger, well-powered studies of newer behavioural counselling interventions for cessation are needed. More studies are also needed that evaluate the benefits and harms of medications to help youth with tobacco cessation. More research is needed on prevention of initiation of use, and cessation of use of e-cigarettes in youth. A brief counselling methodology for paediatricians is to be formulated for prevention of tobacco use initiation in children and adolescents. There should be improvements in screening methods among teenagers for tobacco and nicotine use. A road map is needed on how parents, caregivers, and adolescents who use e-cigarettes can be referred to tobacco cessation counselling and approved pharmacotherapies appropriate to the level of addiction. It is important to address parent and caregiver tobacco dependence as part of the visit with the paediatrician.

CONCLUSION

The use of e-cigarettes was initially marketed as a replacement and preventive strategy for combustible cigarette smoking. However, instead they have been found to bring the reverse effect. The contents of e-cigarettes and other chemicals, including flavouring agents, have proven to be far from safe in many respects. It is clear that e-cigarette use among young adults is a clear risk factor for future use of regular combustible cigarettes. Smoking during pregnancy is a large modifiable risk factor for pregnancy-related morbidity and mortality and is also the most important modifiable risk factor for asthma. In fact, reports have even found lower efficacy of inhaled corticosteroids in asthmatic children of mothers exposed to smoking in pregnancy. Behavioural counselling interventions are found to be useful for those who are involved in vaping, as well as their caregivers.

REFERENCES

1. Zhu SH, Sharon EC, Gary JT, et al. E-cigarette use and associated changes in population smoking cessation; evidence from US current population surveys. BMJ 2017; 358:j3262.

2. Gotts JE, Sven-Eric J, McConnell R, et al. What are the respiratory effects of e-cigarettes? BMJ 2019;366:5275. doi:10.1136/bmj.l5275

3. Sleiman M, Logue JM, Montesinos VN, et al. Emissions from electronic cigarettes: key parameters affecting the release of harmful chemicals. Environ Sci Technol 2016; 50(17):9644–51.

4. Benowitz, NL, Hukkanen J, Jacob P. Nicotine chemistry, metabolism, kinetics and biomarkers. Handb Exp Pharmacol 2009; 192:29–60.

5. D'Alessandro A, Boeckelmann I, Hammwhoner M, et al. Nicotine, cigarette smoking and cardiac arrhythmia: an overview. Eur J Prev Cardiol 2012; 19(3):297–305. [PubMed: 22779085]

6. Kershbaum A, Bellet S, Dickstein ER, et al. Effect of cigarette smoking and nicotine on serum free fatty acids based on a study in the human subject and the experimental animal. Circ Res 1961; 9:631–8. [PubMed: 13752687]

7. Kershbaum A, Osada H, Pappajohn DJ, et al. Effect of nicotine on the mobilization of free fatty acids from adipose tissue in vitro. Experientia 1969; 25(2):128. [PubMed: 5786078]

8. Carlson LA, Oro L, et al. The effect of nicotine acid on the plasma free fatty acids demonstration of a metabolic type of sympathicolysis. J Intern Med 1962; 172(6):641–45.

9. Omvik P. How smoking affects blood pressure. Blood Press 1996; 5(2):71–7. [PubMed: 9162447]

10. Benowitz NL, Henningfield JE. Reducing the nicotine content to make cigarettes less addictive. Tob Control 2013; 22(suppl 1):i14–i7. [PubMed:23591498]

11. Clapp PW, Jasper. I. Electronic cigarettes: Their constituents and potential links to asthma. Curr Allergy Asthma Rep 2017; 17(11):79.

12. Kreiss K, Gomaa A, Kullman G, et al. Clinical bronchiolitis obliterans in workers at a microwave-popcorn plant. N Engl J Med 2002; 347(5):330–8. [PubMed:12151470]

13. Van Rooy FG, Rooyackers JM, Prokop M, et al. Bronchiolitis obliterans syndrome in chemical workers producing diacetly for food flavourings. Am J Respir Crit Care Med 2007; 176(5):498–504. [PubMed:17541015]

14. Barrington-Trimis JL, Samet JM, McConnell R, et al. Flavorings in electronic cigarettes: an unrecognized respiratory health hazard? JAMA 2014; 312(23):2493–4. [PubMed: 25383564]

15. Chetambath R. Popcorn lung – Report of a rare case and its significance in a coffee-growing district of Kerala. Lung India 2019; 36 (4):367–8.

16. Plevkova J, Kollarik M, Poliacek I, et al. The role of trigeminal nasal TRPM8-expressing afferent neurons in the antitussive effects of menthol. J Appl Physiol (1985) 2013; 115(2):268–74. [PubMed: 23640596.

17. Zacharasiewicz A. Maternal smoking in pregnancy and its influence on asthma. ERJ Open Res 2016; 2(3):00042. doi:10.1183/23120541.00042

18. Jankharia B, Rajan S, Angirish B. Vaping associated lung injury (EVALI) as an organizing pneumonia pattern—A case report. Lung India 2020; 37(6):533–35. doi:10.4103/lungindia.

19. Kalininskiy A, Christina TB, Nicholas EN, et al. E-cigarette, or vaping, product use associated lung injury (EVALI): case series and diagnostic approach. Lancet Respir Med 2019; 7:1017–26.

20. Chadi N, Scott EH, Sion KH. Understanding the implications of the "vaping epidemic" among adolescents and young adults: A call for action. Subst Abus 2019; 40(1):7–10. doi:10.1080/08897077.2019.1580241

21. US Preventive Services Task Force. Primary care interventions for prevention and cessation of tobacco use in children and adolescents. JAMA 2020; 323(16):1590–1598. doi:10.1001/jama.2020.467

22. US Department of Health and Human Services. The health consequences of smoking: 50 years of progress: A Report of surgeon general. US Department of Health and Human services, centres for disease control and prevention, National center for chronic Disease prevention and health promotion, Office of smoking on Health, 2014.

23. US Department of Health and Human Services. E-cCigarettes Use among youth and young Adults: A Report of the surgeon general. Office of the Surgeon General, 2016.

24. Goriounova NA, Mansvelder HD. Short- and long-term consequences of nicotine exposure during adolescence for prefrontal cortex neuronsl network function. Cold Spring Harb Perspect Med 2012; 2(12):a012120. doi:10.1101/chsperspect.a012120

25. Musso F, Bettermann F, Vucurevic G, et al. Smoking impacts on prefrontal attentional network function in young adult brain. Psychopharmacology (Berl) 2007; 191(1):159–169. doi:10.1007/s00213-006-0499-8

15 Clinical Presentation of Asthma in Adolescents and Young Adults

Rajesh Swarnakar

CONTENTS

INTRODUCTION

Asthma is a heterogeneous disorder, and age of onset plays a vital role. Asthma is seen in patients across all age groups and has been observed to begin right from childhood. There is in fact a considerable database of studies documenting the origins of allergic asthma starting in childhood. Young adults (18–25 years) are a unique set of patients who have often progressed from childhood asthma to asthma persisting into young adulthood. Asthma is a common chronic condition among young adults. The 2020 Global Initiative for Asthma guidelines state that the underdiagnosis of asthma may be occurring in about 50% of adolescents and young adults in low and middle-income countries (1).

There is a paucity of studies on the risk factors, predictors of successful treatment outcomes, and the impact of asthma on quality of life in young adults. Asthma can have far-reaching consequences for young adults, due to attitudes towards the disease itself,

treatment acceptance, and readiness to accept some limitations in choice of activities in daily life. Understanding risk factors, leading to the development of asthma in young adults and adopting a proactive approach to the problems faced by this set of patients will help improve treatment acceptance, and therefore, also the outcomes of treatment.

RISK FACTORS FOR THE DEVELOPMENT OF ASTHMA IN YOUNG ADULTS

Asthma and allergic rhinitis have been observed in several longitudinal studies to often coexist, especially among the younger generation, but there have been few studies focusing on young adults (2). Allergic rhinitis and asthma-like symptoms are considered to be strong and independent predictors of adult-onset asthma, with a higher association among women in recent generations (3). Several clinical trials have proven that earlier treatment of allergic rhinitis symptoms with immunotherapy, pharmacological therapy, and allergen

DOI: 10.1201/9781003125785-15

Table 15.1: Risk Factors for the Development of Asthma in Young Adults

- Female gender
- Obesity or long-standing elevated body mass index (BMI) since childhood
- Allergic rhinitis
- Persistent wheezing in childhood
- Nocturnal dyspnoea and tightness
- Exposure to cigarette smoke in childhood
- Exposure to moulds and damp living
- Atopy on skin testing, with positive skin tests to Cladosporium, house dust mite, cat and rye grass pollen in childhood
- Maternal asthma
- Hay fever
- Early respiratory infection
- Occupational exposure
- Reduced lung function in early infancy

avoidance may modify the natural evolution of asthma and prevent the development of the more severe form of the disease (4) (Table 15.1).

Almost 3–5% of people who wheeze in childhood continue to wheeze as adults, and this was demonstrated in the Tucson Children's Respiratory Study (5). The results of this study indicated that persistent wheezing in childhood might most likely persist into early adulthood, and that airway hyperresponsiveness at 6 years of age is often predictive of the presence of asthma at 22 years (5). Some researchers have demonstrated that persistent asthma in adulthood had associations with the persistence of airway hyperresponsiveness, atopy, and lower lung function in childhood by the age of 13 (6,7,8).

Studies have demonstrated that symptoms such as diurnal wheezing and nocturnal dyspnoea and chest tightness are the most influential independent predictors of the incidence of asthma (4). Often, in young adults, mild symptoms of wheezing and nocturnal dyspnoea and tightness are disregarded or treated trivially by the patient and are probably not recognised as asthma. Subsequently, after daily symptoms for several years, the diagnosis of asthma is made only when the symptoms and the disease have become worse with frequent exacerbations (4).

Contradictory results have been reported in different studies regarding the risk of smoking and the development of asthma in young adults. A subset of researchers believes that active smoking is not associated with an increase in the risk of asthma in adults, probably due to the fact that susceptible people do not start smoking or quit smoking very quickly. But some longitudinal studies on adolescents found an association between active smoking and the high incidence of

asthma (9). Exposure to parental smoking during childhood was significantly associated with physician-reported asthma in young adults (10). Current smokers were 1.7 times more likely to have current asthma (11).

Exposure to moulds and damp living was also associated with asthma in young adults (10). A serious respiratory infection before 5 years of age caused a 2.3-fold increased risk of asthma. Atopy on skin testing, with positive skin tests to Cladosporium, house dust mites, cats, and rye grass pollen had as strong positive association with the development of asthma in young adults. Other risk factors for development of asthma in young adults include female gender, maternal asthma, hay fever, early respiratory infection, occupational exposure, and atopy (11). The prevalence of probable IgE-mediated food reactions is rare in young adults (12).

Reduced lung function in early infancy is considered predictive of persistent asthma in young adults. Researchers consider that a persistent reduction in lung function is indicative of abnormal lung development during growth in utero or very early in life (13).

Obesity or long-standing elevated body mass index (BMI) since childhood is considered a risk factor for the development of asthma in young adults. Children who are overweight at 6–8 years of age and continue to be overweight at 18 years of age have higher rates of asthma compared with their counterparts who are not overweight at 6–8 years but overweight at 18 years. Longitudinal studies have proven this association of obesity in childhood with adult asthma particularly among males (14) (Table 15.1).

PRESENTING FEATURES OF ASTHMA IN YOUNG ADULTS

The common presenting complaints in young adults with asthma include nasal allergies (41%), nocturnal cough (28.6%), nocturnal chest tightness, dyspnoea and wheeze (28.1%) (11). Young adults with asthma usually have persistent symptoms.

Young adults with asthma, and especially those with coexisting allergic rhinitis, experience a significantly greater incidence of cold temperature-related respiratory symptoms as compared to their healthy young adult counterparts. Hence, young adults with a respiratory disease, form a susceptible subset who require special care and guidance for coping with cold weather (15).

Sleep disturbances have been reported in a high proportion of young adults with asthma (more than 90%). The sleep diaries maintained by these patients in clinical studies have

Table 15.2: Clinical Phenotypes of Asthma in Young Adults

Adult-onset mild asthma	• Female preponderance • No significant history of smoking • High incidence of atopy • Body mass index (BMI) is often low • This milder asthma phenotype may typify transient cases of adult-onset asthma • Can have a milder clinical course and prognosis
Adult-onset obese female preponderant asthma	• Predominantly seen in female patients with a higher BMI • Less atopy • A high symptom expression, in the absence of eosinophilic airway inflammation • In spite of the short duration of asthma, these patients have decreased lung function, report to have taken complicated medical regimens and regular systemic corticosteroids • The patients' symptoms and healthcare utilisation appear to be disproportionate to their degree of airflow obstruction. • The primary treatment should consist of weight reduction, rather than stepping up anti-inflammatory treatment
Adult-onset nonatopic, inflammation-predominant phenotype with fixed airflow limitation	• The most severe adult-onset asthma phenotype • Chiefly seen in males with few daily symptoms and active eosinophilic airway inflammation • Persistent sputum eosinophilia, the key characteristics of this phenotype • Frequent asthma exacerbations, persistent airflow limitation and oral corticosteroid dependence • This phenotype is associated with chronic rhinosinusitis, nasal polyps and aspirin sensitivity • Have more air trapping and reduced diffusion capacity, suggestive of more peripheral airway inflammation • Drugs that inhibit recruitment and activation of eosinophilis might be effective • Anti-interleukin (IL)-5 therapy may be effective
Smoking-related asthma	• Male patients • High percentage of patients have no atopy • Have a relatively well preserved FEV_1

effectively proven this sleep disturbance. Shorter duration of sleep, daytime sleepiness, tiredness, and difficulty in maintaining sleep, along with early morning awakening have been reported by young adults with asthma. This sleep deprivation results in impaired educational and work performance and poor quality of life (16).

Young adults with long-term, controlled asthma have been observed to have dental caries, more gingival inflammation, and a lower stimulated salivary secretion rate as compared to young adults without asthma (17).

PHENOTYPES OF ADULT-ONSET ASTHMA

The identification of specific, clinically well-recognised adult-onset asthma phenotypes by cluster analysis is the first step to better understand the mechanisms of asthma development in adulthood (18) (Table 15.2).

DIAGNOSIS OF ASTHMA

A history of variable respiratory symptoms and evidence of variable expiratory flow limitation will help in the diagnosis of asthma (Table 15.3).

ISSUES IN YOUNG ADULTS WITH ASTHMA

Young adults with asthma present a unique set of dilemmas to the clinician. Young adults are at greater risk of denying symptoms, being careless about dangerous inhalation exposure,

pollution exposure, and the exacerbating effects of cigarette smoke.

Anxiety sensitivity in this population leads to more problematic asthma symptoms and greater functional limitations. Anxiety

Table 15.3: Making the Diagnosis of Asthma

History of variable respiratory symptoms

• Typical symptoms of asthma include wheeze, shortness of breath
• Symptoms vary over time and vary in intensity
• Symptoms occur or are worse at night or on awakening
• Symptoms are triggered by exercise, laughter, cold air, allergens
• Symptoms occur or worsen with viral infections
• Ask about occupational exposure. Do the symptoms get relieved when away from the workplace?
• Ask about hobbies to identify triggers

Evidence of variable expiratory airflow limitation

• Document at least once that the FEV_1/FVC ratio is below the lower limit of normal
• Document that the variation in lung function is greater than that in healthy people
• Testing may need to be repeated during symptoms, in the early morning, or after withholding bronchodilator medications
• Significant bronchodilator reversibility may be absent during severe exacerbations or viral infections

sensitivity has been postulated to foster a greater reactivity to asthma-related physical sensations. Individuals with asthma who are anxious about physiological arousal are a particularly 'at-risk' population for poor asthma outcomes owing to the greater reactivity and could benefit from interventions addressing this anxiety sensitivity (19).

Poor adherence to asthma treatment in young adults results in decreased asthma control and increased number of acute healthcare visits. Uncontrolled asthma was associated with factors such as smoking, use of periodic reliever treatment on most days, and acute healthcare visits (20). The personality trait Negative Affectivity and perceived asthma control have been observed to play a role in the nonadherence to prescribed medications in young adults (21).

IMPACT OF ASTHMA IN YOUNG ADULTS

Asthma may impact the choice of work in some young adults. Over the past decade, there has been a greater appreciation of the importance of occupational asthma and recently, the frequency of work-exacerbated asthma (WEA) has also been recognised. The term 'work-related asthma' (WRA) encompasses both occupational asthma and WEA. Young adults with asthma may need to be advised and counselled about WRA and their career choices before they begin their training.

Career choices are made in young adulthood, and these choices will most likely shape their future. Young adults with asthma must be made aware that there is a risk of asthma worsening if they have exposure to workplace respiratory irritant agents, and there is a probability of development of sensitization to workplace agents that might require long-term alterations in medical management and/or workplace changes. However, few young adults talk or seek counselling from their treating physician about career choices and asthma. This is an area of asthma care that needs to be addressed in young adults with asthma (22).

There is a paucity of studies on the impact of asthma on quality of life in young adults: since most of the studies about quality of life have been carried out in older or much younger populations. The personality of the patient can have a significant influence on how the young adult with asthma will deal with his asthma and a long-term medication protocol and will have a definite impact on the health related quality of life (HRQL). A gender difference has been observed in the impact of asthma on

HRQL. Females may have a greater decrease in asthma-related quality of life as compared to males. Asthmatic females score lower in the physical dimension aspect of HRQL measures. An association has been observed between low FEV_1 and a decline in quality of life in young adults with asthma, i.e. low FEV_1 predicts a decrease in quality of life over a 5-year period, especially in females (23).

TREATMENT PRINCIPLES
Environmental Control

Regular cleaning and dusting of the homes is recommended. Active smoking and exposure to passive smoke must be avoided. Measures to avoid dust mites include use of impervious covers on mattresses or pillows, washing the beddings in hot water, removing carpets from the rooms, reducing the use of upholstered furniture, reducing the number of window blinds, and putting clothing away in closets and drawers. Other measures include minimising the number of soft toys, and washing them weekly or periodically putting them in the freezer. Decreasing room humidity (<50%) can be also helpful.

Animals

The small size (1–20 μm) of dander, saliva, urine, or serum proteins of cats and other animals, makes allergens airborne. Removing animals at least from the bedroom, and washing cats and dogs as often as twice weekly is recommended.

Cockroaches and Moulds

For cockroaches avoidance, use cockroach poison baits and traps, keep food out of the bedroom, and never leave food out in the open.

For indoor moulds (size 1–150 μm), avoidance includes keeping areas dry (e.g., remove carpets from wet floors), removing old wallpaper, cleaning with bleach products, and storing firewood.

Pollen

Pollen (size 1–150 μm) avoidance is difficult or impossible, but reducing exposure can be achieved by closing windows and doors, using air conditioning and high-efficiency particulate air filters in the car and home.

Medical Care

The goal of asthma treatment is to prevent symptoms, minimise morbidity from acute episodes, prevent functional and psychological morbidity, and reduce limitation of lifestyle.

Table 15.4: Treatment Recommendation for Adolescents and Adults (12 years and above) as Adapted from the GINA 2020 Treatment Strategy

Options	Step 1	Step 2	Step 3	Step 4	Step 5
Preferred controller to prevent exacerbations and control symptoms	As needed basis low-dose ICS-formoterol[a]	Daily low-dose inhaled corticosteroid (ICS) or as needed low dose ICS-formoterol[a]	Low dose ICS-LABA	Medium dose ICS-LABA	High-dose ICS-LABA; refer for phenotyping ± add-on therapy, e.g. tiotropium, anti-IgE, anti-IL5/5R; anti-IL-4R
Other controller options	Low-dose ICS whenever SABA is taken[b]	Daily leukotriene receptor antagonist (LTRA), or low dose ICS whenever SABA is taken[b]	Medium-dose ICS or low-dose ICS+ LTRA[d]	High-dose ICS, add-on tiotropium or add-on LTRA[d]	Add low-dose OCS, but consider side effects
Preferred reliever	As-needed low-dose ICS-formoterol[a]	As-needed low-dose ICS-formoterol[a]	As-needed low-dose ICS-formoterol for patients prescribed maintenance and reliever therapy[c]	As-needed low-dose ICS-formoterol for patients prescribed maintenance and reliever therapy[c]	As-needed low-dose ICS-formoterol for patients prescribed maintenance and reliever therapy[c]
Other reliever options	As-needed SABA	As-needed SABA	As-needed SABA	As-needed SABA	As-needed SABA

Abbreviations: SABA, short-acting beta-2 agonist; ICS, inhaled corticosteroid; LTRA, leukotriene receptor antagonist; LABA, long-acting beta agonists; HDM SLIT, house dust mite (HDM) sublingual immunotherapy (SLIT) tablet; FEV_1, forced expiratory volume in 1 second.

[a] Data available only with budesonide-formoterol (bud-form).
[b] Separate or combination ICS and SABA inhalers.
[c] Low dose ICS-form is the reliever only for patients prescribed bud-form or BDP-form maintenance and reliever therapy.
[d] Consider adding HDM SLIT for sensitised patients with allergic rhinitis and $FEV_1 > 70\%$ predicted.

Both acute asthmatic episodes and control of chronic symptoms, including nocturnal and exercise-induced asthmatic symptoms, are encompassed in medical care. Pharmacologic management includes the use of controller drugs such as inhaled corticosteroids, long-acting bronchodilators (beta-agonists and anticholinergics), theophylline, leukotriene modifiers, and the use of anti-immunoglobulin E (IgE) antibodies (omalizumab), anti–IL5 antibodies, and anti–IL4/IL13 antibodies in some selected patients. Relief medications include short-acting bronchodilators, systemic corticosteroids, and ipratropium.

In all patients, quick-relief medications such as rapid-acting beta-2 agonists are recommended on an as needed basis for symptoms. The severity of symptoms determines the intensity of treatment. In case the patient has to use rapid-acting beta-2 agonists more than 2 days a week for symptom relief, step up of treatment may be considered. The preferred controller medication of choice for children and adults are inhaled corticosteroids. After initiation of treatment, patients should be assessed every 1–6 months for asthma control. At every visit, adherence, environmental control, and comorbid conditions must be evaluated. When the patient has good control of their asthma for at least 3 months, treatment step down may be considered but the patient must be reassessed in 2–4 weeks to ensure that control is maintained with the new treatment.

In young adults, treatment guided by fractional concentration of exhaled nitric oxide was associated with a significant reduction in the number of patients with ≥1 exacerbations (1). The step-care approach suggested by the Global Initiative for Asthma (GINA) guidelines must be adopted to manage asthma in young adults (Table 15.4).

ASSESSMENT OF A PATIENT WITH ASTHMA

Assess Symptom Control

■ Asses symptom control over the last 4 weeks

■ Identify any modifiable risk factors for poor outcomes

■ Measure lung function before starting treatment, 3–6 months later, and then periodically at least every year

Comorbid Conditions

- Allergic rhinitis, gastroesophageal reflux disease, obesity, obstructive sleep apnoea, depression, diabetes, and anxiety

Treatment Adherence

- Ask about side effects
- Watch the patient using the inhaler—check the technique
- Have an empathetic discussion about adherence
- Check the written action plan of the patient
- Ask the patient about their goals and preferences about treatment

Risk Factors for Poor Asthma Control

Assess the risk factors at diagnosis and periodically every 1–2 years in patients with exacerbations.

- Uncontrolled asthma symptoms present
  - Medications: Inhaled corticosteroids (ICS) not prescribed; incorrect inhaler technique; high short-acting beta-2 agonist (SABA) use (mortality increases if >1 × 200 dose canister/month is used)
- Comorbidities: obesity, chronic rhinosinusitis, GERD, confirmed food allergy, anxiety, depression, allergen exposure if sensitised, air pollution (Table 15.5)
- Setting: Major socioeconomic problems
- Lung function: low FEV_1, especially if <60% predicted; high reversibility
- Other tests: Sputum/blood eosinophilia, elevated FeNO in allergic adults on ICS

Other Major Independent Risk Factors for Exacerbations

Ever been intubated or intensive care for asthma required; having ≥1 severe exacerbations in the last 12 months.

Table 15.5: Treatment of Comorbid Illnesses

Comorbid Disease	Treatment
GERD	Treatment with proton pump inhibitors, antacids, or H2 blockers may improve asthma symptoms or unexplained chronic cough.
Sinusitis	Treatment of acute sinusitis requires at least 10 days of antibiotics to improve asthma symptoms.

Risk Factors for Developing Fixed Airflow Limitation

- Preterm birth, low birth weight, greater infant weight gain
- Lack of ICS treatment
- Exposures to tobacco smoke, noxious chemicals, occupational experience
- Low FEV_1
- Chronic mucus hypersecretion
- Sputum or blood eosinophilia

Risk Factors for Medication Side Effects

- Systemic: frequent oral corticosteroids, high dose and or potent ICS, also taking CYP450 inhibitors
- Local: High-dose or potent ICS; poor inhaler technique

MONOCLONAL ANTIBODY THERAPY

Monoclonal antibodies such as omalizumab are indicated for adults and children aged 6 years or older with moderate-to-severe persistent asthma who have a positive skin test result or in vitro reactivity to a perennial aeroallergen and whose symptoms are inadequately controlled with inhaled corticosteroids. Patients should have IgE levels between 30 and 700 IU and must not weigh more than 150 kg. In the age group of 6–12 years IgE of up to 1300 may be acceptable. Omalizumab is a humanised murine IgG antibody against the Fc component of the IgE antibody, which prevents IgE from binding directly to the mast cell receptor, thus preventing cell degranulation without causing degranulation itself. It decreases free IgE antibody levels by 99% and cell receptor sites for IgE antibody by 97%. This results in a reduced histamine production (90%), reduced early phase bronchospasm (40%), and reduction of late-phase bronchospasm (70%), as well as a decrease in the number, migration, and activity of eosinophils. Levels drop quickly and remain low for at least a month. It is also effective for allergic rhinitis. Other monoclonal antibodies developed include IgG kappa monoclonal antibodies that inhibits IL-5 such as mepolizumab, reslizumab and benralizumab (24,25).

DETERMINANTS OF OUTCOMES OF TREATMENT

In prospective, randomised clinical trials, pulmonary function below predicted, severity of disease expressed by asthma score and use of ICS and/or long-acting beta agonists (LABA) have been observed to be determinants for persistent early onset asthma. Use of ICS and/or LABA was observed to be a determinant in late-onset asthma. A high asthma score was indicative of insufficient disease control in a substantial proportion of these patients (26).

APPROACH TO MANAGEMENT OF ASTHMA IN YOUNG ADULTS

- Use spirometry to assess lung function objectively and to confirm the diagnosis, even if the person had asthma during childhood

- Consider objective tests (e.g. exercise testing, bronchial provocation (challenge tests) or referral to investigate the possibility of non-asthma causes such as dyspnoea due to poor cardiopulmonary fitness, hyperventilation, or upper airway obstruction

- Ask about smoking and exposure to other people's tobacco smoke

- In females, consider whether asthma symptoms are affected by the menstrual cycle

PROGNOSTIC FEATURES

Adult onset asthma has been observed to have a poorer prognosis and poorer response to treatment as compared to childhood onset asthma (27).

The presence of asthma attacks and nocturnal asthma symptoms such as tightness and dyspnoea in young adults results in a two fold increase in the risk of dying in the subsequent 7 years, as compared to asymptomatic patients. The presence of asthma attacks and/or nocturnal asthma symptoms is associated with an increased overall mortality risk.

Young adult asthmatics have a five to six fold greater risk of dying from accidents than the general population, especially those patients who have a history of asthma attacks and nocturnal symptoms which make them even more susceptible to this hazard. Interference with diurnal attentiveness could cause fatal occupational accidents, as well as car accidents. Moreover, since these patients have high rates of anxiety disorders and major depression they may be more prone to accidents. Often, asthmatic patients also take antihistaminic drugs for their symptoms, and the sedative effects of these drugs could further alter their diurnal concentration, resulting in accidents (4).

CONCLUSION

Young adults are a unique set of patients who have often progressed from childhood asthma to asthma that has persisted in young adulthood. The underdiagnosis of asthma may be reduced by increasing patient awareness and counselling. Counselling of young adults can alter the patient's own attitude to asthma, impact treatment acceptance and adherence, as well as the readiness to accept some limitations in choice of activities in daily life. Treatment of asthma based on guideline recommendations and improving adherence to treatment can improve outcomes in this population of young adults with asthma.

REFERENCES

1. https://ginasthma.org/wp-content/uploads/2020/04/Main-pocket-guide_2020_04_03-final-wms.pdf

2. Kimura H, Konno S, Isada A, Maeda Y, Musashi M, Nishimura M. Contrasting associations of body mass index and measles with asthma and rhinitis in young adults Allergy Asthma Proc 2015; 36(4):293–9.

3. Passalacqua G, Ciprandi G, Canonica GW. United airways disease: therapeutic aspects. Thorax 2000; 55(Suppl 2):26–7.

4. deMarco R, Locatelli F, Cazzoletti L, et al. Incidence of asthma and mortality in a cohort of young adults: a 7-year prospective study. Respir Res 2005; 6:95. https://doi.org/10.1186/1465-9921-6-95

5. Stern DA, Morgan WJ, Halonen M, Wright AL. Wheezing and bronchial hyper-responsiveness in early childhood as predictors of newly diagnosed asthma in early adulthood: a longitudinal birth-cohort study. Lancet 2008; 372:1058–64. doi:10.1016/S0140-6736(08)61447-6

6. Sears MR, Greene JM, Willan AR, Wiecek EM, Taylor DR, Flannery EM, et al. A longitudinal, population-based, cohort study of childhood asthma followed to adulthood. N Engl J Med 2003; 349:1414–22. doi:10.1056/NEJMoa022363

7. Tai A, Tran H, Roberts M, Clarke N, Gibson AM, Vidmar S, et al. Outcomes of childhood asthma to the age of 50 years. J Allergy Clin Immunol 2014; 133:1572–8 e3. doi:10.1016/j.jaci.2013.12.1033

8. Andersson M, Hedman L, Bjerg A, Forsberg B, Lundback B, Ronmark E. Remission and persistence of asthma followed from 7 to 19 years of age. Pediatrics 2013; 132:e435–42. doi:10.1542/peds.2013-0741

9. Larsson L. Incidence of asthma in Swedish teenagers: relation to sex and smoking habits. Thorax 1995; 50:260–4.

10. Hu FB, Persky V, Flay BR, Richardson J. An epidemiological study of asthma prevalence and related factors among young adults. J Asthma 1997;34(1):67–76.

11. Abramson M, Kutin JJ, Raven J, Lanigan A, Czarny D, Walters EH. Risk factors for asthma among young adults in Melbourne, Australia. Respirology 1996;1(4):291–7.

12. Woods RK, Thien F, Raven J, Haydn Walters, E, Abramson M. Prevalence of food allergies in young adults and their relationship to asthma, nasal allergies, and eczema Ann Allergy Asthma Immunol 2002;88(2):183–9.

13. Owens L, Laing IA, Zhang G, Le Souëf PN. Infant lung function predicts asthma persistence and remission in young adults. Respirology 2017;22(2):289–294.

14. Porter M, Wegienka G, Havstad S, et al. Relationship between childhood body mass index and young adult asthma. Ann Allergy Asthma Immunol. 2012 Dec; 109(6): 408–11.e1.

15. Hyrkäs H, Jaakkola MS, Ikäheimo TM, Hugg TT, Jaakkola JJK. Asthma and allergic rhinitis increase respiratory symptoms in cold weather among young adults. Respir Med 2014 Jan; 108(1):63–70.

16. Molzon ES, Bonner MS, Hullmann SE, et al. Differences in sleep quality and health-related quality of life in young adults with allergies and asthma and their healthy peers. J Am Coll Health 2013; 61(8):484–9.

17. Stensson M, Wendt L-K, Koch G, Oldaeus G, Ramberg P, Birkhed D. Oral health in young adults with long-term, controlled asthma. Acta Odontol Scand 2011 May; 69(3):158–64. doi:doi.org/10.3109/00016357.2010.547516

18. de Nijs SB, Venekamp LN, Bel EH. Adult-onset asthma: is it really different? Eur Respir Rev 2013; 22:44–5.

19. McLeish AC, Luberto CM, O'Bryan EM. Anxiety sensitivity and reactivity to asthma-like sensations among young adults with asthma. Behav Modif 2016; 40(1-2):164–77.

20. Selberg S, Hedman L, Jansson S-A, Backman H. Stridsman C. Asthma control and acute healthcare visits among young adults with asthma-A population-based study. J Adv Nurs 2019 Dec; 75(12):3525–3534.

21. Axelsson M. Personality and reasons for not using asthma medication in young adults. Heart Lung 2013; 42(4):241–6.

22. Bhinder S, Cicutto L, Abdel-Qadir HM, Tarlo SM. Perception of asthma as a factor in career choice among young adults with asthma. Can Respir J 2009; 16 (6):e69–e75

23. Sundberg R, Palmqvist M, Tunsäter A, Torén, K. Health-related quality of life in young adults with asthma. Respir Med 2009; 103:1580–5.

24. Wechsler ME, Laviolette M, Rubin AS, Fiterman J, Lapa E, Silva JR, Shah PL, et al. Bronchial thermoplasty: long-term safety and effectiveness in patients with severe persistent asthma. J Allergy Clin Immunol 2013 Dec; 132(6):1295–302.

25. Boggs W. Bronchial Thermoplasty Effective for Severe Persistent Asthma. Available at http://www.medscape.com/viewarticle/811113. Accessed: September 30, 2013.

26. Krogh Traulsen L, Halling A, Bælum J, Rømhild Davidsen J, Miller M, Omland O, et al. Determinants of persistent asthma in young adults. Eur Clin Respir J 2018; 5(1):1478593.

27. Lindsay Withers A, Green R. Transition for adolescents and young adults with asthma. Front Pediatr 2019; 7:301.

16 Diagnosis of Asthma

George A D'Souza

CONTENTS

INTRODUCTION

Asthma is one of the most common non-communicable respiratory diseases affecting people of all ages across the globe. Over 300 million people are affected worldwide with approximately 4.3% of adults reporting physician-diagnosed asthma. In children, the prevalence is high but varies widely (1,2). It is both an overdiagnosed (33%) and underdiagnosed condition (19–73%). This is because of its heterogeneity at the time of presentation. Both underdiagnosis and overdiagnosis have tremendous socioeconomic costs and potential to expose patients to unwanted drug side effects. It may also result in delay in reaching an alternate diagnosis (3,4). The heterogeneity at presentation and the inadequate use of tools to establish the diagnosis has resulted in this state. Hence it is important to establish asthma diagnosis as accurately as possible (5).

BASIS OF DIAGNOSING ASTHMA

The basis of the diagnosis of asthma rests in the definition: Asthma is a heterogenous disease, usually characterized by chronic inflammation. It is defined by the history of respiratory symptoms such as wheeze, shortness of breath, tightness of chest and cough, that vary over time and in intensity, together with variable expiratory airflow limitation (6). Based on this definition, the diagnosis of asthma hinges on the presence of respiratory symptoms suggestive of asthma, demonstration of airflow limitation, and demonstration of variable airflow with or without treatment. Evidence of airway inflammation will substantiate the diagnosis and may also help in management. It is imperative that a positive diagnosis of asthma be made at some stage in the course of a patient's illness, preferably early on, to avoid

significant overdiagnosis and underdiagnosis with its attendant consequences. Further, it is useful to revisit the diagnosis in very stable patients so as to be able to scale down or stop the treatment while continuing to monitor (4,5).

The symptoms of asthma are cough, chest tightness, wheeze and shortness of breath, which often disturb sleep (7). As can be seen, these symptoms are present in many other respiratory illnesses and even in cardiac illness (Table 16.1). The characteristics of these symptoms are their variability with or without treatment. Asthma is often precipitated by characteristic triggers like allergens, irritants, exercise, cold air, climate change, and infections, particularly viral ones. It can be present only in the day (38.8%) or in the night (32.3%), or both (6,7).

Cough in asthma is usually not productive or productive of minimal mucoid expectoration. During an exacerbation, tenacious sputum and even mucous plugs may be expectorated. Cough tends to be present more towards the night or early morning. Rarely, the cough presents as the lone symptom and is called cough variant asthma. This presentation is more often in children. In adults, other causes of cough should be ruled out when cough is the only symptom (6).

Wheeze (49.7%), breathlessness (50.31%), or chest tightness (50.41%) are the more important symptoms. Most often (71.26%) they are not isolated but appear together (Table 16.2). Associated nasal stuffiness (61%) and associated history suggestive of atopy are common. Disturbance in sleep is seen in over half the asthmatics (7). Features that are against the diagnosis of asthma are significant and chronic sputum production, dyspnoea with noisy inspiration during exertion, chest pain and breathlessness with lightness of head and tingling of peripheries (6).

DOI: 10.1201/9781003125785-16

Table 16.1: Differential Diagnosis of Asthma

Children

Inhaled foreign particle
Inducible laryngeal obstruction
Ciliary dyskinesia
Chronic upper airway cough syndrome
Bronchiectasis
Cystic fibrosis
Bronchopulmonary dysplasia
Congenital heart disease

Adults

Inhaled foreign particle
Vocal cord dysfunction (VCD)
Bronchiectasis
Chronic obstructive pulmonary disease (COPD)
Heart failure
Chronic pulmonary hypertension
Chronic pulmonary thromboembolism
Gastroesophageal reflux disease
Habitual cough

Associated history of atopy (allergic rhinitis or eczema) or family history helps strengthen the possibility of the symptoms being due to asthma. Family history is most useful, particularly in those less than 27 years of age and the association is highest when both parents are asthmatic (8). The presence of association with known triggers increases the probability of the patient having asthma. In children, symptoms when the child does not have a cold or respiratory infection, or a definite association with triggers increases the probability of the child having asthma (9). Common triggers are allergens (e.g. dust mites, animal dander, pollen, cockroach droppings, etc.), irritants like air pollution and tobacco smoke, exercise and emotions, weather (including cold air and humidity), viral and bacterial infections, medicines like NSAIDs, and acid reflux. The next step in the diagnosis of asthma is to demonstrate airway obstruction and variability of airflow.

Table 16.2: Common Symptoms in Asthma and Their Frequency

Symptoms	Frequency (%)
Cough	39.3
Wheezing	46.9
Breathlessness	50.3
Chest tightness	50.4
Nasal congestion	61.5
Sleep disturbance	56.5

DEMONSTRATION OF AIRFLOW OBSTRUCTION

Spirometry is the investigation of choice to demonstrate obstruction to airflow. A reduced FEV_1 (forced expiratory volume in the 1st second) along with a reduced FEV_1/FVC (forced vital capacity) ratio is used to demonstrate obstruction (6). In normal adults, the ratio of FEV_1/FVC is 0 .75–0.8 and >0.9 in children. For practical purposes, a ratio <0.7 is considered as obstruction. But one must be aware that this may lead to an over diagnosis of obstruction in elderly as the ratio falls with age. On the flip side, in the young it may be underdiagnosed. Hence, some guidelines have suggested to use lower limits of normal (LLN), i.e. less than the lowest 5% of the population, to avoid this pitfall (10).

DEMONSTRATION OF REVERSIBLE AIRFLOW

Airflow reversibility is demonstrated by showing variable airflow at different time points or reversible airflow with treatment. Variability in FEV_1 or peak expiratory flow rate (PEFR) is used to demonstrate variability. A peak flow metre is a portable device that is not expensive and hence is useful both for diagnosis and monitoring. It is also a good tool in resource limited settings.

The most convenient way to demonstrate reversibility is to do FEV_1 or PEFR before and after inhalation of a bronchodilator at the time of a clinical visit. If done at the time of spirometry, both airway obstruction and reversibility can be demonstrated in one sitting. The spirometry is done before and 10–15 minutes after inhalation of a beta-2 agonist (usually 200–400 micrograms of salbutamol). A 12% increase in FEV_1 and an absolute increase of 200 ml are consistent with reversible airway disease. A change by 400 ml is definitive of a diagnosis of asthma. If PEFR is being used, the improvement should be 20%. The test should be done at least 4 hours after taking a short-acting beta-2 agonist and at least 15 hours after taking a long-acting beta-2 agonist.

The other method of demonstrating variability is to measure lung function over a period of time and demonstrate variability. The first reading is best taken in the clinic so as to make sure the patient understands how to use it. Recordings are made of the peak expiratory rate over 7–14 days. The daily variability (maximum minus minimum divided by maximum) averaged by the number of days of recording gives the average airflow variability. An average variability >10% in adults and >13% in children is consistent with a diagnosis of asthma (6).

Similarly, variability in FEV_1 of 12% and 200 ml between different visits is also consistent with reversible airflow. Reversibility after treatment with inhaled/oral steroids is also adequate to confirm asthma.

Often a patient who is already on treatment at the time of evaluation, the spirometry is normal. In such circumstances repeated measurements may be useful to demonstrate obstruction and variability. If the patient is asymptomatic and on treatment a gradual reduction in the dose of inhaled corticosteroids should be done. It is also important that the diagnosis of asthma be based on good spirometry manoeuvres which are reproducible. But in all patients an objective diagnosis of asthma should be established.

In patients where it has not been possible to establish the diagnosis of asthma, and where the probability of asthma is significant, demonstrating airway hyper reactivity may be the option (6). This is done by doing a bronchial provocative test (BPT).

BRONCHIAL PROVOCATION TESTING

This test is to be done when confronted with a high suspicion of asthma, but the spirometry is normal. It is also useful when evaluating cough variant asthma. The principle is to provoke bronchial constriction either by non-pharmacological means or by the inhalation of provocative agents and measuring the change in FEV_1 or PEFR. An exaggerated response as compared to normal is considered positive and suggestive of asthma. The sensitivity is high, but the specificity and positive predictive value are low.

The non-pharmacological agents are exercise and eucapnic hyperventilation. They act by causing the release of endogenous mediators that trigger airway smooth muscle contraction (11). A fall in FEV_1 of 10% and 200ml in adults and a fall of 12–15% in children is considered positive. There are many limitations to using exercise test as a routine. There is a need for exercise testing equipment which is not available in most centres. In addition, there are many variables including type of exercise protocol, prior exposure to drugs or allergens and the like which can affect the results. Last but not least, there is a significant variability (up to 50%) in the test making it necessary to repeat the test if it is negative. Eucapnic hyperventilation is the other non-pharmacological stimulus that can be used. Here, the patient achieves target ventilation over 6 minutes (usually 21–30 times the FEV_1) and the FEV_1 measured over the next 5 minutes. A fall >10% and sustained over 2 readings is considered diagnostic. This again is difficult to do as the baseline FEV_1 should be >1.5 l, and the CO_2 needs to be monitored and maintained over a wide range of ventilation. These tests are particularly useful when evaluating patients with symptoms only of exercise-induced asthma (EIA).

Pharmacologic agents used for BPT can be directly acting agents like histamine or methacholine or indirectly acting agent like hypertonic saline or mannitol. The latter acts by inducing the release of endogenous mediators of bronchoconstriction. A fall in FEV_1 of 20% with the inhalation of a concentration of <4 mg/ml of methacholine or histamine is considered positive. With mannitol or hypertonic saline, a fall of 15% is considered positive (11).

FRACTIONAL EXHALED NITRIC OXIDE (FeNO)

NO is produced in the lung when there is eosinophilic inflammation of the airways. It is hence elevated in patients with asthma particularly atopic asthma. It is not recommended by most guidelines. But the NICE guidelines suggest that it may be useful, particularly in children when other tests are equivocal (12). The test involves exhalation for 10 seconds into the measuring device. A level of 19–21 ppm in children and 20–47 ppm in adults is suggestive of asthma. A normal level does not rule out asthma. Smoking is a confounder and is associated with low levels. A recent study suggested that in children a history of wheeze, particularly with triggers like pollen or pets, and a positive FeNO or BPT to methacholine were better in diagnosing asthma than FEV_1 and FEV_1/FVC (13). A suggested algorithm for diagnosis of asthma is given in Figure 16.1.

DIAGNOSING ASTHMA PHENOTYPES

It is increasingly being recognized that asthma is a heterogenous disease with different biological mechanisms resulting in similar clinical presentation; cough, breathlessness, tightness of the chest and wheeze. While the majority of asthmatics will respond well to standard care, a small majority (5%) will not be controlled. Understanding what drives the disease in them becomes important to be able to tailor treatment individually. With increasing knowledge of the pathophysiology and pathobiology of asthma and the development of treatment targeted at these mechanisms, diagnosis will include the identification of these mechanisms. Looking at the type of airway inflammation is one of the first steps (Figure 16.2).

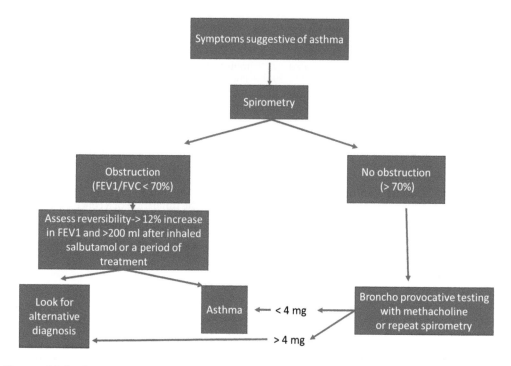

Figure 16.1 Diagnostic algorithm for asthma.

It is well known that in the vast majority of patients, the asthma (50%) is characterized by an eosinophilic inflammation. It has now been shown that eosinophilic airway disease can be IgE mediated and associated with elevated IgE or can be non-atopic driven by interleukins 4, 5, and 13 secreted by innate type 2 lymphoid cells. Allergic asthma is usually seen in the young, while eosinophil mediated asthma not associated with allergy is seen in older patients. They are often male and often associated with persistent airway obstruction and chronic

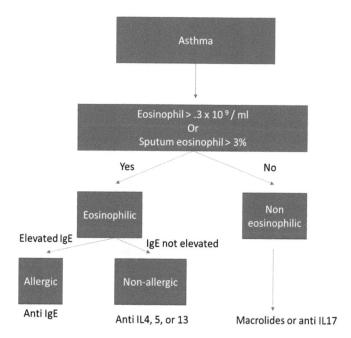

Figure 16.2 Diagnosing asthma phenotypes.

rhinosinusitis with nasal polyps. The former can be targeted by anti-IgE (omalizumab), and the latter by anti-IL 4, 5 (mepolizumab, reslizumab) and 13 (duplizumab). Non eosinophilic inflammation may respond to azithromycin (14).

An induced sputum specimen is used to assess the airway inflammation. Sputum is induced using hypertonic saline. A count greater than 3% is considered eosinophilic inflammation. A surrogate for eosinophilic asthma is the peripheral eosinophil count with a count greater than 0.3×10^9/ml, suggestive of an eosinophilic phenotype. This has a specificity of 84–97% (15). In India because of other causes for eosinophilia, like helminthiasis, this needs to be validated. Eosinophilic asthma can then be grouped further into atopic and non-atopic driven, based on clinical features and the presence or absence of elevated IgE. Those with elevated IgE will benefit from anti-IgE therapy (omalizumab), and those with normal IgE levels with anti-IL4 or Il-5.

CONCLUSION

It is important to make a positive diagnosis of asthma to avoid the high levels of under or overdiagnosis. The diagnosis hinges on the presence of appropriate symptoms and demonstration of reversible airflow. Identifying asthma phenotypes is becoming important as treatment may have to be tailored in specific phenotypes. As the pathophysiology and pathobiology becomes better understood, newer targeted therapy are likely to be identified in the future and may be part of the diagnosis of a patient with asthma. One such phenotype is the eosinophilic phenotype.

REFERENCES

1. Papi A, Brightling C, Pederson SE, Reddel Helen KH. Asthma. Lancet 2018; 391:783–800.

2. Ashler MI, Montefort S, Birksten B, et al. Worldwide time trends in the prevalence of asthma, allergic rhinoconjunctivitis and eczema in childhood: ISAAC phase one and three repeat multicountry cross sectional surveys. Lancet 2006; 368:733–743.

3. Aron SD, Philippe B, Reddel HK, et al. Underdiagnosis and overdiagnosis of asthma. AJRCCM 2018; 198:1012–1020.

4. Aneeshkumar S, Singh RB. Economic burden of asthma among patients visiting a private hospital in South India. Lung India 2018; 35:312–315.

5. Kavanah J, Jackson DJ, Kent BD. Over- and under-diagnosis of asthma. Breathe 2019; 15:e20–e27.

6. GINA guidelines. https://ginasthma.org/wp-content/uploads/2020/06/GINA-2020-report_20_06_04-1-wms.pdf. Pg 20

7. Zengguang H, Feng J, Xia J, et al. Frequency of signs and symptoms of asthma. Respir Care 2020; 65:252–264.

8. Paaso EMS, Jaakkola MS, Lajunen TK, et al. The importance of family history in asthma during the first 27 years of life. AJRCCM 2013; 188:624–626.

9. de Jong CCM, Pederson ESL, Mozun R, Goutaki M, et al. Diagnosis of asthma in children: the contribution of detailed history and test results. Eur Respir J 2019; 54:1901326. Doi:10.1183/1399003.01326-2019.

10. Pellegrino R, Viegi G, Brusasco V, et al. Interpretive strategies for lung function tests. Eur Respir J 2005; 26:948–968.

11. Anderson SD. Bronchial challenge test: usefulness, availability and limitations. Breathe 2011; 8:53–59.

12. National Institute for Health and Care Excellence. Measuring Fractional Exhaled Nitric Oxide Content in Asthma: NIOX MINO, NIOX, VERO, and NObreath 2014. https://www.nice.org.uk/guidance/dg12/resources/measuring-fractionalexhaled-nitric-oxide-concentration-in-asthma-nioxmino-niox-vero-and-nobreath-1053626430661.

13. de Jong CCM, Pederson ESL, Mozun R, et al. Diagnosis of asthma in children: the contribution of a detailed history and test results. Eur Respir J 2019; 54:1901326.DOI: 10.1183/13993003.01326-2019

14. Jones TL, Neville DM, Chauhan AJ. Diagnosis and treatment of severe asthma: a phenotype-based approach. Clin Med 2018; 18:s36–s40.

15. Coumou H, Bel EH. Improving the diagnosis of eosinophilic asthma. Expert Rev Respir Med 2016; 10(10):1093–1103. doi: 10.1080/17476348.2017.1236688.

17 Asthma in Children: What Happens When They Grow?

Lisha Pallivalappil and Ravindran Chetambath

CONTENTS

INTRODUCTION

Asthma is one of the most common chronic childhood illnesses[1]. Physicians who treat asthma in children face different clinical challenges. Some patients have early onset of asthma in infancy and regress completely. Others have a later onset and continue to be symptomatic throughout their life, progressing to the stage of irreversible airflow obstruction. The clinical course is therefore extremely variable. In most patients, asthma begins in childhood. The frequency of wheezing is greater up to 11 years of age. Remission is more common in those who had their first episode of wheezing before 5 years of age and in those who have fewer episodes of wheezing in late childhood. The late-onset wheezers have more episodes of wheezing in late childhood that then continued to the adolescent age. It has been found that the genetic predisposition and exposure to infectious agents were the major early determinants associated with the development of asthma. Acute respiratory infections in early childhood were found to increase the risk of asthma onset at any time in life. The female sex has lesser asthma attacks in childhood as against their adult counterparts.

NATURAL HISTORY OF ASTHMA

An increasing prevalence and severity of asthma has been reported worldwide[2]. There was an increasing incidence reported among children and adolescents during the 20-year-period from 1964 to 1983[3]. The incidence was higher in males from infancy to 9 years of age, and in the older than 50 years age group. The incidence of asthma in children was found to be 284 per 100,000 population[3].

Evaluation of children and adults has shown a low prevalence rate of asthma (2–4%) in Asian countries compared to western countries (15–20%)[4]. Indian studies done on school-age children reported that the prevalence of asthma varies from 7.0–29.5%[5]. The median age of onset was 3 years in males and 8 years in females. Before the age of 14 years, the prevalence of asthma is nearly two times greater in boys than in girls. As they get older this gap narrows, and in adults the prevalence of asthma is greater in women than in men.

The Tucson Children's Respiratory Prospective Birth Cohort study[6] is the most significant study in throwing light on the natural history of asthma. This study began in 1980 and followed up 1246 children and their family members from birth. This was a long-term longitudinal study to investigate the relationship of many potential risk factors and lower respiratory tract infections in childhood—especially during the first 3 years of life—to the subsequent development of chronic lung disorders.

The study provided extensive and longitudinal information about various aspects of asthma in children. Children were grouped into four clinical subtypes such as never wheeze, transient early wheeze, late-onset wheeze at 6 years of age and persistent wheeze. The transient early wheezers had low initial lung function that persisted until the age of 16 years. Their wheezing episodes stopped by that age, whereas the late onset and persistent wheezers had more episodes of wheezing in the late childhood and adolescent age group. The frequency of wheezing was greater up to 11 years of age. Remission was more frequent among those who had their first episode of

DOI: 10.1201/9781003125785-17

wheezing before 5 years of age and in those who had fewer episodes of wheezing in late childhood[7]. These children had an association between early sensitization and bronchial hyperresponsiveness. One-third of children age 3 years of age or younger had LRTI associated with wheezing, and almost 60% of these children stopped wheezing by the age of 6 years.

A study by Kurukulaaratchy R.J. et al. included 1456 children recruited at birth and assessed for atopic sensitization by the skin prick test (SPT) to common allergens at 4 years. They were then reviewed at 1, 2, 4 and 10 years of age by lung function, bronchial challenge, serum IgE and skin prick testing. Atopic phenotypes were defined, by sensitization pattern, for children with SPT at both 4 and 10 years of age. The phenotypes identified were never atopic, early childhood atopic, late childhood atopic and chronic atopic based on skin test sensitivity[8]. The study showed that chronic childhood atopics showed the highest prevalence of lifetime wheeze. They also reported more persistent wheeze, eczema, rhinitis and bronchial hyperresponsiveness than other phenotypes.

A study of 18,873 subjects carried out in Italy from 1998 to 2000 aimed at assessing the incidence and remission of asthma in subjects from birth up to 44 years of age[9]. This study found an overall remission rate of 45.8% (41.6% in women and 49.5% in men, $P < .001$). Asthmatic patients in remission had an earlier age at onset (7.8 vs 15.9 years, $P < .001$) and a shorter duration of the disease (5.6 vs 16.1 years, $P < .001$) than patients with current asthma. The probability of remission was strongly and inversely related to the age at onset (62.8% and 15.0% in the <10- and > or equal to 20-years age-at-onset groups, respectively).

Follow up of asthmatic children[10] for 20 years pointed to favorable prognosis for early onset asthma (before 3 years of age). The presence of atopic disease in first-degree relatives significantly affected the prognosis and probability of persistent wheezing in adulthood. A positive skin test also indicated more severe outcome in asthma.

LUNG FUNCTION DECLINE IN CHILDHOOD ASTHMATICS

Lung function growth has been tracked from infancy to adulthood in asthmatics in various trials across race, gender and ethnic groups. Various growth patterns and factors associated with them have been identified.

It was found that baseline bronchodilator response, airway responsiveness, and level of forced expiratory volume (FEV_1) are independent predictors of subsequent level of FEV_1 in childhood asthma. This may have treatment-specific prognostic significance for persistence of symptoms into early adulthood[11]. Those with asthma have a slower growth of MMEF and FEV_1. The Tucson Children's Respiratory Study has recognized four patterns of longitudinal changes in FEV_1. They are normal growth, reduced growth and early decline, reduced growth only, normal growth and early decline. All these patterns are possible in children with or without asthma.

Dysanapsis—or small airways for lung volume—may have its origin in utero due to factors like maternal smoking[12]. Many additional factors may affect the progression of lung function. Some of these factors are inherited, but most are acquired. Various environmental agents have been implicated in recurrent and persistent wheezing in childhood leading to decreased lung function in adulthood. Factors such as female gender, smoking, sensitization to house dust mites, airway hyperresponsiveness and early age of onset predicted persistence of asthma symptoms or relapse of asthma[13]. Potentially avoidable environmental exposures such as teenage smoking can modify the trajectories of lung function decline. Not all children with lower lung functions grow up to be asthmatics with persistent symptoms.

Even if they become asymptomatic in adulthood, children with asthma and repeated exacerbations in early childhood may be at risk of chronic obstructive pulmonary disease (COPD) in adulthood, especially if they reach a lower peak lung function in early adulthood. But there is also enough evidence to support the fact that improving air pollution, not taking up smoking and standard of care medical treatment for asthma in children will improve airway symptoms even in those with lower lung function growth rates.

AGE OF ONSET PHENOTYPES IN ASTHMA

Based on the age of onset of symptoms, three separate phenotypes are identified[14]. They are:

1. **Infant wheezes:**

   These are children with onset of wheezing in the first year of life. There are multitudes of causes, including laryngomalacia, and infant wheeze has no correlation with outcome at 10 years of age. This may be because many noises made by infants are misrecognised as wheezes or because actual wheezing is under recognized by the inexperienced parents.

Table 17.1: Tucson Study Group Epidemiological Phenotypes[6]

	Number (%)	Lung Function Shortly after Birth	Wheeze Age 3	Lung Function Age 6	Wheeze Age 6
Normal subjects	425 (51%)	Normal	–	Normal	–
Transient wheeze	164 (20%)	Obstructed	+	Some catch up, still obstructed	–
Persistent wheeze	113 (14%)	Normal	+	Obstructed	+
Late onset wheeze	124 (15%)	Normal	–	Normal	+

2. **Preschool (1–6 years) wheezes:**

This phenotype includes children between ages 1 and 6 years. Apart from asthma, there are other causes for wheeze such as bronchiolitis and respiratory viral infections.

3. **Late childhood wheezes:**

These children develop wheeze during the school years. Most of them are atopic, having sensitization to one or more allergens.

The Tucson study provided the classical epidemiological phenotypes of childhood asthma (Table 17.1).

The Avon Longitudinal Study of Parents and Children (ALSPAC) described six phenotypic patterns; namely, (1) never or infrequent wheeze, (2) transient early wheeze, (3) prolonged early wheeze, (4) intermediate-onset wheeze, (5) late-onset wheeze and (6) persistent wheeze[15]. This classification can be considered as an extension of the four classical groups reported in the Tucson study.

These epidemiological phenotypes throw light on the mechanisms of the disease. In the transient wheezers lung function is impaired at birth. Various etiological factors have been identified for this. Cigarette smoke exposure in utero has been found to result in significantly greater mean distance between alveolar attachments in intraparenchymal airways, leading to abnormal airway functioning due to a reduction in the forces opposing airway narrowing[16]. The distance between alveolar attachments was greater in infants exposed to maternal smoking in utero when compared to those infants exposed to cigarette smoking after birth.

The fetal risk of maternal smoke exposure is greater in Glutathione S transferase isoforms M1 and T1 deficiency[17]. Maternal atopy, maternal diabetes, preeclampsia, use of antibiotics during pregnancy, amniocentesis, chorionic villous sampling and environmental pollution have been associated with transient early wheezing and impaired lung function at birth[18,19].

Children with persistent wheeze appear to have normal lung function at birth but develop airway obstruction at age 4–6 years. Children followed up from birth to 13 years of age showed that sensitization to perennial allergens developing in the first 3 years of life was associated with loss of lung function by school age[20]. So the chronic course of asthma with airflow limitation at adolescence was associated with persistent allergic airway inflammation in early childhood. A study on immigrant populations has also shown the importance of environmental factors in early life in the development of persistent wheezing. It is to be noted that a large proportion of transient early wheezers grow out of their symptoms and attain normal lung function by school age.

ATOPY AND ASTHMA IN CHILDREN

The atopic march which begins as eczema in infancy, followed by allergic rhinitis in childhood and asthma in adulthood holds true[21]. Association with atopy can also be used as a phenotypic marker in childhood asthma. The Tasmanian Longitudinal Health (TLH) Study investigated the influence of eczema on the development of asthma from childhood to adult life and found that childhood eczema was significantly associated with new-onset asthma in three separate life stages between 8 and 44 years: pre-adolescence, adolescence and adult life[22].

Early sensitization and sensitization to multiple allergens are considered to be stronger predictors of asthma persistence in childhood and into adulthood. The Manchester Asthma and Allergy Study showed that those with early sensitization to multiple allergens that formed more than 10.6% of the cohort were more likely to have severe asthma and decreased lung function[23].

Food allergy has also been associated with atopic dermatitis. It is unclear whether the progression from IgE mediated food allergy to asthma in subjects without eczema is causal or a result of shared environment and/ or shared genetics. Because eczema and food allergy can co-exist in infants, it is also unclear whether the observed association is related to co-manifestation of other allergic conditions such as eczema and allergic rhinitis that predict asthma or whether it is the consequence of food allergy itself[24]. In the preschool years, the association between atopy and asthma is not well described. Atopy takes some time to manifest in infancy. The two events of wheezing and atopy may not be connected even if both occur together. Therefore, atopy may not be useful as a phenotypic marker or a marker of response to inhaled glucocorticoid therapy[25].

PHENOTYPE BASED ON SYMPTOM PATTERN

There are two clinical phenotypes for childhood asthma[26].

1. Episodic wheeze associated with viral infections. This is described as wheezing during discrete time periods, often in association with clinical evidence of a viral cold, with absence of wheeze between episodes.

2. Multiple trigger wheezes caused by triggers in addition to viral infections. This is described as wheezing that shows discrete exacerbations, but also involves having symptoms between episodes. Triggers include dust, cold air, exercise, laughter, etc.

Transition from episodic to multiple trigger wheezes may occur over time and depend on genetic and environmental factors. Episodic wheeze is more common in the preschool age group and responds to inhaled corticosteroid (ICS) and oral leukotriene receptor antagonists (LTRA) used intermittently. Multiple trigger wheezing will respond to ICS in all instances, but viral-induced wheezing episodes effectively convert them to episodic wheezing. So this phenotypic classification has an impact on treatment decisions as well.

ASTHMA PREDICTIVE INDEX

Several studies have dealt with markers or predictors of subsequent development of adult asthma or progression of childhood asthma into adulthood. The Tucson Children's Respiratory Study group,[6] described earlier in this chapter, developed an Asthma Predictive Index. This includes major and minor criteria (Table 17.2).

More than three-fourths of all children with a positive index had symptoms consistent with active asthma at least once from the ages of 6 to

Table 17.2: Asthma Predictive Index[6]

Obligatory	Major Criteria	Minor Criteria
Recurrent episodes of wheezing during the previous year	Atopic dermatitis as diagnosed by a physician	Peripheral blood eosinophilia
	Physician-diagnosed parental asthma	Wheezing apart from colds
		Physician-diagnosed allergic rhinitis
Positive API	Obligatory plus one major or two minor criteria	

13 years, whereas 68% of those with a negative index never had symptoms consistent with active asthma during the school years.

ASTHMA IN ADOLESCENTS: HOW DOES IT DIFFER FROM CHILDHOOD ASTHMA?

Asthma may change to a great extent during adolescence. Although cross sectional studies have demonstrated that significant changes occur in the asthmatic population in adolescents, individual factors that influence prognosis have not been identified. The higher incidence of asthma in boys tends to reverse after adolescence, and females become more susceptible in adulthood than men. This may be due to being of the male sex is a risk factor for late onset atopy and female sex a risk factor for late onset bronchial hyperreactivity[27]. This could also be due to a higher rate of onset of asthma in puberty in females or a lower remission rate of asthma in females after puberty[28]. It may also reflect a better response to treatment in childhood in males with increased likelihood of resolution.

Atopy acquired in childhood is associated with the onset of asthma during adolescence and early adulthood. It has been confirmed in other studies that atopy defined by skin prick tests is an important risk factor for diagnosis of new onset asthma in the adolescent age group. The rates of atopy and recent onset wheeze are higher than remission rates during adolescence and young adulthood. It is found to be rare for patients who were atopic at 8–12 years of age to become non-atopic during adolescence or early adulthood[28].

Remission of asthma can also occur during adolescence. But it is not known whether remission would really mean that underlying pathology reverses or continues undetected.

The observations of a longitudinal Dutch cohort[29] suggest that the underlying airway pathology does not resolve despite remission of symptoms, as asymptomatic patients still had abnormal lung function and/or persisting airway hyperresponsiveness.

Asthma which has resolved in childhood may relapse later in life, even if asymptomatic as adolescents or young adults. Relapse of symptoms in adulthood was associated with smoking and atopy and those asymptomatic with airway hyperresponsiveness at 13 years of age. In a study that assessed remission objectively using lung function studies to assess FEV_1 and bronchial hyperreactiveness, along with clinical and subjective assessment of remission, it was found that 57% of subjects in clinical remission had bronchial hyperresponsiveness or a low lung function. Therefore, defining remission of asthma in childhood solely based on clinical parameters like absence of symptoms and not requiring inhalers will lead to missing those subjects with continuing airway inflammation and remodelling[29,30].

TRANSITION OF CARE FROM CHILDREN TO ADOLESCENTS AND YOUNG ADULTS

Adolescents and young adults (AYA) form a large group of patients with asthma. The medical care in this group is complicated by the biological, psychological and social changes in this age group. As AYA gain increasing autonomy, they also have to become more socially and financially independent, while their primary relationships switch from family to peer-based interactions. These changes may continue up to 25 years of age.

The EAACI Guidelines[31] on the effective transition of adolescents and young adults with allergy and asthma have put forth the following points while managing transition of care from childhood to adolescents and young adults:

- Preparation for transition may be considered from early adolescence (11–13 years) in accordance with the patient's developmental stage.

- Transition Readiness Assessment Questionnaire,"Ready, Steady, Go" and TR(x) ANSITION Scale can be used for assessing readiness for transition.

- It has been shown that AYA are more likely to follow treatment plans and attend adult service medical appointments when they have a good knowledge of their disease and the reasons for treatment and good family support.

- Developing skills related to self-management of allergy and/or asthma, within current and future education or work should be considered.

- Adherence recommendations include medication reminders, mobile applications and web-based applications can be recommended to improve adherence, symptom control and quality of life

- Empowering AYA with self-management skills can help them become autonomous, expert patients, minimizing their dependency on parents and health care providers. It is therefore essential that AYA have the knowledge and skills to ensure they can self-manage their allergies and/or asthma effectively and confidently.

- Many AYA with allergy and/or asthma have co-existing psychological issues, including anxiety, depression, suicidal ideation and relational difficulties. These problems may magnify the complexities of self-management, care coordination and treatment planning in AYA with allergy and/or asthma.

- From early adolescence onwards, along with growing independence, relationships de-centralize from the core family to peers, friends and other social networks. Social comparison and being part of the group become increasingly important. As a result, the AYA may feel embarrassed about their allergy and/or asthma due to fear of being perceived as different from their peers. To prevent this, it may be recommended to encourage AYA to let their friends know about their allergy and/or asthma and how they can help in an emergency.

CONCLUSION

Wheezing in children is a heterogeneous group of disorders that includes asthma, as well as many other conditions presenting with wheeze. Children below 3 years of age usually have respiratory viral infections presenting as wheeze. These transient wheezers do not develop asthma in late childhood. At the same time, late onset wheezers, especially those having an atopic background transform to persistent wheezers and have asthma in adolescence and early adult life. This suggests that childhood asthma have different phenotypes, each having different outcomes as the child grows. Environmental factors, especially parental smoking, play a vital role in the development and persistence of asthma in children. Early identification of the phenotype and providing standard of care helps in adequate control of symptoms and prevents deterioration in pulmonary function.

REFERENCES

1. The International Study of Asthma and Allergies in Childhood (ISAAC) steering committee. Worldwide prevalence of symptoms of asthma, allergic rhino-conjunctivitis and atopic asthma. Lancet 1998; 351:1225–1235.

2. Amir M, Kumar S, Kumar Gupta R, Singh GV, Kumar R, Anand S, et al. An observational study of bronchial asthma in 6–12 years school going children of Agra District. Ind J Allergy, Asthma and Immunol 2015; 29:62–69.

3. Yunginger JW, Reed CE, O'Connell EJ, Melton III LJ, O'Fallon WM, Silverstein MD. A community-based study of the epidemiology of asthma: incidence rates, 1964–1983. Am Rev Respir Dis 1992; 146(4):888–8894.

4. Peat JK. Vandenberg RH, Curien WF. Changing prevalence of sthma in Australian children. BMJ 1994; 308:1591–1596.

5. Paramesh H. Epidemiology of asthma in India. Indian J Pediatr 2002; 69:309–312.

6. Taussig LM, Wright AL, Holberg CJ, Halonen M, Morgan WJ, Martinez FD. Tucson Children's Respiratory Study: 1980 to present. J Allergy Clin Immunol 2003; 111:661–675.

7. Rhodes HL, Thomas P, Sporik R, Holgate ST, Cogswell JJ. A birth cohort study of subjects at risk of atopy: twenty-two-year follow-up of wheeze and atopic status. Am J Respir Crit Care Med 2002; 165:176–180.

8. Kurukulaaratchy RJ, Matthews S, Arshad SH, Matthews S. Defining childhood atopic phenotypes to investigate the association of atopic sensitization with allergic disease. Allergy 2005; 60:1280–1286.

9. De Marco R, Locatelli F, Cerveri I, Bugiani M, Marinoni A, Giammanco G; Italian Study on Asthma in Young Adults study group. Incidence and remission of asthma: a retrospective study on the natural history of asthma in Italy. J Allergy Clin Immunol. 2002 Aug; 110(2):228–235.

10. Blair H. Natural history of childhood asthma 20-year follow-up. Arch Dis Childhood 1977; 52:613–619.

11. Tantisira KG, Fuhlbrigge AL, Tonascia T, Szesfler SJ, Weiss ST, et al. Bronchodilation and bronchoconstriction: predictors of future lung function in childhood asthma. J Allergy Clin Immunol 2006; 117(6):1264–1271. https://doi.org/10.1016/j.jaci.2006.01.050

12. Speizer FE, Tager IB. Epidemiology of chronic mucus hypersecretion and obstructive airways disease. Epidemiol Rev. 1979; 1:124–142. https://doi.org/10.1056/NEJMOA022363

13. Sears MR, Greene JM, Willan AR, Wiecek EM, Taylor DR, Flannery EM, et al. A longitudinal, population-based, cohort study of childhood asthma followed to adulthood. N Engl J Med 2003; 349:1414–1422. https://doi.org/10.1056/NEJMoa022363

14. Bush A, Menzies-Gow A. Phenotypic differences between pediatric and adult asthma. Proc Am Thorac Soc 2009; 6(8):53–56.

15. Henderson J, Granell R, Heron J, Sherriff A, Simpson A, Woodcock A, et al. Associations of wheezing phenotypes in the first 6 years of lifewith atopy, lung function and airway responsiveness in mid-childhood. Thorax 2008;63:974–980.

16. John G Elliot JG, Carroll NG, James AL, Robinson PJ. Airway alveolar attachment points and exposure to cigarette smoke in utero. Am J Respir Crit Care Med 2003; 167(1):45–49.

17. Kabesch M, Hoefler C, Carr D, Leupold W, Weiland SK, von Mutius E. Glutathione S transferase deficiency and passive smoking increase childhood asthma. Thorax 2004; 59(7):569–573.

18. Rusconi F, Galassi C, Forastiere F, Bellasio M, De Sario M, Ciccone G, et al. Maternal complications and procedures in pregnancy and at birth and wheezing phenotypes in children. Am J Respir Crit Care Med 2007; 175:16–21.

19. Gilliland FD, Li YF, Dubeau L, Berhane K, Avol E, McConnell R,et al. Effects of glutathione S-transferase M1, maternal smoking during pregnancy, and environmental tobacco smoke on asthma and wheezing in children. Am J Respir Crit Care Med 2002; 166:457–463.

20. Illi S, von Mutius E, Lau S, Niggemann B, Grüber C, Wahn U; Multicentre Allergy Study (MAS) group. Perennial allergen sensitiztion early in life and chronic asthma in children: a birth cohort study. Lancet 2006 Aug 26; 368(9537):763–770. https://doi.org/10.1016/S0140-6736(06)69286-6. Erratum in: Lancet. 2006 Sep 30;368(9542):1154. PMID: 16935687

21. Bantz SK, Zhu Z, Zheng T. The atopic march: Progression from atopic dermatitis to allergic rhinitis and asthma. J Clin Cell Immunol 2014 Apr; 5(2):202–208.

22. van der Hulst AE, Klip H, Brand PL. Risk of developing asthma in young children with atopic eczema: a systematic review. J Allergy Clin Immunol 2007 Sep; 120(3):565–569.

23. Belgrave DC, Buchan I, Bishop C, Lowe L, Simpson A, Custovic A. Trajectories of lung function during childhood. Am J Respir Crit Care Med 2014; 189(9): 1101–1109. https://doi.org/10.1164/rccm.201309-1700OC

24. Saarinen KM, Pelkonen AS, Mäkelä MJ, Savilahti E. Clinical course and prognosis of cow's milk allergy are dependent on milk-specific IgE status. J Allergy Clin Immunol 2005; 116(4):869–875.

25. Castro-Rodriguez JA, Rodrigo GJ. Efficacy of inhaled corticosteroids in infants andpre-schoolers with recurrent wheezing and asthma: a systematic review with meta-analysis. Pediatrics 2009;123:e519–e525.

26. Brand PL, Baraldi E, Bisgaard H, Boner AL, Castro-Rodriguez JA, Custovic A, et al. Definition, assessment and treatment of wheezing disorders in preschool children: an evidence-based approach. Eur Respir J 2008; 32: 1096–1110.

27. Russell G. Asthma in the transition from childhood to adulthood. Thorax 2002; 57:96–7. https://doi.org/10.1136/thorax.57.2.96

28. Xuan W, Marks GB, Toelle BG, Belousova E, Peat JK, Berry G, et al. Risk factors for onset and remission of atopy, wheeze, and airway hyperresponsiveness. Thorax 2002; 57:104–109. 10.1136/thorax.57.2.104

29. Vonk JM, Postma DS, Boezen HM, Grol MH, Schouten JP, Koeter GH, et al.Childhood factors associated with asthma remission after 30 year follow up. Thorax 2004; 59:925–929.

30. Strachan DP, Butland BK, Anderson HR. Incidence and prognosis of asthma and wheezing illness from early childhood to age 33 in a national British cohort. BMJ 1996; 312:1195–1199. https://doi.org/10.1136/bmj.312.7040.1195

31. Roberts G, Vazquez-Ortiz M, Knibb R, Khaleva E, Alviani C, Angier, E, et al. EAACI Guideline on the effective transition of adolescents and young adults with allergy and asthma. Allergy 2020; 00:1–19. https://doi.org/10.1111/all.14459

18 Asthma in Pregnancy

Priti Nair

CONTENTS

INTRODUCTION

Asthma is the most common respiratory condition affecting women in pregnancy. The incidence of asthma has increased worldwide for a variety of reasons. Asthma involves episodic reversible airway obstruction characterised by bronchoconstriction, inflammation, airway remodelling and mucous plugging. If not controlled properly, asthma can seriously affect the outcome in pregnancy in a number of ways including pregnancy-induced hypertension, preterm deliveries, interventions in pregnancies and perinatal mortality[1]. There are many short- and long-term risks of having uncontrolled asthma during pregnancy, both to the fetus and the mother. There is increasing evidence that controlling asthma during pregnancy leads to better maternal and fetal outcomes[1].

Although women with mild asthma are unlikely to have problems, those with severe asthma are at the highest risk of deterioration. The deterioration risk is highest in the last weeks of pregnancy. Severe and poorly controlled asthma has been associated with numerous poor perinatal outcomes, including preeclampsia, pregnancy-induced hypertension, uterine haemorrhage, preterm labour, premature birth, congenital anomalies, fetal growth restriction, low birth weight, small size for gestational age, perinatal mortality, neonatal hypoglycemia, seizures, tachypnea, childhood respiratory diseases and neonatal intensive care unit admissions[1,2].

Using data from an Ontario Asthma Surveillance Study, babies born to women from a cohort of 103,424 singleton pregnancies with asthma exacerbation during pregnancy had an

DOI: 10.1201/9781003125785-18

elevated risk of asthma and pneumonia in the first five years of life. Asthma exacerbation in pregnant women with asthma was associated with a higher incidence of preeclampsia, pregnancy-induced hypertension, low birth weight and congenital malformations[2].

Despite these risks, there is suboptimal control of asthma in pregnancy due to a lack of sufficient knowledge regarding usage of medications and their safety during pregnancy.

EPIDEMIOLOGY

According to the World Health Organization, an estimated 235 million people have asthma worldwide. Despite the advances in the management of asthma with inhalational treatment, there were 383,000 asthma-related deaths in 2015[3].

Asthma has been reported to affect 3.7–8.4% pregnant women globally, making it potentially the most common serious medical problem in pregnancy[4]. Multiple exacerbations can increase the risks in pregnancy, while well controlled asthma decreases the risks[5].

Physiological Changes in the Lung in Pregnancy

The changes in the course of bronchial asthma are due to changes in hormonal function, volume of the abdomen and immunological functions. In pregnancy changes in hormones and the mechanical effects of abdominal distension causes changes in lung function. This was studied in a cohort of 100 healthy white women with singleton pregnancy in an antenatal clinic at Oslo University Hospital[6]. The main finding of the study was that forced vital capacity (FVC) and peak expiratory flow (PEF) increase progressively after 14–16 weeks of gestation (Table 18.1).

Table 18.1: Changes in Lung Function during Pregnancy

Lung capacity measurement	Physiological changes of pregnancy
Functional residual capacity	Decrease by 17–20% [300–500 ml]
Residual volume	Decreased by 20–25% [200–300 ml]
Tidal volume	Increased by 30–50%
Expiratory reserve volume	Decreased by 5–15% [100–300 ml]
FEV_1	Unchanged
PEFR	Unchanged or increased
Minute ventilation	Increased by 30–50%
PaO_2	Increased
$PaCO_2$	Decreased
Bicarbonate	Decreased
pH	Slightly increased
Level of diaphragm	Higher

The parous women were found to have higher FVC compared to primigravida women, and the change seems to be permanent. This has significant implications in the management of pregnant women with pre-existing lung disease[6]. Previous studies have shown that minute ventilation and tidal volumes are increased in pregnancy, while functional residual capacity and expiratory reserve volume are decreased[6,7]. The functional residual capacity is decreased because of the increasing size of the uterus and changes in the diaphragm. The widening of the sub costal angle compensates for the increasing size of the uterus and the flattening of the diaphragm. The FEV_1 remains unchanged in pregnancy, so any changes in FEV_1 can be attributed to disease. Studies have showed that pulmonary function tests do not change much in a normal pregnancy compared to the non-pregnant control group or to the post-partum state[6,7]. The progressive increase in PEF during pregnancy is probably due to bronchodilatation, which is probably attributed to reduced vagal efferent activity and progesterone mediated alteration in airway smooth muscle tone[8]. The increase in minute ventilation in pregnancy is because of an increase in tidal volume and not because of an increase in respiratory rate. Healthy pregnant women show very little change in FEV_1 and only a mild rise in FVC (about 1/10 of a litre) and no change in FEV_1/FVC[6].

The increased weight in pregnancy can cause shortening of the neck and oropharyngeal changes that can affect the mechanics of breathing[9].

The cardiovascular changes in pregnancy are mainly to meet the metabolic demand of the mother, fetus and placenta to prepare for delivery, where there is an increase in cardiac output, stroke volume and heart rate. There is a significant fall in cardiac output in the supine position but it is better in the left lateral position[8,10].

The hormonal effects exerted during pregnancy—particularly that of progesterone—are immunomodulatory, improve lung function and have properties of repair after influenza illness[11]. Progesterone is a respiratory stimulant that can increase the sensitivity of the respiratory centre to carbon dioxide. Several host immunological factors play a role in improving pulmonary function and promoting a pulmonary repair environment[11].

Arterial Blood Gas in Pregnant Women

The maternal pCO_2 should ideally be low, as any rise in pCO_2 will cause a rise in fetal acidosis. Hence, a normal pCO_2 level in the ABG analysis is indicative of a degree of CO_2 retention and possible early respiratory failure[12].

Effect of Pregnancy on Asthma

Exacerbations are more likely to occur between the 24th and 36th weeks of pregnancy[13]. Some of the common triggers found were viral infections in 34% and non-adherence to medications in 29% of the cases. Asthma is more likely to deteriorate in severe asthma (52–65% of the time) than in mild asthma (8–13% of the time)[13].

It has been found that one-third of patients with asthma symptoms in pregnancy become better, one-third become worse and one-third remain the same (Figure 18.1). There is an increase in free cortisol, which may have anti-inflammatory role, and an increase in bronchodilator hormones such as progesterone. An increase in the level of prostaglandin F2 alpha may promote bronchoconstriction. Modification of cell mediated immunity alters maternal response to infection[14].

Effect of Asthma on Pregnancy

Initial asthma severity classified as mild, moderate and severe was significantly related to subsequent asthma morbidity, hospitalizations, unscheduled visits, corticosteroid requirements and asthma symptoms during labour and delivery[15]. Exacerbation in pregnancy occurred in 12.6% of patients initially classified as mild, 25.7%

classified as moderate and 51.9% classified as severe[15]. During pregnancy, exacerbations of asthma which require medical intervention occur in about 20% of women, and 6% are admitted in hospitals[16].

Asthma severity is associated with poor obstetric outcome with an increased need for caesarean delivery[16]. Studies have suggested a strong increase in the incidence of childhood asthma in the babies born after caesarean sections, which cannot be explained only by genetic factors. There is a moderately increased risk of asthma, atopy and hay fever in children delivered by caesarean section[17].

Maternal asthma is associated with an increased risk of gestational diabetes and pulmonary embolism and an increased risk of viral illness, particularly influenza. Spontaneous abortion was more common in uncontrolled asthma in pregnancy as shown in a Canadian study[18]. Murphy et al. showed the relative risk of preterm delivery among asthmatics, which can be effectively reduced by active management and control of asthma[19]. There is growing evidence that uncontrolled asthma causes placental insufficiency, causing decreased fetal growth and low birth weight in babies[20]. Several studies have shown a correlation between low birth weight and or gestational age and childhood asthma. There is a growing amount of data showing that intrauterine growth retardation (IUGR) causes an increased risk for respiratory deficiencies

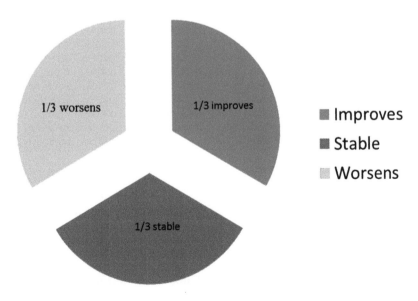

Figure 18.1 Effects of asthma in pregnancy.

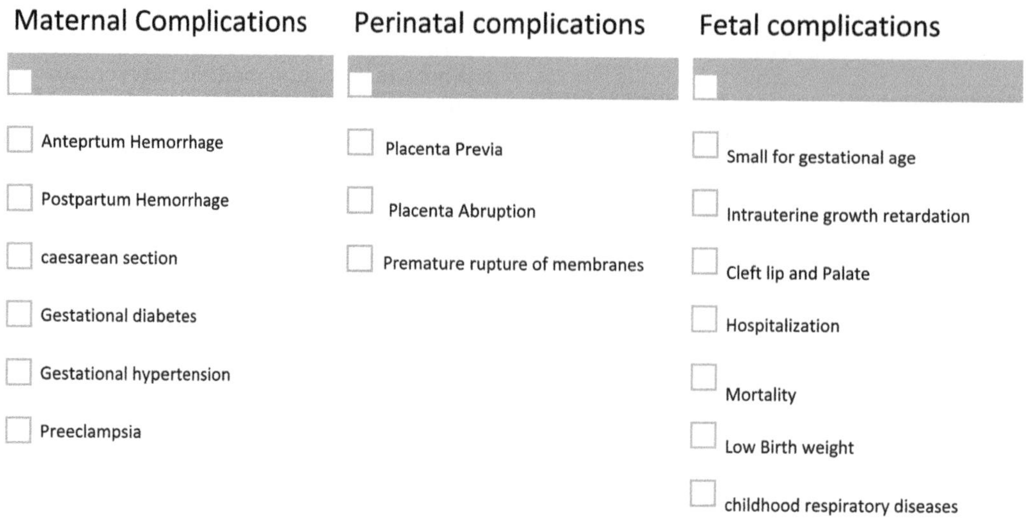

Maternal Complications

- [ ] Anteprtum Hemorrhage
- [ ] Postpartum Hemorrhage
- [ ] caesarean section
- [ ] Gestational diabetes
- [ ] Gestational hypertension
- [ ] Preeclampsia

Perinatal complications

- [ ] Placenta Previa
- [ ] Placenta Abruption
- [ ] Premature rupture of membranes

Fetal complications

- [ ] Small for gestational age
- [ ] Intrauterine growth retardation
- [ ] Cleft lip and Palate
- [ ] Hospitalization
- [ ] Mortality
- [ ] Low Birth weight
- [ ] childhood respiratory diseases

Figure 18.2 Complications of uncontrolled asthma in pregnancy.

after birth. Babies who are small for their gestational age can have adversely affected lung function, thus calling into question the widely held concept that IUGR accelerates lung maturity[21] (Figure 18.2).

There are insufficient studies on how asthma control before pregnancy affects pregnancy. In a large number of pregnant asthmatics, pregnancy-induced hypertension is seen in moderate to severe asthmatics. Many studies have suggested that maternal hypoxia, placental hypoxia, smoking and altered placental function can result in poor outcomes[22,23].

INVESTIGATIONS

Regular monitoring of lung function has been an important aspect of treating asthma in pregnancy. FEV_1 is the single best measure of obstruction in pregnancy; when the value is less than 80%, it is found to be significantly associated with preterm delivery before 32 weeks and before 37 weeks and birth weight below 2500 g.

Pre- and post-bronchodilator spirometry is necessary for the diagnosis of asthma. Impaired pulmonary function during pregnancy has been associated with adverse perinatal outcomes, including gestational hypertension and prematurity[23]. After the initial measures of pulmonary function follow up measures are done by spirometry, and subsequently, it is enough to measure the peak expiratory flow[24]. An alternative to monitoring pulmonary function test is to monitor airway

inflammation, such as sputum eosinophils and fraction of expired nitric oxide[25]. These measure airway inflammation, which is the target of inhaled corticosteroids. A Cochrane review of the use of inhaled corticosteroids based on FeNO did not show much advantage in the use of FeNO for titrating the dose of inhaled corticosteroids in non-pregnant asthmatics[26]. NAEPP 2020 guidelines give us only a conditional recommendation for the use of FeNO as an adjunct in the diagnosis of asthma. The review for use of sputum eosinophils for tailoring inhaled corticosteroid doses supports the benefit of the use of sputum eosinophils as a marker[26].

Fractional exhaled nitric oxide-based asthma management reduces the number of exacerbations of asthma in pregnancy by 50% and reduces the incidence of bronchiolitis in the first few years of life of the fetus[27]. A study has been conducted to find whether it is possible to implement the use of FeNO in asthma management in antenatal care in New South Wales.

Phenotype and Genotype of Asthma in Pregnancy

It is generally accepted that asthma is a heterogeneous condition, and phenotyping of asthma patients has become mandatory for all patients not satisfactorily responding to standard therapy with inhaled corticosteroids[28]. A study showed that allergic phenotypes of asthma and hay fever had no significant increase in the adverse outcomes in pregnancy, whereas the non-atopic phenotype of asthma without hay fever had more adverse outcomes[29].

Medication in Pregnancy
Controller Medication in Asthma

The effectiveness of medications is assumed to be the same in the non-pregnant and in the pregnant state, though there are no studies. The 1993 National Asthma Education and Prevention Program working group initial classification of asthma has been mild, moderate and severe, based on symptoms and spirometry and was related to subsequent asthma morbidity during pregnancy; that is hospitalization, unscheduled visits, use of corticosteroids and asthma symptoms during pregnancy and labour[28].

Studies show that 65% of patients have poor control of asthma during pregnancy, inhaler technology is not correct in 64.4% of cases and only 17% of patients have had a spirometry in the past 5 years.

Inhaled corticosteroids are needed at all stages of pregnancy. Corticosteroids are anti-inflammatory and reduce the hyper responsiveness of the airways. There had been concerns of teratogenicity with the use of corticosteroids, which have not been shown in various observational studies[30]. This has been extensively reviewed by the National Asthma Education and Prevention Program guidelines[31].

Budesonide is the preferred steroid in pregnant asthmatics, as it is considered category B in pregnancy as per FDA from human gestational studies. The rest of the inhaled corticosteroids like fluticasone, and also theophyllines and cromolyn, are considered category C. However if an asthmatic had been using a different medication prior to pregnancy, it would be advisable to continue using it[30].

Inhaled beta-2 agonist and ICS are safe in pregnancy[30]. If a patient is on oral medication, it is better to switch to inhaled steroids. The use of short-acting beta-2 agonist, long-acting beta-2 agonist, inhaled corticosteroid and oral theophyllines with the checking of levels is necessary as per guidelines. Oral corticosteroids and leukotriene receptor antagonists should be used when needed.

The NAEPP 2020 guideline recommends ICS and formoterol in a single inhaler, both as a daily controller and as quick relief inhaler. Formoterol is the recommended long-acting beta-agonist (LABA). Good asthma control with treatment based on guidelines is the key to a successful outcome.

GINA Guidelines has categorised asthma on the basis of severity. With increasing severity of asthma, a low dose of inhaled corticosteroids or a combination of long-acting beta agonists and low dose inhaled corticosteroids is recommended, with stepping up the doses as needed and re-evaluation and stepping down as warranted, maintaining the lowest possible dose.

Treatment of Asthma with Preventive Medications

The main goal in asthma is titration of medications of inhaled corticosteroids and long-acting beta agonists and oral corticosteroids to prevent exacerbation and achieve adequate control during pregnancy.

Management of Acute Asthma in Pregnancy

Standard treatment includes nebulised bronchodilators and intravenous corticosteroids, magnesium and use of non-invasive or invasive ventilation. Additional considerations include neuromuscular blockade, inhaled anaesthetics and sedatives[32]. The medications should be given as for a non-pregnant patient with systemic steroids and magnesium sulphate. High flow oxygen should be given immediately to maintain the saturation of 94–98%.

Acute severe asthma is an emergency and should be treated vigorously in the hospital. For those with poorly controlled asthma, there should be coordination between the pulmonologist and the obstetrician[33]. There should be continuous fetal monitoring.

Difficult-to-treat asthma is managed by first confirming diagnosis and looking for differential diagnosis and factors contributing to poor quality of life. Management should be optimised with an asthma controller and reliever, with biologicals if required; review of response should be made after 3–6 months.

Short-Acting Beta Agonists

During pregnancy short-acting beta agonist are used as reliever medications for all types of mild, moderate and severe asthma with low dose ICS, whereas long-acting beta agonists are used for moderate and severe asthma with low or moderate dose of ICS. One study found an increased risk of side effects with SABA; others showed no increase. It has been reported that 40–70% of asthmatic women use SABA and 8–13% use LABA. Salbutamol has been found to be the preferred beta agonist in pregnancy and has been found to be safe in pregnancy[34].

Long-Acting Beta Agonist

The data from one experimental and six human studies done was reassuring regarding the safety of beta agonists. The data available was mainly for albuterol. Two LABAs (salmeterol and formoterol) have been available since 1993. However, there is limited data regarding their use in pregnancy. The pharmacological and toxicological profile is similar to short-acting ones[34].

Inhaled Corticosteroids

The preferred inhaled corticosteroid is budesonide because of the evidence on its safety though if a pregnant patient's symptoms have been controlled by other inhaled corticosteroids, this should be continued. A retrospective study of more than 5000 pregnancies exposed to inhaled corticosteroids in the first trimester did not show any greater risk of congenital malformation with fluticasone propionate compared to other steroids[35].

Four studies investigating the association between use of corticosteroids in pregnancy and increased perinatal mortality did not show much difference[36]. Using controller therapy during pregnancy is important. Because the risks are greater than the adverse effects, it is important to continue controller medications[36].

In a prospective observational study of 504 pregnant asthmatic patients, an 18% incidence of acute asthmatic attacks was noticed in patients not on inhaled corticosteroids compared with a 4% attack rate in those on inhaled corticosteroids[36]. Wendel and colleagues studied 58 women hospitalised for 65 acute attacks of asthma in pregnancy. Eleven had received intravenous methyl prednisone and tapering oral corticosteroids. The patients were randomised to receive inhaled corticosteroids and inhaled long-acting beta-2 agonist or inhaled beta-2 agonist alone. Those receiving inhaled corticosteroid had 12% readmission, whereas those who had not, had 33% readmission[37].

For the patients using ICS before pregnancy, the rate of asthma related physician visits decreased and emergency department (ED) visits were unchanged, whereas physician and ED visits increased after pregnancy in those patients not on ICS earlier[38]. Overall the data suggests that asthma is undertreated in those contemplating pregnancy and in those who are pregnant.

ICS should be used in pregnancy in low to moderate doses sufficient to control symptoms and prevent exacerbation. The effect of higher doses is not fully studied. The low dose inhaled budesonide is safe in pregnancy and seems to be safe for both mother and fetus[39].

Patient education for the proper administration of ICS and adherence and compliance is to be ensured, particularly in the first trimester.

Asthmatic pregnant women tend to decrease use of medication during pregnancy, which tends to increase exacerbations and increase them post-delivery[40].

THEOPHYLLINES

Theophylline has been used in pregnancy for years and has demonstrated clinical effectiveness. However it has the potential for toxicity and drug interactions. There is a need for titration and measurements to keep the levels in the range of 5–12 mcg/ml[41].

ORAL CORTICOSTEROIDS

A meta-analysis from 1975 to 2012 found that maternal oral corticosteroid use was associated with low birth weight and preterm delivery. It also found moderate to severe asthma was associated with small for gestational size babies. Also, a recent prospective control study showed uncontrolled asthma as a greater predictor for poor perinatal outcomes than exacerbations. This study also defined recurrent uncontrolled asthma as an Asthma Control Questionnaire (ACQ) score > 1.5 on two or more occasions. The same study showed a remarkable effect of gender of the fetus affecting outcomes, with the female fetus being small for its gestational age and the male fetus being more often preterm[1].

BIOLOGICALS

In pregnancy with asthma the risk of using biologics is unknown and should not be started. Cessation of biologics for a planned pregnancy is inadvisable due to the effect on the disease and placental insufficiency in uncontrolled asthma. Monoclonal antibody should not be started in pregnancy due to risk of anaphylaxis. Omalizumab Pregnancy Registry data (Xolair Pregnancy Registry–EXPECT) indicate no increase in congenital malformations or small for gestational age births or prematurity[1].

Clinicians caring for pregnant women will need to be specifically aware of the heightened risk of infections and type 4 immune or cytokine imbalance syndrome. All biologicals are potent suppressors of various components of pathways to immune system. A women commencing a biological agent in pregnancy should undergo the same screening for infections and vaccinations prior to starting a biologic, with the exceptions of live vaccines.[14,25]

IMMUNOTHERAPY

Immunotherapy should not be initiated during pregnancy due to the risk of anaphylaxis. If already on immunotherapy, this should be continued and the dose not escalated.[42]

Leukotriene Receptor Antagonist

The leukotriene receptor antagonists montelukast and zafirleukast are considered safe in pregnancy due to animal data and no significant congenital malformations in humans, while in tests with zileuton teratogenicity has been reported in animal studies[43].

Treatment of Exacerbations of Asthma during Pregnancy

A study found that pregnant patients presenting to the emergency with asthma exacerbations were less likely to receive steroids and were more likely to come back to emergency after discharge[44].

The management of asthma with controller medications in pregnancy is important. When asthma occurs in the primary care setting, it is necessary to transfer to acute care setting to undergo oxygen therapy, nebulised therapy and possible NIV in selected cases. In cases not responding to nebulised short-acting beta-2 agonists and ipratropium bromide, it is necessary to consider Noninvasive Positive-Pressure Ventilation (NPPV) to mitigate hypoxia and hypercapnia in a few subsets of asthma. The number of randomised controlled trials are very limited and in the range of 10–20 patients[44].

There have been studies with the use of NPPV in asthma exacerbation in pregnancy with successful results[45].

The patient selection has to be careful. NPPV was mainly used to alleviate dyspnoea in pregnant patients with asthma with low oxygen saturation and dyspnoea to prevent intubation and invasive ventilation. The NPPV was used on the grounds that using positive airway pressure would cause bronchodilatation and decrease the airway resistance[46].

PEFR monitoring should be done in those women who are prone to exacerbations. They should be given an individualised action plan. They should seek medical advice if fetal movement is decreased or there is a poor response to rescue medication. In patients with status asthmaticus, delivery should be considered and a caesarean section if emergent.

Antenatal fetal surveillance is necessary in pregnant asthmatics who are poorly controlled at 32 weeks of pregnancy with ultrasound or with intrauterine fetal growth retardation[1].

Differential Diagnosis of Dyspnoea in Pregnancy

It is important to consider the differential diagnosis of dyspnoea in pregnancy, one of them being bronchial asthma and the asthma mimics. The others are physiological dyspnoea of pregnancy, pulmonary embolism, amniotic fluid embolism, peripartum cardiomyopathy and pulmonary edema. They may be coexisting causes of dyspnoea in pregnancy that must be treated accordingly.

Management of Asthma during Labour and Delivery

Asthma medications should be continued during labour and delivery. Asthmatic attack is rare during labour. If there is no acute attack of asthma during delivery the indication for caesarean is the same as for obstetric indication. It would be preferable to use regional anaesthesia instead of general anaesthesia in case inhaled anaesthetic agents cause bronchoconstriction. Those taking oral corticosteroids at a dose of more than 7.5 mg for 2 weeks prior to delivery should be started on parenteral hydrocortisone. Neuraxial anaesthesia decreases the oxygen requirement and thus minute ventilation. Parenteral hydrocortisone 100 mg IV 6–8 hourly prior to labour can be helpful in controlling asthma symptoms during labour, and if continued 24 hours post-partum and then stopped. Tapering of steroids is not required. If steroids have been used previously then stress dose steroids have to be used. Medications used for tocolysis, induction of labour or cervical ripening can have an effect on medication-sensitive asthma. Prostaglandin E2 or E1 can be used for cervical ripening, for post-partum haemorrhage or to induce abortion without adverse reactions. Carboprost (prostaglandin f2 alpha), ergonovine and methyl ergonovine can cause bronchospasms, especially in the aspirin sensitive patients. In these cases, misoprostol, which is an E1, is more appropriate[47]. Magnesium sulphate is a bronchodilator and should not cause adverse effects.

Ketamine is pregnancy class B drug. For procedural sedation and for intubation, doses are 1–2 mg/kg IV. For asthma exacerbation doses such as 0.2 mg/kg followed by an infusion of 0.5 mg/kg/hr are often used. Ketamine can be safely used for patients with possible hypovolemia or asthma who are undergoing induction of general anaesthesia in undergoing caesarean section.

Preventing Asthma Attacks during Pregnancy

Preventing asthma attacks is mainly achieved by avoiding triggers, smoking, contact with sick patients and stress. Some of the major triggers of asthma like rhinitis, chronic rhinosinusitis, obesity, obstructive sleep apnoea, depression and GERD have to be addressed and treated.

Allergic rhinitis and asthma are the two principal closely related allergic diseases. Intranasal corticosteroids are the most effective for allergic rhinitis in pregnancy and have a lower risk of systemic effects. The choice in second-generation antihistaminics during pregnancy is loratidine or cetirizine.

Obesity is associated with increased exacerbations of asthma in pregnancy. Also it is associated with complications like obstructive sleep apnoea and obesity hypoventilation and right heart failure[48]. Anxiety and depression are common disorders that affect a large part of the population. The prevalence is 6–15% among pregnant women with asthma.

These conditions not only affect the psychological wellbeing of patients but also affect other diseases. Depression and anxiety are associated with asthma and adverse fetal outcomes[49]. Exercise is important in controlling asthma, and using a short-acting inhaler prior to simple exercises like swimming is helpful.

Control Measures for Environmental Triggers

Control measures for environmental triggers that can make asthma worse are important aspects in preventing asthma exacerbation. Measures of controlling animal dander have to be instituted by removing animals from the house and covering the air ducts with filters. House dust comprised of organic and inorganic substances such as mites, mite faeces, fibres, mould and pollen are abundant on mattresses and control measures include encasing beddings. Avoiding pollen by staying indoors on high pollen count days and shutting the windows could prevent exposure to pollen. Avoiding second hand smoke, quitting smoking, avoiding wood burning stoves, adding vents and avoiding perfumes and spray are the measures for preventing environmental allergies.

Allergic diseases are more common in urban areas, which may suggest a causal link between outdoor and indoor pollution and allergies and asthma. High indoor pollution [particulate matter] PM 2.5 exposures were associated with smoking and gas appliances. Exposure to particulate matter may cause increased allergies and asthma exacerbation and can affect asthma status in pregnancy[50].

Assessment and Monitoring of Asthma in Pregnancy

Objective measures of pulmonary function tests and monthly evaluation, including history and physical examination with the aid of validated asthma questionnaires is needed. PEFR also may be sufficient for monitoring the status of asthma. Fetal ultrasound monitoring is important after 32 weeks in patients with asthma who are suboptimally controlled and those with moderate to severe asthma.

Childhood asthma risk is lessened when asthma is well controlled in the mother during pregnancy. Avoiding stress, using fewer antibiotics during pregnancy, the mode of delivery and supplemental vitamin D are also factors leading to less asthma risk in children. It is mainly passed onto the child due to genetics. Studies investigating asthma in mothers during pregnancy have found increased incidence of wheezing at 15 months of age in the infants[51].

Non-Pharmacological Methods in Preventing Asthma Exacerbations in Pregnant Asthmatics

Pregnant asthmatics should be provided with asthma education, a definite asthma action plan and good communication between their pulmonologist and obstetrician. This should include educating asthmatic women prior to pregnancy and teaching inhaler techniques. Part of the action plan includes monitoring the fetal movements. It should be emphasised that if an asthma attack is associated with reduced fetal movements, it is imperative to reach a health care facility.

Vaccination in Pregnancy

Protection against influenza with vaccination is essential and is possible in all trimesters. The recommendations are to obtain an influenza vaccine before the influenza season since pregnant women with asthma tend to develop severe illness from influenza because of changes in immunity, and in heart and lung function.

Management of Asthma during Breastfeeding and Post-Partum

It is important to continue asthma medication post-partum, possibly with peak flow monitoring. Breastfeeding from 1–6 months in infancy is protective from atopy later in childhood, though it is not protective from asthma.

CONCLUSION

It is extremely important to control asthma during pregnancy in order to prevent the complications of uncontrolled asthma. Asthma is a chronic respiratory condition and the most common respiratory condition in pregnancy. Adequate treatment could enable better fetal and maternal outcomes. It is safer for an asthmatic to take all asthma medication than have symptoms and exacerbations that may compromise oxygenation—and hence oxygenation to the fetus—that can cause perinatal mortality and morbidity.

REFERENCES

1. Bonham CA, Patterson KC, Strek ME. Asthma outcomes and management during pregnancy. Chest 2018; 153(2):515–527. https://doi.org/10.1016/j.chest.2017.08.02

2. Abdullah K, Zhu J, Gershon A, Dell S, To, T. Effect of asthma exacerbation during pregnancy in women with asthma: A population based cohort study. Eur Respir J 2019; 1901335. https://doi.org/10.1183/13993003.01335-2019

3. World Health Organization. Asthma. 2017. http://www.who.int/mediacentre/factsheets/fs307/en/.

4. Kwon HL, Belanger K, Bracken MB. Asthma prevalence among pregnant and childbearing-aged women in the United States: estimates from national health surveys. Ann Epidemiol 2003; 13(5):317–324.

5. Källén B, Rydhstroem H, Åberg A. Asthma during pregnancy—a population based study. Eur J Epidemiol 2000; 16(2):167–171.

6. Grindheim, G., Toska, K., Estensen, M-E, et al. Changes in pulmonary function during pregnancy: a longitudinal cohort study. BJOG 2012; 119:94–101.

7. Kolarzyk E, Szot WM, Lyszczarz J. Lung function and breathing regulation parameters during pregnancy. Arch Gynecol Obstet 2005; 272:53–58.

8. Avery ND, Wolfe LA, Amara CE, Davies GA, McGrath MJ. Effects of human pregnancy on cardiac autonomic function above and below the ventilatory threshold. J Appl Physiol 2001; 90:321–328.

9. Annamraju H, Mackillop L. Respiratory disease in pregnancy. Obstet Gynaecol Reprod Med 2017; 27 (4):105–111.

10. Petersen JW, Liu J, Chi YY, et al. Comparison of multiple non-invasive methods of measuring cardiac output during pregnancy reveals marked heterogeneity in the magnitude of cardiac output change between women. Physiol Rep 2017; 5(8): e13223.

11. Hall OJ, Limjunyawong N, Vermillion MS, et al. Progesterone-based therapy protects against influenza by promoting lung repair and recovery in females. PLoS Pathog 2016; 12(9):e1005840. https://doi.org/10.1371/journal.ppat.1005840

12. Omo-Aghoja L. Maternal and fetal acid-base chemistry: a major determinant of perinatal outcome. Ann Med Health Sci Res 2014; 4(1):8–17. https://doi.org/10.4103/2141-9248.126602

13. Murphy VE. Managing asthma in pregnancy. Breathe (Sheff) 2015; 11(4):258–267. https://doi.org/10.1183/20734735.007915

14. Wang H, Li N, Huang H. Asthma in pregnancy: pathophysiology, diagnosis, whole-course management, and medication safety. Can Respir J 2020, Article ID 9046842, https://doi.org/10.1155/2020/9046842

15. Schatz M, Dombrowski MP, Wise R, et al. Asthma morbidity during pregnancy can be predicted by severity classification. J Allergy Clin Immunol 2003; 112(2):283–288. https://doi.org/10.1067/mai.2003.1516

16. Wang G, Murphy VE, Namazy J, et al. The risk of maternal and placental complications in pregnant women with asthma: a systematic review and meta-analysis. J Matern Fetal Neonatal Med 2014; 27:934–942.

17. Tollånes MC, Moster D, Daltveit AK, Irgens LM. Cesarean section and risk of severe childhood asthma: a population-based cohort study. J Pediatr 2008; 153(1):112–116. doi:10.1016/j.jpeds.2008.01.02

18. Blais L, Kettani FZ, Forget A. Relationship between maternal asthma, its severity and control and abortion. Hum Reprod 2013; 28:908–915.

19. Murphy VE, Schatz M. Asthma in pregnancy: a hit for two. Eur Respir Rev 2014; 23(131): 64–68.

20. Meakin AS, Saif Z, Jones AR, Valenzula Aviles PF, Clifton VL. Review: placental adaptations to the presence of maternal asthma during pregnancy. Placenta 2017; 54:17–23.

21. Despina DB, Malamitsi-Puchner A. Small for gestational age birth weight: impact on lung structure and function. Paediatr Respir Rev 2013; 14 (4):256–262.

22. Schatz M, Dombrowski MP, Wise R, et al. Asthma morbidity during pregnancy can be predicted by severity classification. J Allergy Clin Immunol 2003; 112(2):283–288. https://doi.org/10.1067/mai.2003.1516

23. Namazy JA, Schatz M. Current guidelines for the management of asthma during pregnancy. Immunol Allergy Clin North Am 2006; 26(1):93–102. https://doi.org/10.1016/j.iac.2005.10.003. PMID: 16443145.

24. National Heart, Lung, and Blood Institute; National Asthma Education and Prevention Program Asthma Pregnancy Working Group NAEPP expert panel report. Managing asthma during pregnancy: recommendations for pharmacologic treatment-2004 update. J Allergy Clin Immunol 2005; 115(1):34–46.

25. Petsky HL, Cates CJ, Lasserson TJ, Li AM, Turner C, Kynaston JA, Chang AB. A systematic review and meta-analysis: tailoring asthma treatment on eosinophilic markers (exhaled nitric oxide or sputum eosinophils). Thorax 2012; 67(3):199–208. https://doi.org/10.1136/thx.2010.135574. Epub 2010 Oct 11. PMID: 205

26. Petsky HL, Cates CJ, Li A, Kynaston JA, Turner C, Chang AB. Tailored interventions based on exhaled nitric oxide versus clinical symptoms for asthma in children and adults. Cochrane Database Syst Rev 2009 Oct 7;(4):CD006340. https://doi.org/10.1002/14651858.CD006340.pub3. PMID: 19821360.

27. Morten M, Collison A, Murphy VE, et al. Managing asthma in pregnancy (MAP) trial: FeNO levels and childhood asthma. J Allergy Clin Immunol 2018; 142(6):1765–1772.e4. doi:10.1016/j.jaci.2018.02.039

28. Schatz M, Rosenwasser L. The allergic asthma phenotype. J Allergy Clin Immunol Pract 2014; 2(6):645–8; quiz 649. doi: 10.1016/j.jaip.2014.09.004. Epub 2014 Nov 6. PMID: 25439351.

29. Turkeltaub PC, Cheon J, Friedmann E. The influence of asthma and/or hay fever on pregnancy: Data from the 1995 National Survey of Family Growth 2017; 5 (6):1679–1690.

30. Gluck JC, Gluck PA. Asthma controller therapy during pregnancy. Am J Obstet Gynecol 2005; 192(2):369–380.

31. National Heart, Lung, and Blood Institute; National Asthma Education and Prevention Program Asthma Pregnancy Working Group NAEPP expert panel report. Managing asthma during pregnancy: recommendations for pharmacologic treatment—2004 update. J Allergy Clin Immunol 2005; 115(1):34–46.

32. Elsayegh D, Shapiro JM. Management of the obstetric patient with status asthmaticus. J Intensive Care Med 2008; 23(6):396–402.

33. Racusin DA, Fox KA, Ramin SM. Severe acute asthma. Semin Perinatol 2013; 37(4):234–245. https://doi.org/10.1053/j.semperi.2013.04.003. PMID: 23916022.

34. Eltonsya K, Kettani F-Z, Blais L. Beta2-agonists use during pregnancy and perinatal outcomes: A systematic review. Respir Med 2014; 108(1):1–228.

35. Charlton RA, Snowball JM, Nightingale AL, Davis, KJ. Safety of fluticasone propionate prescribed for asthma during pregnancy: a UK population-based cohort study. J Allergy Clin Immunol Pract 2015; 3:772–779.e3

36. Breton MC, Beauchesne MF, Lemière C, et al. Risk of perinatal mortality associated with inhaled corticosteroid use for the treatment of asthma during pregnancy. J Allergy Clin Immunol 2010; 126(4): 772–777.e2. https://doi.org/10.1016/j.jaci.2010.08.018

37. Campbell LA, Klocke RA. Implications for the pregnant patient. Am J Respir Crit Care Med 2001 Apr; 163(5):1051–4. https://doi.org/10.1164/ajrccm.163.5.16353. PMID: 11316633

38. Schatz M, Leibman C. Inhaled corticosteroid use and outcomes in pregnancy. Ann Allergy Asthma Immunol 2005; 95(3):234–238. https://doi.org/10.1016/S1081-1206(10)61219-7

39. Smy L, Chan AC, Bozzo P, Koren G. Is it safe to use inhaled corticosteroids in pregnancy? Can Fam Physician 2014; 60(9):809–e435.

40. Koo SM, Kim Y, Park C, et al. Effect of pregnancy on quantitative medication use and relation to exacerbations in asthma. Biomed Res Int 2017;8276190. doi:10.1155/2017/8276190

41. Frederiksen MC, Ruo TI, Chow MJ, Atkinson Jr AJ. Theophylline pharmacokinetics in pregnancy. Clin Pharmacol Ther 1986; 40(3):321–8. https://doi.org/10.1038/clpt.1986.183. PMID: 3742937.

42. Pali-Schöll I, Namazy J, Jensen-Jarolim E. Allergic diseases and asthma in pregnancy, a secondary publication. World Allergy Organ J 2017; 10(1):10. https://doi.org/10.1186/s40413-017-0141-8. PMID: 28286601; PMCID: PMC5333384.

43. Bracken MB, Triche EW, Belanger K et al. Asthma symptoms, severity, and drug therapy: a prospective study of effects on 2205 pregnancies. Obstet Gynecol 2003; 102(4):739–752. https://doi.org/10.1016/s0029-7844(03)00621-5. PMID: 14551004.

44. Cydulka RK, Emerman CL, Schreiber D. et al. Acute asthma among pregnant women presenting to the emergency department. Am J Respir Crit Care Med 1999; 160(3):887–892.

45. Sekiguchi H, Kondo Y, Fukuda T, et al. Noninvasive positive pressure ventilation for treating acute asthmatic attacks in three pregnant women with dyspnea and hypoxemia. Clin Case Rep 2019; 7(5):881–887. Published 2019 Mar 22. https://doi.org/10.1002/ccr3.2117

46. Dalar L, Caner H, Eryuksel E, Kosar F. Application of non-invasive mechanical ventilation in an asthmatic pregnant woman in respiratory failure: a case report. J Thorac Dis 2013; 5:97–100.

47. Goldie MH, Brightling CE. Asthma in pregnancy. TOG 2013; 15: 241–245.

48. Hendler I, Schatz M, Momirova V, et al. Association of obesity with pulmonary and nonpulmonary complications of pregnancy in asthmatic women. Obstet Gynecol 2006; 108(1):77–82.

49. Rejnö G, Lundholm C, Öberg S, et al. Maternal anxiety, depression and asthma and adverse pregnancy outcomes - a population based study. Sci Rep 2019; 9(1):13101. Published 2019 Sep 11. https://doi.org/10.1038/s41598-019-49508-z

50. Cockcroft DW. Treatment of asthma during pregnancy. Ann Allergy Asthma Immunol 2005; 95(3):213–214. https://doi.org/10.1016/S1081-1206(10)61215-X

51. Fazel N, Kundi M, Jensen-Jarolim E, et al. Prospective cohort study of pregnancy complications and birth outcomes in women with asthma. Arch Gynecol Obstet 2018; 298(2):279–287. https://doi.org/10.1007/s00404-018-4800-y

19 Asthma and Obesity

Ravindran Chetambath

CONTENTS

INTRODUCTION

Obesity is both a major risk factor and a disease modifier of asthma in children and adults. In adults, obesity is defined as a body mass index (BMI) of 30 kg/m² or more. Adipose tissue inflammation is increased in obese individuals with asthma compared with obese controls.[1] IL-6 produced by macrophages in adipose tissue acts as a marker of metabolic health and is also a marker of asthma severity.

Asthma affects approximately 6.5 million children (~9% prevalence) in the United States.[2] Likewise, 17% of children in this country are obese and another 15% are overweight.[3] Obesity-induced increases in asthma risk may start in utero. In a meta-analysis of over 108,000 participants, it was found that maternal obesity and weight gain during pregnancy are independently associated with a 15–30% increased risk of asthma in the offsprings.[4] Mechanisms involved may include inflammatory or other changes during pregnancy or early post-natal life.[5-7] These mechanisms may explain why excessive weight gain in infancy has also been linked to recurrent wheezing and asthma. The prevalence of asthma in lean adults is 7.1% and in obese adults 11.1%. This relationship is greater among women. The prevalence of asthma in lean versus obese women is 7.9 and 14.6%, respectively.[8]

Asthma and obesity cannot be considered as two conditions of chance coexistence. There is an obese-asthma phenotype in which obesity modifies asthma[9]. Obese children with asthma tend to have Th1-skewed responses, particularly in response to inflammatory stimuli, which is mediated by systemic inflammation, insulin resistance, and/or alterations in lipid metabolism. Obese children tend to have increased asthma severity, poorer disease control, and a lower quality of life (Figure 19.1). These children and adolescents also tend to have a decreased response to asthma medications.

CLINICAL FEATURES

Obese adults present with more severe asthma than do lean adults, and there is a 4–6-fold higher risk of being hospitalized due to severe exacerbation. Obese patients also have worse asthma control and a lower quality of life. These patients do not respond well to standard controller medications, such as inhaled corticosteroid (ICS) and combination of ICS and long-acting beta agonists (LABA).[10]

There are many phenotypes within the obese asthma syndrome. The obese asthmatics with early onset disease tend to have higher markers of Th2 inflammation and present with more severe disease. There is also a group with later-onset disease, most often female, with significant inflammation in adipose tissue and increased airway oxidative stress. Obese individuals appear to have increased susceptibility to air-pollutants.

OBESITY AND LUNG FUNCTION

Obesity has a significant effect on lung function. Childhood obesity is associated with normal or higher forced expiratory volume (FEV_1) and forced vital capacity (FVC), but a lower FEV_1/FVC ratio.[11] There is an inverse relationship between the growth of the lung parenchyma and that of the caliber of the airways which is reflected in normal or supra-normal FEV_1 and FVC. This effect is much more with FVC that lead to a low FEV_1/FVC ratio. Obese children with asthma had increased symptoms, medication use, and asthma exacerbations. Den Dekker et al showed that greater birth weight and faster infant weight gain were associated with higher FEV_1 and FVC, but lower FEV_1/FVC,

DOI: 10.1201/9781003125785-19

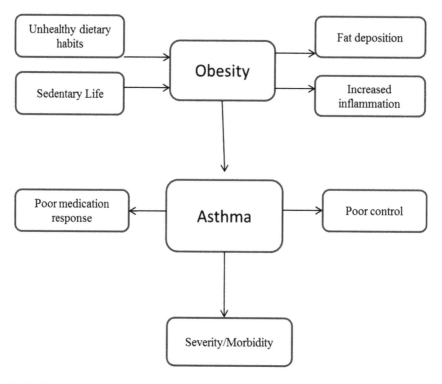

Figure 19.1 Relationship between obesity and asthma.

in school-age children.[12] Obese patients with early-onset asthma have more severe airflow limitations than obese adults with late-onset asthma. It is not clear whether obesity leads to changes in airway hyper-responsiveness (AHR) in children; some studies have reported higher AHR.[13]

Excessive accumulation of fat in the thoracic and abdominal cavities leads to lung compression and an attendant reduction in lung volume in adults. Obesity increases the collapsibility of the peripheral airways and parenchyma, especially among asthmatics with late-onset disease. A prospective longitudinal cohort study that investigated the relationship between obesity and AHR reported that the risk for AHR increases with BMI and weight gain was a risk factor for developing AHR.[14]

DIET AND OBESE ASTHMA

Specific micronutrients may be involved in the association between obesity and asthma. Vitamin D deficiency may be a risk factor for the development of both obesity and asthma. Prenatal vitamin D insufficiency has been associated with obesity in the offspring,[15] and prenatal vitamin D supplementation has led to a small decrease in the risk of wheezing illness by 3 years of age.[16] There is an association between vitamin D deficiency and the risk of

respiratory infections, asthma exacerbations, and corticosteroid resistance;[17] thus, vitamin D deficiency may predispose to the development of obesity, and then to severe asthma and corticosteroid resistance. The efficacy of vitamin D supplementation on asthma in obesity is not well studied.

Diets high in saturated fatty acids, low in fibre, low in anti-oxidants, and high in sugars like fructose promote obesity. Ingestion of a meal which is high in saturated fatty acids increases neutrophilic airway inflammation and decreases bronchodilator responsiveness.[18] Studies in a mouse model of asthma suggest that a diet high in fructose promotes systemic metabolic dysfunction, and increases AHR and airway oxidative stress.[19]

Specific dietary and nutritional risk factors may affect children. Breastfeeding has been associated with lower risks of both obesity and asthma. High-sugar containing beverages are a risk factor for asthma,[20] as is a diet poor in vegetables and grains but rich in sweets and dairy products.[21] Omega-3 fatty acid has been associated with a lower incidence of asthma, whereas omega-6 fatty acids are associated with a higher risk of asthma in the pediatric age group.[22]

Dietary changes may lead to alterations in the gut microbiome, and diets which promote obesity may also help in the development of allergic airway disease. Bacterial colonization of the gut plays a key role in the fermentation of dietary fibre and in the generation of short-chain fatty acids (SCFA). A low-fibre diet decreases levels of the SCFA propionate. A low-fibre diet with low circulating propionate was associated with exaggerated allergic airway inflammation in a mouse model. Increasing propionate decreased the ability of dendritic cells to promote Th2 responses and so attenuated allergic airway inflammation.[23] A high-fibre diet increases levels of acetate, which inhibits the development of allergic airway inflammation in a mouse model through effects on histone deacetylase. Many studies have suggested that diets low in fibre lead to changes in the gut microbiome, which can promote both obesity and allergic asthma.

The airway microbiome may be altered in obese asthma. A recent study in bronchial brushings from severe asthmatics showed that BMI was associated with changes in airway microbial composition and with fewer lung tissue eosinophils.[24] It is unclear whether these microbiome changes cause the reduced eosinophils or are simply an unrelated consequence of obesity.

INFLAMMATION IN OBESE ASTHMA

Obesity-related asthma is a non Th2 phenotype. It is reported that obesity was associated with asthma only among individuals with normal or low exhaled nitric oxide (FeNO). Other markers of Th2 inflammation, such as peripheral eosinophilia and elevated serum IgE are also not consistently present in obese asthmatics. Obesity skews CD4 cells towards Th1 polarization, which is associated with worse asthma severity and control and abnormal lung function.[25] These asthmatic respond poorly to corticosteroids. Zheng et al. reported increased sputum neutrophils in "non-atopic obese asthmatics", while subjects with "atopy-obesity overlap" exhibited higher sputum macrophage counts, suggesting the importance of these innate pathways in obesity-related asthma.[26] Innate immune responses involving Th17 pathways and innate lymphoid cells (ILCs) have also been implicated.[27] Macrophage activation by ILCs and other pathways may constitute an important link between adiposity and worse asthma outcomes (Figure 19.1).

Adipokines and other cytokines produced or induced by adipose tissue may also affect the lungs and the airways. Higher leptin levels in obese adolescents correlate inversely with FEV_1, FVC, and FEV_1/FVC.[28] Visceral fat leptin expression also correlates with airway reactivity in adults. Leptin and adiponectin have also been associated with exercise-induced changes in lung function.

Many complications of obesity, including asthma are explained by metabolic dysregulation.[29] Hyperglycemia and hyperinsulinemia associated with obesity may lead to AHR and remodelling through epithelial damage and airway smooth muscle proliferation.[30] Insulin resistance and the metabolic syndrome are associated with lower lung function in adolescents with and without asthma.[31] Obesity-related pro-inflammatory cytokines like IL-6 may play a crucial role in the relationship between the metabolic syndrome, lung function, and asthma severity (Figure 19.2). Increased oxidative stress occurs in obesity, and increased airway oxidative stress has been found particularly in obese adults with late onset asthma.[32]

LIFESTYLE INTERVENTIONS IN OBESE ASTHMA

Various lifestyle interventions and weight loss strategies have demonstrated significant improvements in asthma control and spirometric

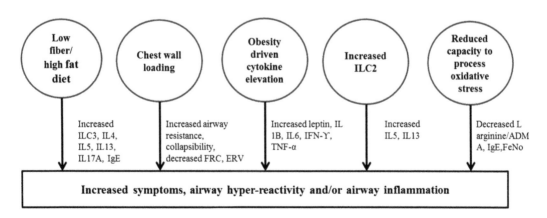

Figure 19.2 Molecular mechanisms of airway inflammation and airway resistance in asthma.

lung function. In adults, a weight loss of at least 5% is required to produce a significant improvement in asthma control.[33] This is associated with improvements in peak flow, spirometric lung function, and ERV. Few studies have reported the effects on markers of airway inflammation. Non-controlled studies in obese children have reported improvements in FEV_1, ERV and TLC that correlate with BMI.[34] In a recent randomized control trial (RCT), a dietary intervention resulted in significant improvements in ERV, although the difference with the control group was not significant.[35] Conversely, another RCT in children with asthma reported a greater improvement in FVC in the intervention group compared to the control group.

BARIATRIC SURGERY

Bariatric surgery is the most effective intervention for producing sustained and significant weight loss, and all studies have reported highly significant improvements in asthma control, airway reactivity, and lung function. Bariatric surgery also has significant effects on asthma exacerbations. Bariatric surgery reduced the risk of having an asthma exacerbation by 60%.[36] Reduced exacerbations may be related to effects on lung mechanics and airway reactivity.

CONCLUSION

Obesity is an important risk factor for asthma, as well as asthma exacerbations both in children and adults. Asthma in the obese is complex and multifactorial. Potential underlying mechanisms include a shared genetic component, dietary and nutritional factors, alterations in the gut microbiome, systemic inflammation, metabolic abnormalities, and changes in lung anatomy and function. There is growing evidence that weight loss interventions also help improve asthma outcomes.

REFERENCES

1. Sideleva O, Suratt BT, Black KE, Tharp WG, Pratley RE, Forgione P, et al. Obesity and asthma: an inflammatory disease of adipose tissue not the airway. Am J Respir Crit Care Med. 2012; 186:598–605. [PMC free article] [PubMed] [Google Scholar]

2. Asthma Data, Statistics, and Surveillance. 2016 Available from http://www.cdc.gov/asthma/most_recent_data.htm.

3. Childhood Obesity. 2016 Available from https://www.cdc.gov/obesity/childhood/index.html.

4. Forno E, Young OM, Kumar R, Simhan H, Celedon JC. Maternal obesity in pregnancy, gestational weight gain, and risk of childhood asthma. Pediatrics. 2014; 134:e535–46. [PMC free article] [PubMed] [Google Scholar]

5. Malti N, Merzouk H, Merzouk SA, Loukidi B, Karaouzene N, Malti A, et al. Oxidative stress and maternal obesity: feto-placental unit interaction. Placenta. 2014; 35:411–416. [PubMed] [Google Scholar]

6. Wilson RM, Marshall NE, Jeske DR, Purnell JQ, Thornburg K, Messaoudi I. Maternal obesity alters immune cell frequencies and responses in umbilical cord blood samples. Pediatr Allergy Immunol. 2015; 26:344–351. [PubMed] [Google Scholar]

7. Costa SM, Isganaitis E, Matthews TJ, Hughes K, Daher G, Dreyfuss JM, et al. Maternal obesity programs mitochondrial and lipid metabolism gene expression in infant umbilical vein endothelial cells. Int J Obes (Lond). 2016 [PMC free article] [PubMed] [Google Scholar]

8. Akinbami LJ, Fryar CD. NCHS data brief, no 239. Hyattsville, MD: National Center for Health Statistics; 2016. Asthma prevalence by weight status among adults: United States, 2001–2014. NCHS Data Brie. Hyattsville, MD: National Center for Health Statistics, 2016. [PubMed] [Google Scholar]

9. Lang JE, Hossain J, Dixon AE, Shade D, Wise RA, Peters SP, et al. Does age impact the obese asthma phenotype? Longitudinal asthma control, airway function, and airflow perception among mild persistent asthmatics. Chest. 2011; 140:1524–1533. [PubMed] [Google Scholar]

10. Boulet LP, Franssen E. Influence of obesity on response to fluticasone with or without salmeterol in moderate asthma. Respiratory medicine. 2007; 101:2240–2247. [PubMed] [Google Scholar]

11. Forno E, Han YY, Mullen J, Celedon JC. Overweight, obesity, and lung function in children and adults – a meta-analysis. 2017 [PMC free article] [PubMed] [Google Scholar]

12. den Dekker HT, Sonnenschein-van der Voort AM, de Jongste JC, Anessi-Maesano I, Arshad SH, Barros H, et al. Early growth characteristics and the risk of reduced lung function and asthma: A meta-analysis of 25,000 children. J Allergy Clin Immunol. 2016; 137:1026–1035. [PubMed] [Google Scholar]

13. Karampatakis N, Karampatakis T, Galli-Tsinopoulou A, Kotanidou EP, Tsergouli K, Eboriadou-Petikopoulou M, et al. Impaired glucose metabolism and bronchial hyperresponsiveness in obese prepubertal asthmatic children. Pediatr Pulmonol. 2016 [PubMed] [Google Scholar]

14. Litonjua AA, Sparrow D, Celedon JC, DeMolles D, Weiss ST. Association of body mass index with the development of methacholine airway hyperresponsiveness in men: the Normative Aging Study. Thorax. 2002; 57:581–585. [PMC free article] [PubMed] [Google Scholar]

15. Boyle VT, Thorstensen EB, Thompson JMD, McCowan LME, Mitchell EA, Godfrey KM, et al. The relationship between maternal 25-hydroxyvitamin D status in pregnancy and childhood adiposity and allergy: An observational study. Int J Obes (Lond). 2017 [PubMed] [Google Scholar]

16. Litonjua AA, Carey VJ, Laranjo N, Harshfield BJ, McElrath TF, O'Connor GT, et al. Effect of prenatal supplementation with vitamin D on asthma or recurrent wheezing in offspring by age 3 years: the VDAART Randomized Clinical Trial. JAMA. 2016; 315:362–370. [PMC free article] [PubMed] [Google Scholar]

17. Lan N, Luo G, Yang X, Cheng Y, Zhang Y, Wang X, et al. 25-Hydroxyvitamin D3-deficiency enhances oxidative stress and corticosteroid resistance in severe asthma exacerbation. PLoS One. 2014; 9:e111599. [PMC free article] [PubMed] [Google Scholar]

18. Wood LG, Garg ML, Gibson PG. A high-fat challenge increases airway inflammation and impairs bronchodilator recovery in asthma. J Allergy Clin Immunol. 2011; 127:1133–1140. [PubMed] [Google Scholar]

19. Singh VP, Aggarwal R, Singh S, Banik A, Ahmad T, Patnaik BR, et al. Metabolic syndrome is associated with increased oxo-nitrative stress and asthma-like changes in lungs. PLoS One. 2015; 10:e0129850. [PMC free article] [PubMed] [Google Scholar]

20. Berentzen NE, van Stokkom VL, Gehring U, Koppelman GH, Schaap LA, Smit HA, et al. Associations of sugar-containing beverages with asthma prevalence in 11-year-old children: the PIAMA birth cohort. Eur J Clin Nutr. 2015; 69:303–308. [PubMed] [Google Scholar]

21. Han YY, Forno E, Brehm JM, Acosta-Perez E, Alvarez M, Colon-Semidey A, et al. Diet, interleukin-17, and childhood asthma in Puerto Ricans. Ann Allergy Asthma Immunol. 2015; 115:288–293. e1. [PMC free article] [PubMed] [Google Scholar]

22. Li J, Xun P, Zamora D, Sood A, Liu K, Daviglus M, et al. Intakes of long-chain omega-3 (n-3 PUFAs and fish in relation to incidence of asthma among American young adults: the CARDIA study. Am J Clin Nutr. 2013; 97:173–178. [PMC free article] [PubMed] [Google Scholar]

23. Trompette A, Gollwitzer ES, Yadava K, Sichelstiel AK, Sprenger N, Ngom-Bru C, et al. Gut microbiota metabolism of dietary fiber influences allergic airway disease and hematopoiesis. Nat Med. 2014; 20:159–166. [PubMed] [Google Scholar]

24. Huang YJ, Nariya S, Harris JM, Lynch SV, Choy DF, Arron JR, et al. The airway microbiome in patients with severe asthma: Associations with disease features and severity. J Allergy Clin Immunol. 2015; 136:874–884. [PMC free article] [PubMed] [Google Scholar]

25. Rastogi D, Fraser S, Oh J, Huber AM, Schulman Y, Bhagtani RH, et al. Inflammation, metabolic dysregulation, and pulmonary function among obese urban adolescents with asthma. Am J Respir Crit Care Med. 2015; 191:149–160. [PMC free article] [PubMed] [Google Scholar]

26. Zheng J, Zhang X, Zhang L, Zhang HP, Wang L, Wang G. Interactive effects between obesity and atopy on inflammation: A pilot study for asthma phenotypic overlap. Ann Allergy Asthma Immunol. 2016; 117:716–717. [PubMed] [Google Scholar]

27. Kim HY, Lee HJ, Chang YJ, Pichavant M, Shore SA, Fitzgerald KA, et al. Interleukin-17-producing innate lymphoid cells and the NLRP3 inflammasome facilitate obesity-associated airway hyperreactivity. Nat Med. 2014; 20:54–61. [PMC free article] [PubMed] [Google Scholar]

28. Huang F, Del-Rio-Navarro BE, Torres-Alcantara S, Perez-Ontiveros JA, Ruiz-Bedolla E, Saucedo-Ramirez OJ, et al. Adipokines, asymmetrical dimethylarginine, and pulmonary function in adolescents with asthma and obesity. J Asthma. 2017; 54:153–161. [PubMed] [Google Scholar]

29. Suratt BT, Ubags NDJ, Rastogi D, Tantisira KG, Marsland BJ, Petrache I, et al. an official American Thoracic Society Workshop Report: Obesity and Metabolism. An emerging frontier in lung health and disease. Ann Am Thorac Soc. 2017; 14:1050–1059. [PMC free article] [PubMed] [Google Scholar]

30. Agrawal A, Mabalirajan U, Ahmad T, Ghosh B. Emerging interface between metabolic syndrome and asthma. Am J Respir Cell Mol Biol. 2011; 44:270–275. [PubMed] [Google Scholar]

31. Forno E, Han YY, Muzumdar RH, Celedon JC. Insulin resistance, metabolic syndrome, and lung function in US adolescents with and without asthma. J Allergy Clin Immunol. 2015; 136:304–311. e8. [PMC free article] [PubMed] [Google Scholar]

32. Holguin F, Comhair SA, Hazen SL, Powers RW, Khatri SS, Bleecker ER, et al. An association between L-arginine/asymmetric dimethyl arginine balance, obesity, and the age of asthma onset phenotype. Am J Respir Crit Care Med. 2013; 187:153–159. [PMC free article] [PubMed] [Google Scholar]

33. Ma J, Strub P, Xiao L, Lavori PW, Camargo CA, Jr, Wilson SR, et al. Behavioral weight loss and physical activity intervention in obese adults with asthma. A randomized trial. Ann Am Thorac Soc. 2015; 12:1–11. [PMC free article] [PubMed] [Google Scholar]

34. van Leeuwen JC, Hoogstrate M, Duiverman EJ, Thio BJ. Effects of dietary induced weight loss on exercise-induced bronchoconstriction in overweight and obese children. Pediatr Pulmonol. 2014; 49:1155–1161. [PubMed] [Google Scholar]

35. Jensen ME, Gibson PG, Collins CE, Hilton JM, Wood LG. Diet-induced weight loss in obese children with asthma: a randomized controlled trial. Clin Exp Allergy. 2013; 43:775–784. [PubMed] [Google Scholar]

36. Hasegawa K, Tsugawa Y, Chang Y, Camargo CA., Jr Risk of an asthma exacerbation after bariatric surgery in adults. J Allergy Clin Immunol. 2015; 136:288–294. e8. [PubMed] [Google Scholar]

20 Difficult-to-Control Asthma

Ravindran Chetambath

CONTENTS

INTRODUCTION

Difficult-to-control asthma, which is also called therapy resistant asthma, is diagnosed when patients with asthma do not respond to maximum doses of inhaled corticosteroids. Around 5–6% of people with asthma have 'difficult-to-control' asthma, and about 4% of asthmatics are categorized as having severe asthma. Because asthma varies significantly from person to person, some patients need a different approach to achieve asthma control. A person with difficult-to-control asthma will need to be diligent about adhering to the medication schedule, following the proper inhaler technique and avoiding triggers and allergens that exacerbate asthma symptoms. Management of difficult-to-control asthma involves identifying and addressing various factors leading to poor control. Severe asthma is a subcategory of difficult-to-control asthma. Patients with severe asthma require a more aggressive approach to treatment, such as controller medications, high-dose corticosteroids and biologic therapies. The following are important factors that may lead to poor control of asthma.

- Inaccurate diagnosis

- Poor adherence to treatment schedule

- Continuous exposure to allergens and triggers

- Concomitant diseases acting as exacerbators

- Sociocultural factors

- Psychological disturbances

Diagnostic Accuracy

When there is a lack of response to standard therapy, the diagnosis of asthma should be reconfirmed. There are multiple conditions that mimic asthma, and clinical suspicion without objective evidence may lead to unnecessary medication (Table 20.1). Pulmonary function testing with documented reversible airway obstruction or airway hyper-responsiveness is the standard practice to establish a definitive diagnosis. A methacholine challenge test should be performed to establish airway hyper-responsiveness. Hyperventilation and vocal cord dysfunction are two frequent mimics of asthma and may coexist with asthma. Nocturnal symptoms can be an indication of uncontrolled asthma; although they can also exist in congestive heart failure or chronic obstructive pulmonary disease (COPD). Obstructive sleep apnea, giving rise to symptoms at night, may be mistaken for asthma. Cardiac asthma is diagnosed in the presence of nocturnal dyspnea, with or without cough, especially in the setting of cardiac dysfunction or coronary artery disease.

DOI: 10.1201/9781003125785-20

Table 20.1: Clinical Conditions That Mimic Asthma

- Hyperventilation
- Vocal cord dysfunction
- Cardiac asthma/congestive heart failure
- Chronic obstructive pulmonary disease
- Gastroesophageal reflux disease
- Restrictive lung disease
- Sleep apnea
- Cystic fibrosis
- Endobronchial lesions

COPD affects long-time smokers and generally has irreversible airflow obstruction. COPD and asthma can have significant overlapping clinical characteristics. COPD typically shows a generally progressive airflow obstruction, with less of airway hyper-reactivity. The distinction is important in deciding the optimal therapy and long-term follow-up[1,2]. A restrictive pattern on pulmonary function tests should lead to a diagnosis of restrictive lung disease. Upper airway obstruction usually manifests with stridor. It can be diagnosed with a proper history and careful examination. In a child with wheezing cystic fibrosis is a possibility, especially in the setting of failure to thrive or persistent diarrhea. Localized obstruction of a major airway arising from endobronchial lesions is a rare but potential cause of wheezing.

HYPERVENTILATION

Symptoms of hyperventilation are often unrecognized and may frequently be attributed to asthma. It was reported that a majority of pseudo-steroid resistant asthmatics had hyperventilation as a potential cause of their disease[3]. In these patients there is difficulty with inhaling. They will struggle to get a good breath without any objective sign of respiratory distress. The methacholine challenge test will be invariably negative. For these patients, it may be beneficial to monitor peak expiratory flow rate (PEFR) before and after hyperventilation episodes to make patients aware of their breathing and to retrain their breathing pattern[4].

VOCAL CORD DYSFUNCTION

Vocal cord dysfunction (VCD) is one condition which can masquerade as mild or severe asthma. This condition often coexists with asthma, making the diagnosis more complex. It is reported that up to one-third of these patients may also have coexisting asthma, making recognition of vocal cord dysfunction difficult[5]. Some patients with VCD may be on aggressive medical regimens and may even be classified as having corticosteroid-resistant asthma[6]. These patients experience difficulty in inhaling rather than exhaling. The episode occurs mostly without any obvious trigger[7]. On auscultation, wheezing is loudest over the larynx. Flow volume loop shows an inspiratory cutoff, which is characteristic of VCD. Direct visualization of the vocal cords, during an acute attack, will show paradoxical movement during inspiration[8]. VCD manifests following physical or psychological trauma[9]. Physician awareness and patient awareness are important, with some patients responding to reassurance, speech therapy and as-needed β-agonist use.

Poor Adherence

Once the diagnosis of asthma is made, it is important to ensure adherence to the medication regimen. Poor adherence is surprisingly common, and this is more so with MDIs compared with oral medications. Some studies documented 10% and 46% adherence to inhaled medication[10]. Adolescents and young adults are notorious for noncompliance. The reasons often quoted are forgetfulness, denial, embarrassment, inconvenience, fear of side effects, a lack of efficacy of medicines and social stigma[11]. Even in a compliant patient, improper inhaler technique may prevent delivery of an adequate quantity of the drug. Patient education and demonstration of proper techniques during each visit can improve treatment outcome.

Exacerbating Factors

Exposure to allergens and other triggers are the most important cause of asthma exacerbations. Identifying and eliminating these factors may help in proper control of asthma. Although dust mite control measures are relatively easy to implement for those with dust mite allergy, it is not so with pollens and moulds. Patients with a history of asthma that improves on weekends or holidays should raise the concern for exposure to occupational allergens or irritants. Such patients require vocational counseling or removal from the workplace. Extensively used drugs such as non-steroidal anti-inflammatory drugs (NSAIDs) and β-blockers may act as significant precipitators of life-threatening asthma[12]. Aspirin and NSAIDs may be a component in many over-the-counter medications and are often overlooked. Identifying the aspirin-sensitive individual with aspirin-exacerbated respiratory disease or aspirin triad will help guide therapy[13]. Cigarette smoking acts both as a trigger to acute attacks, as well as a cause of poor response to asthma medications. In a study of adults presenting to emergency departments with acute asthma, 35% were cigarette smokers[14]. Moreover asthmatic who are long time smokers develop asthma-COPD overlap (ACO), which is more difficult to treat.

One important cause for adult-onset asthma is exposure to irritants at the workplace (occupational asthma). Occupational asthma accounts for 9–15% of all cases of adult asthma[15]. More than 300 agents have been reported to cause occupational asthma. The diagnosis should be confirmed by objective testing for asthma and by establishing the relation between asthma and exposure to triggers at workplace. Removal of the patient from the exposure is an ideal way to control occupational asthma.

CONCOMITANT DISEASES

Difficult-to-control asthma is sometimes associated with another undiagnosed or untreated illness that worsens asthma, such as allergic bronchopulmonary aspergillosis, eosinophilic pneumonia, eosinophilic granulomatosis with polyangitis (Churg–Strauss syndrome), α1-antitrypsin deficiency, carcinoid syndrome, thyrotoxicosis or obstructive sleep apnea (Table 20.2). These conditions, if present, require specific therapy along with management of asthma. Obesity is associated with asthma, especially in women and young adults, and will intensify the inflammatory process making asthma difficult to control[16].

GASTROESOPHAGEAL REFLUX DISEASE

Gastroesophageal reflux disease (GERD) is associated with asthma in multiple ways. It is reported that GERD is a causative factor for asthma. At the same time, there are reasons to believe that asthma or its medication can induce GERD. The estimated prevalence of GERD among asthmatics varies from 34–80%[17]. To confirm the diagnosis, a 24-hour pH monitoring dual-probe study should be done

Table 20.2: Concomitant Diseases Exacerbating Asthma

- Gastroesophageal reflux disease
- Allergic rhinitis
- Chronic rhino-sinusitis
- Hyperventilation
- Endocrinopathies (e.g. hyperthyroidism, carcinoid syndrome)
- Allergic bronchopulmonary aspergillosis
- Aspirin-exacerbated respiratory disease
- Eosinophilic granulomatosis with polyangitis (Churg–Strauss syndrome)
- Eosinophilic pneumonia
- Obstructive sleep apnoea
- Obesity

to correlate episodes of reflux with symptoms of asthma. A therapeutic trial of medical therapy for GERD may be both diagnostic and therapeutic. Correction of GERD with proton pump inhibitors and lifestyle modifications are recommended for better control of asthma.

HYPERVENTILATION AND DYSFUNCTIONAL BREATHING DISORDERS

Hyperventilation and other forms of dysfunctional breathing disorders may exist concomitantly with asthma[18]. Recognizing the coexistence of these conditions and providing proper counselling can prevent the unnecessary step-up of asthma therapy.

CHRONIC RHINO-SINUSITIS

There is increasing evidence that the upper and lower airways are part of a one continuous airway. One airway-one disease concept is given more importance especially when allergic diseases are treated. Therefore, uncontrolled allergic rhinitis or chronic rhino-sinusitis can influence asthma control. Unless coexisting rhinitis or rhinosinusitis are controlled, asthma control becomes difficult. It is shown that treatment of allergic rhinitis with nasal corticosteroids improves symptoms of asthma and airway hyper-responsiveness[19]. Identifying and managing upper respiratory inflammation is therefore important, especially in the group of difficult-to-control asthmatics.

ENDOCRINOPATHIES

Endocrinopathies such as hyperthyroidism or hypocorticism may lead to exacerbations of asthma and require proper treatment. Carcinoid syndrome is also known to precipitate bronchospasm and lead to poor control of asthma.

ALLERGIC BRONCHOPULMONARY ASPERGILLOSIS

An elevated immunoglobulin E level in an uncontrolled asthma with evidence of centrilobular bronchiectasis should lead to a suspicion of allergic bronchopulmonary aspergillosis (ABPA). If not treated and controlled, ABPA will lead to irreversible fibrosis. Treatment is with oral corticosteroid until remission and gradually tapering the dose to identify the lowest effective dose.

ASPIRIN-EXACERBATED RESPIRATORY DISEASE

In some individuals, the use of aspirin exacerbates asthma, which then will not respond to usual medications. These patients may have rhinitis and nasal polyposis as part of the syndrome. Peripheral eosinophilia is always reported. These patients respond to systemic steroids and leukotriene modifiers.

EOSINOPHILIC GRANULOMATOSIS WITH POLYANGIITIS (CHURG–STRAUSS SYNDROME)

Patients with Churg–Strauss vasculitis may also have particularly severe and difficult-to-control asthma, the presence of which should be suspected in the setting of serum eosinophilia or a mononeuritis multiplex.

SOCIOECONOMIC FACTORS

When there are no identifiable and correctable medical reasons for asthma to remain uncontrolled, socioeconomic issues of the patient must be verified (Table 20.3). These include issues of poverty, poor access to medical care, poor adherence, racial issues and psychosocial issues. These factors particularly affect the inner-city population of adolescents and young adults[20]. Poverty appears to be an important cause leading to poor medical attention and non-adherence to prescribed medication. The specific role that race plays is less certain, but marginalized societies are much affected due to poor access to standard medical care, poverty and ignorance. For those attempting to access the proper services, there are multiple barriers for proper care, such as lack of transportation, loss of work hours, financial restrictions and language issues[21]. Non-adherence to scheduled follow-up visits and medications can affect treatment outcome. Adherence can be a problem in any population, but additional barriers exist among socioeconomically disadvantaged individuals. Lack of education, low household income, racial or ethnic minority status and poor patient–physician communication are all factors associated leading to non-adherence.

The psychosocial risk factors that exist in certain societies can have a large impact on asthma control. Drug abuse, smoking, alcoholism, unemployment, a poor work environment and broken families contribute to stress, which may indirectly affect adherence to treatment protocol. Additionally, aggression, anxiety and depression can be important issues in difficult living conditions and are considered risk factors for childhood asthma mortality[22]. Differing cultural practices in certain communities act as barriers to effective care, as they frequently seek unconventional remedies for cure or search for quacks instead of seeking standard medical care.

Environmental exposure to allergen and irritants is also a major risk. Poor housing standards and overcrowding may expose inmates to indoor allergens, environmental smoking and viral infections. In highly polluted and industrial environments, limiting outdoor exposure to chemicals such as sulphur dioxide and ozone can be particularly difficult[23].

PSYCHOLOGICAL FACTORS

Treatment and control of asthma become difficult if the patient is suffering from psychological disorders (Table 20.4). Emotional disturbances, even in normal patients, can influence the symptoms and management of asthma and should be addressed along with management of asthma. Asthma is often associated with anxiety and panic. Approximately 6–30% of patients with asthma meet the criteria for panic disorder[24]. In such patients increased panic and anxiety are associated with the use of more intensive corticosteroid regimens, overuse of bronchodilators and more frequent hospitalizations. A functional component should be suspected when a patient presents with atypical symptoms or does not respond to medications as expected. Asthmatics with comorbid depression are especially difficult to treat. Psychiatric analysis and management approaches are essential to address these issues for the successful control of asthma[25].

Other Causes of Difficult-to-Control Asthma

■ Steroid-dependent asthma is seen in a group of patients who need recurring bursts of systemic corticosteroid therapy. These

Table 20.3: Socioeconomic Risk Factors for Difficult-to-Control Asthma

- Poverty
- Race
- Access to medical care
- Adherence
- Psychosocial issues
- Environment (indoor and outdoor allergens and passive smoking)
- Differing cultural practices

Table 20.4: Psychological Risk Factors for Difficult-to-Control Asthma

- Negative emotions
- Functional symptoms
- Anxiety/panic disorders
- Depression

patients are treated during exacerbations with high doses of steroids for a longer period to achieve control.

- Steroid-resistant asthmatics are defined as those patients with persistent symptoms despite treatment with 40 mg prednisone per day for more than 14 days. This can be 'pseudo resistance' as some patients may respond to higher doses of steroids[26]. True steroid resistances are of two types. The first type is less common and is believed to result from a reduction in the number of existing and functioning glucocorticoid receptors. Patients with this type do not respond to steroid therapy, nor do they experience any side effects from the steroids. The second type is more common and involves a reversible binding defect of the steroid to its receptor.

- Premenstrual worsening of asthma is seen in some females and is typically poorly responsive to glucocorticoids but may respond to aggressive hormonal therapy.

- Brittle asthma is an extremely unstable variant and may be due to a lack of perception of symptoms and disease severity. Patients with this variant may require individualized therapy[27].

MANAGEMENT

Patients with difficult-to-control asthma require high-dose inhaled corticosteroids and long-acting inhaled β2 agonists as therapy[28]. Along with this aggressive therapy, patients may require frequent bursts of oral corticosteroids or chronic daily therapy. Regular education sessions during each visit regarding the correct use of inhalers and spacer devices are essential for positive results.

Additional therapy is indicated either to control the disease or prevent the need for long-term systemic corticosteroid therapy. Frequently used drugs in clinical practice are leukotriene modifiers, anti-IgE therapy and methotrexate. The leukotriene modifier montelukast decreases airway eosinophilic inflammation and improves asthma control. It is particularly useful in aspirin exacerbated respiratory syndrome. In patients with allergic asthma with an elevated IgE level, monoclonal antibody against IgE (omalizumab) is effective. Treatment with omalizumab results in decreased airway inflammation and improved asthma control, facilitating withdrawal of oral corticosteroids[29]. Methotrexate, gold, and cyclosporine have been proposed as steroid-sparing agents in patients with difficult-to-control asthma treated with long-term systemic steroids.

The benefit of therapy will be evident only when the patient strictly adheres to the treatment. Both patient and physician have an important role to play to improve adherence. Strategies include early identification of non-adherence, convincing the patient of the benefits of therapy, providing clear instructions and regular monitoring[30].

CONCLUSION

Difficult-to-control asthma is identified when a patient is refractory to inhaled β2 agonists and high-dose inhaled corticosteroids. When such a situation is encountered, a systematic and logical approach should be adopted. The first step is to establish a proper diagnosis of asthma and to exclude potential conditions mimicking asthma, such as hyperventilation, VCD or COPD. The next step is to ascertain adherence as well as proper inhalational techniques. Identifying concomitant diseases acting as exacerbating factors are to be identified and corrected. Another important issue is continuous exposure to provoking stimuli such as allergens or irritants, either at home or the workplace. Environmental tobacco smoke is an important reason, especially among children and adolescents, for poor control of their asthma. Knowledge of any underlying socioeconomic or psychological factors may help in a subset of patients who are otherwise devoid of any other identifiable cause for exacerbations. Identifying and addressing these issues in a systematic manner will help the patient to avoid unnecessary and inefficient therapy.

REFERENCES

1. Sutherland ER, Martin RJ. Airway inflammation in chronic obstructive pulmonary disease: comparisons with asthma. J Allergy Clin Immunol. 2003; 112: 819–827. https://doi.org/10.1016/S0091-6749(03)02011-6. Article PubMed Google Scholar

2. Sutherland EF. Outpatient treatment of chronic obstructive pulmonary disease: comparisons with asthma. J Allergy Clin Immunol. 2004, 114:715–724. https://doi.org/10.1016/j.jaci.2004.07.044. Article PubMed Google Scholar

3. Thomas PS, Duncan MG, Barnes PJ. Pseudosteroid resistant asthma. Thorax. 1999, 54:352–356. 1https://doi.org/0.1136/thx.54.4.352. PubMed Central CAS Article PubMed Google Scholar

4. De Peuter S, Van Diest I, Lemaigre V. Can subjective asthma symptoms be learned?. Psychosom Med. 2005; 67:454–461. https://doi.org/10.1097/01.psy.0000160470.43167.e2. Article PubMed Google Scholar

5. Barnes PJ, Woolcock AJ. Difficult asthma. Eur Respir J. 1998; 12:1209–1218. Crossref, Medline, Google Scholar

6. O'Connell MA, Sklarew PR, Goodman DL. Spectrum of presentation of paradoxical vocal cord motion in ambulatory patients. Ann Allergy. 1995; 74:341–344. Google Scholar

7. Christopher KL, Wood RP, Eckert RC. Vocal-cord dysfunction presenting as asthma. N Engl J Med. 1983; 308:1566–1570. https://doi.org/10.1056/NEJM198306303082605. CAS Article PubMed Google Scholar

8. Newman KB, Mason UG, Schmaling KB. Clinical features of vocal cord dysfunction. Am J Respir Crit Care Med. 1995; 152:1382–1386. CAS Article PubMed Google Scholar

9. Gavin LA, Wamboldt M, Brugman S. Psychological and family characteristics of adolescents with vocal cord dysfunction. J Asthma. 1998; 35:409–417. https://doi.org/10.3109/02770909809048949. CAS Article PubMed Google Scholar

10. Celano M, Geller RJ, Philips KM. Treatment adherence among low-income children with asthma. J Pediatr Psychol. 1998; 23:345–348. https://doi.org/10.1093/jpepsy/23.6.345. CAS Article PubMed Google Scholar

11. Buston KM, Wood SF. Non-compliance amongst adolescents with asthma: listening to what they tell us about self-management. Fam Pract. 2000; 17:134–138. https://doi.org/10.1093/fampra/17.2.134. CAS Article PubMed Google Scholar

12. Ind PW, Dixon CMS, Fuller RW. Anticholinergic blockade of β blocker induced bronchoconstriction. Am Rev Respir Dis. 1989; 139:1390–1394. CAS Article PubMed Google Scholar

13. Szczeklik A, Stevenson DD. Aspirin-induced asthma: advances in pathogenesis, diagnosis, and management. J Allergy Clin Immunol. 2003; 111:913–921. https://doi.org/10.1067/mai.2003.1487. CAS Article PubMed Google Scholar

14. Silverman RA, Boudreaux ED, Woodruff PG, Clark S, Camargo CA Jr. Cigarette smoking among asthmatic adults presenting to 64 emergency departments. Chest. 2003; 123:1472–1479. Crossref, Medline, Google Scholar

15. Mapp CE, Boschetto P, Maestrelli P, Fabbri LM. Occupational asthma. Am J Respir Crit Care. Med. 2005; 172:280–305. Abstract, Medline, Google Scholar

16. Weiss ST, Shore SS. Obesity and asthma. Am J Respir Crit Care. Med. 2004; 169:963–968.Abstract, Medline, Google Scholar

17. Simpson WG. Gastroesophageal reflux disease and asthma: diagnosis and management. Arch Intern Med. 1995; 155:798–804. https://doi.org/10.1001/archinte.155.8.798. CAS Article PubMed Google Scholar Google Scholar

18. Morgan MDL. Dysfunctional breathing in asthma: is it common, identifiable and correctable? Thorax. 2002; 57:ii31–5. PubMed Central PubMed Google Scholar.

19. Aubier M, Levy J, Cleici C. Different effects of nasal and bronchial glucocorticoid administration on bronchial hyperresponsiveness in patients with allergic rhinitis. Am Rev Respir Dis. 1992; 146:122–126. CAS Article PubMed Google Scholar

20. Pongracic J, Evans R. Environmental and socioeconomic risk factors in asthma. Immunol Allergy Clin North Am. 2001; 21:413–426. https://doi.org/10.1016/S0889-8561(05)70218-6. Article Google ScholarCAS Article PubMed Google Scholar

21. Evans R. Prevalence, morbidity, and mortality of asthma in the inner city. Pediatr Asthma Allergy Immunol. 1994; 8:171–177. https://doi.org/10.1089/pai.1994.8.171. Article Google Scholar

22. Strunk R, Mrazek D. Deaths from asthma in childhood: can they be predicted?. N Engl Regional Allergy Proc. 1986; 7:454–461. https://doi.org/10.2500/108854186778984691. CAS Article Google Scholar

23. Peden D. The effect of air pollution in asthma and respiratory allergy–the American experience. Allergy Clin Immunol News. 1995; 7:1–5. Google Scholar

24. Smoller JW, Pollack MH, Otto MW, Rosenbaum JF, Kradin RL. Panic anxiety, dyspnea, and respiratory disease. Am J Respir Crit Care. Med. 1996; 154:6–17. Abstract, Medline, Google Scholar

25. Rietveld S, Creer TL. Psychiatric factors in asthma: implications for diagnosis and therapy. Am J Respir Med. 2003; 2:1–10. Article PubMed Google ScholarCAS Article PubMed Google Scholar

26. Woolcock AJ. Steroid resistant asthma: what is the definition? Eur Respir J. 1993; 6:743–747. CAS PubMed Google Scholar

27. Ayres JG, Miles JF, Barnes PJ. Brittle asthma. Thorax. 1998; 53:315–321. https://doi.org/10.1136/thx.53.4.315. PubMed Central

28. National Asthma Education and Prevention Program. Expert Panel Report: guidelines for the diagnosis and management of asthma: update on selected topics 2002. Bethesda, MD; National Institutes of Health; 2003. NIH Publication No. 02–5074.Google Scholar

29. Djukanović R, Wilson SJ, Kraft M, Jarjour NN, Steel M, Fan Chung K, Bao W, Fowler-Taylor A, Matthews J, Busse WW, et al. Effects of treatment with anti-immunoglobulin E antibody omalizumab on airway inflammation in allergic asthma. Am J Respir Crit Care. Med. 2004; 170:583–593. Abstract, Medline, Google Scholar Crossref, Medline, Google Scholar

30. Osterberg L, Blaschke T. Adherence to medication. N Engl J Med. 2005; 353:487–497.

153

21 Acute Severe Asthma: Diagnosis and Management

Priyank Jain and Deepak Talwar

CONTENTS

INTRODUCTION

Asthma is a heterogeneous disease, characterized by chronic inflammation of the airways and respiratory symptoms that vary over time and in intensity, along with variable expiratory airflow limitation[1]. Airway inflammation, bronchial hyperresponsiveness (BHR), and airway remodelling are the main pathophysiological mechanisms of asthma[2]. The term flare-up, attacks, episodes, status asthmaticus, and acute severe asthma are often used to describe exacerbations. The term 'flare-up' is preferred by GINA as it conveys meaning to laymen better than exacerbation[1]. Status asthmaticus is now replaced by the term acute severe asthma. Exacerbations of asthma are defined as the increase in respiratory symptoms with a decrease in respiratory function that leads to a change in treatment[3]. Exacerbations may occur in already diagnosed patients or as the first presentation of asthma.

Acute severe asthma occurs due to various triggers in patients usually having risk factors for it. Many factors are correlated regarding their risk with acute severe asthma including poor asthma control or adherence to medications[4], female gender[5], smoking, comorbidities[6], older age, and most importantly history of near-fatal asthma/hospitalizations[7]. Exposure to external agents in already sensitized patients produces an inflammatory response leading to exacerbation. These triggers include allergen[8], environmental pollutants[8], respiratory tract infections[9], exercise[10], weather changes[11], and allergies to food and drugs[12].

It is of utmost importance to identify early patients of acute severe asthma or patients at risk, as acute severe asthma is associated with serious consequences such as hospitalization and even death. Early identification and effective management also reduces the health care burden and resource utilization.

DEFINITION OF ACUTE SEVERE ASTHMA

Different societies have given different criteria for defining acute severe asthma (Table 21.1). Although these definitions are not identical, considerable overlap suggests that identifying an exacerbation is necessary, as it correlates with the patient's morbidity and mortality.

The term Critical Asthma Syndromes (CAS) is defined as conditions that can cause respiratory fatigue/arrest and includes acute

DOI: 10.1201/9781003125785-21

Table 21.1: Definition of Acute Severe Asthma

GINA 2020[1]

According to GINA, a patient with severe asthma shows the following:

- talks in words
- leans forward, is agitated
- uses accessory respiratory muscles
- has a respiratory rate > 30/min
- heart rate > 120/min
- O_2 saturation on room air <90%
- and PEF ≤ 50% of their best or predicted value is having acute severe asthma or severe exacerbation

British Guidelines for Asthma 2014[13]

According to the British Guidelines for Asthma, acute severe asthma is defined as an asthma exacerbation in patients with any of the following:

- PEF33–50% best or predicted
- respiratory rate ≥ 25/min
- heart rate ≥ 110/min
- an inability to complete sentences in one breath

ATS/ERS Task Force[3]

According to the ATS/ERS task force, severe asthma is defined as an exacerbation on the basis that these patients require urgent action to prevent a serious outcome. According to the task force, the definition of a severe asthma exacerbation includes at least 1 of the following:

- use of systemic corticosteroids or an increase from a stable maintenance dose, for at least 3 days
- a hospitalization or emergency department visit requiring systemic corticosteroids

severe asthma, refractory asthma, status asthmaticus, and near-fatal asthma[14].

EPIDEMIOLOGY

Asthma affects a large number of people, around 334 million people worldwide, although its prevalence varies among countries. It causes decreased QOL, reduction in pulmonary functions, psychological restraints, absenteeism from work, socioeconomic burden, and an increased health care resource utilization[15]. According to WHO, there are 15–20 million asthmatics in India. The AP-AIM study revealed that in 40% of patients, asthma was uncontrolled, and around 8.4% exacerbations were reported in asthmatic patients every year in India[16].

RISK FACTORS FOR ASTHMA EXACERBATIONS

Many factors are described for their association with the risk of acute severe asthma and related death (Table 21.2).

Table 21.2: Risk Factors for Severe Asthma Exacerbations and Asthma-Related Death

- History of near-fatal asthma/Invasive mechanical ventilation (IMV)[7]
- ≥ 1 severe exacerbation in previous year[7]
- Uncontrolled asthma[17]
- Medications – Inadequate ICS[7], High SABA use[18], Poor adherence and incorrect inhaler technique[4]
- Exposures – Smoking, Allergen[8], Air pollution[8]
- Comorbidities – Obesity, Chronic rhinosinusitis, GERD, Food allergy, Psychosocial problems[6]
- Female gender[5], Older age
- Poor perception of symptoms[19]
- Lack of written asthma action plan[4]

TRIGGERS FOR ASTHMA EXACERBATIONS

Exposure to external agents in already sensitized patients triggers an inflammatory response leading to exacerbation (Table 21.3).

GENETICS AND ASTHMA EXACERBATIONS

Studies on genetic associations with asthma have revealed the role of polymorphisms for IL33, IL1R1/IL18R1, HLA-DQ, SMAD3, and locus on 17q21[20]. The complex-restricted T cell-associated molecule gene (CTARM) was found to associate with increased asthma exacerbation in children[21]. ORMDL3 and GSDMB genes on the 17q12-21 locus are also implicated in affecting asthma risk. The TT allele compared to the CC allele at rs7216389, is associated with increased risk of exacerbation[22].

PATHOGENESIS

Asthma results from complex host-environmental interactions and is classified according to observed characteristics (phenotype) and according to mechanisms (endotype). Inflammatory cells, including eosinophils, neutrophils, mast cells, T-lymphocytes, macrophages, and airway structural cells are responsible for airway inflammation

Table 21.3: Triggers for Asthma Exacerbation

- Respiratory infections (primarily viral)[9]
- Allergen exposure[8]
- Outdoor air pollution[8]
- Tobacco smoke
- Weather change[11],
- Exercise[10]
- Drug and food allergy[12]
- Poor adherence to ICS[4]

and remodelling. Depending on the type of predominant immune cell responses, asthma is categorized as type 2 or non-type 2. Asthma exacerbations triggered by viral infections occur due to a deficient IFN-b response and by allergic sensitization in allergen-induced asthma.

BIOMARKERS

Based on the pathogenesis of asthma, biomarkers were identified to predict exacerbations. Sputum and blood eosinophil counts, serum total IgE, FeNO, and serum periostin are found to be associated with severity of asthma and exacerbations in Th2 asthma patients. Exhaled Breath Condensate (EBC) can also be used in predicting exacerbations[23].

PATHOPHYSIOLOGY

Abnormal gas exchange presents as arterial hypoxemia due to V/Q mismatch and hypercapnia from alveolar hypoventilation because of respiratory muscle fatigue[24]. There is increased airway resistance, decreased lung recoil, mucous impaction, compression of small airways, and hyperinflation, which leads to low flow rates and increased work of breathing. RV, FRC, and TLC may increase, while there is a decrease in the FEV_1 and PEFR. In acute severe asthma, pulsus paradoxus occurs due to the development of positive intrathoracic pressure[25].

CLINICAL ASSESSMENT

Asthma exacerbations are medical emergencies and should be managed in acute care settings. History taking and a physical examination should be done concurrently with initiation of treatment. A brief history includes assessment of triggers, risk factors for exacerbations and asthma related death, time of onset and severity of symptoms, and medications history[1]. In the physical examination, assessment of exacerbation severity (vital signs) should be done, along with evaluation of complicating factors (anaphylaxis, pneumonia, pneumothorax and pneumomediastinum) and signs indicative of alternative diagnosis (heart failure, pulmonary embolism, foreign body and vocal cord dysfunction syndrome)[26]. For assessment of exacerbation severity, objective assessment is also needed along with the history and physical examination. Objective assessment includes measurement of lung function, oxygen saturation (pulse oximetry), chest X-ray and blood gases, whenever needed[1]. PEF or FEV_1 should be measured before starting the treatment, after 1 hour and until

there is clear response to treatment. ABG measurements should be done in patients having $FEV_1 < 50\%$, clinical deterioration or drowsiness[27]. Chest X-ray is useful if a complicating factor or alternative diagnosis is suspected[28]. The patient's management is guided according to exacerbation severity (Figure 21.1).

MANAGEMENT

In acute care settings, therapy for acute severe asthma includes bronchodilators, systemic corticosteroids, controlled oxygen and respiratory support if needed (Table 21.4). Magnesium sulphate should be considered if the patient is not responding to standard treatment (Figure 21.1).

Bronchodilators

SABAs are the choice of bronchodilators. Combination of SABA along with ipratropium bromide should be used in all patients with severe asthma exacerbations[29]. It should be given from pMDI with a spacer[30]. If the patient is too sick to take MDI, bronchodilators should be delivered with a nebulizer in the form of continuous nebulization. The role of ICS-LABA combinations in acute asthma is unclear, and there is limited evidence to support its use[31].

Corticosteroids

Systemic corticosteroids should be given to all patients with severe exacerbation and should be considered in non-severe exacerbations not responding to bronchodilators, patient already on OCS or those having a history of exacerbation requiring OCS[1]. Corticosteroids fasten improvement and also prevent relapse[32]. Oral administration is equally effective as the parental route except in sick patients[33]. ICS are not routinely recommended in acute asthma, as they don't provide any additional benefit. However, their dose should be increased for 2–4 weeks at discharge[34].

Antibiotics

Antibiotics are not given routinely unless the patient is having signs or symptoms suggestive of infection (viz., purulent expectoration, fever or pneumonia)[35].

Magnesium Sulphate

IV magnesium sulphate is not routinely given to patients with acute asthma. It should be considered in severe exacerbations patients, those not responding to the standard therapy or with FEV_1 <30% predicted at presentation[36].

Mechanical Ventilation

There is no recommendation regarding the use of NIV in acute asthma because of the paucity of data[37]. A trial of NIV should be given before invasive mechanical ventilation, if no contraindication is present[38]. Indication to IMV includes cardiac or respiratory arrest, coma, severe and refractory hypoxemia, hemodynamic instability, and exhaustion leading to progressive respiratory acidosis superimposed on metabolic acidosis[39]. Endotracheal intubation done using rapid sequence intubation (RSI) includes pre-oxygenation, induction with anaesthetic agents (ketamine, propofol), and tube placement. The goals of mechanical ventilation are to maintain oxygenation, to reduce the work of breathing, and to prevent/decrease dynamic hyperinflation, along with a lung-protective strategy (to prevent VILI)[40].

Oxygen Therapy

Oxygen is given to patients of acute severe asthma to maintain an arterial oxygen saturation of 93–95%[1]. Oxygen delivery can be done through nasal cannula, a face mask, or any of the other oxygen delivery devices, depending on the clinical need[41]. High Flow Nasal Cannula (HFNC) is a new modality that can be tried in patients not responding to conventional therapies[42]. There is a paucity of data on the role of HFNC in asthmatic adults.

ECLS (Extra Corporeal Life Support)

ECLS for patients of acute severe asthma includes ECMO (extracorporeal membrane oxygenation) and $ECCO_2R$ (extracorporeal carbon dioxide removal). There is a lack of evidence for the use of ECMO & $ECCO_2R$ in patients with exacerbation—limited evidence suggests that it could be given as additional support in patients whose gas exchange abnormality persists, despite being given optimized conventional therapy[43].

Other Therapies

1. IM epinephrine should be used in case of anaphylaxis or angioedema complicating exacerbation, along with standard treatment or if there is no response to standard therapy[44].

2. Methylxanthines should not be used routinely in asthma exacerbations because of potentially harmful side effects and they have no additional benefit over standard therapy[45].

3. Heliox is not recommended for routine use. It may be given to the patients who do not improve or deteriorate on standard therapy[46].

4. There is limited evidence for use of LTRAs in acute asthma[47].

5. Sedation should not be used during the period of acute asthma.

6. Anaesthetic agents such as Halothane, Isoflurane, and sevoflurane act as bronchodilators, probably not only through a direct relaxation effect on airway smooth muscles but also by attenuating cholinergic tone. But there are no randomized controlled trials to evaluate and confirm their efficacy in near-death adult asthmatic patients. Hence, their usage is a last resort measure[48].

7. Enoximone is an intravenous selective phosphodiesterase III inhibitor, bronchodilator agent that can be used in severe asthma exacerbation in adults. It has been shown to have an immediate bronchodilator effect. But further studies are needed to confirm enoximone efficacy and safety[49].

Prevention and Risk Reduction

1. ICS containing controller treatment should be given to all patients of asthma.

2. Asthma treatment should be optimised.

3. Adherence to treatment and use of the correct inhaler technique must be checked.

4. Comorbidities should be assessed and managed accordingly.

5. Modifiable risk factors (smoking, allergen and environmental exposure, medications) should be assessed.

6. Nonpharmacological interventions (smoking cessation, vaccination, weight loss, and exercise) should be utilised.

7. Phenotypic assessments should be done and considered for add-on therapy in severe, refractory asthma.

8. Written asthma action plan and guided self-management education, including monitoring of lung function and symptoms should be provided to all asthma patients.

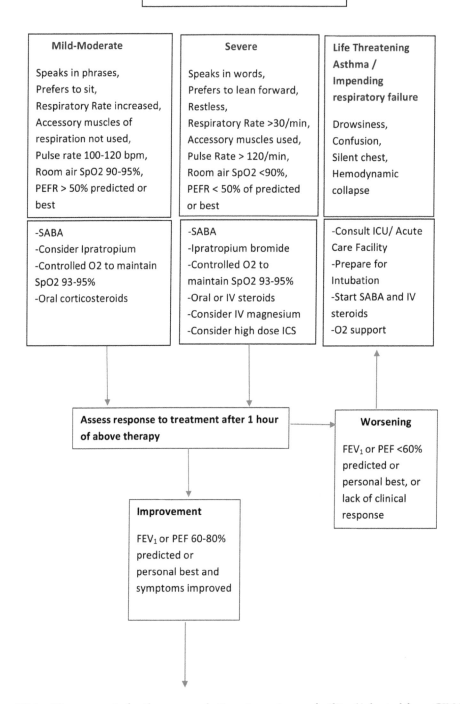

Figure 21.1 Management of asthma exacerbations in acute care facility. (Adapted from GINA 2020 Recommendations.) PEF: Peak expiratory flow; FEV$_1$: forced expiratory volume in 1 second; SABA, short-acting beta-2 agonists; ICU, intensive care unit; ED, emergency department. (*Continued*)

Discharge assessment	Arrange at discharge
-Clinically improving with no further SABA requirement -PEF/FEV$_1$ improving, and 60-80% of personal best or predicted -Room air SpO$_2$ >94% -Adequate care available at home	-Reliever: Continue as needed -Controller: Start or step up. Check inhaler technique, adherence. -Prednisolone: continue, usually for 5-7 days -Provide a written asthma action plan

Follow-up with in first week of discharge

Review symptoms and signs
Reliever: reduce to as needed
Controller: continue higher dose for initial two weeks or long term (3 months) depending on background to exacerbation
Risk factors: check and correct modifiable risk factors

Figure 21.1 (*Continued*)

CONCLUSION

Acute severe asthma causes significant morbidity and mortality in asthma patients and results in functional impairment and increased health care utilization. Asthma exacerbation can occur irrespective of underlying disease severity, phenotype, or even in patients having optimized treatment and well-controlled asthma. Prevention of exacerbations remains a major goal in asthma management. Early identification of patients at risk of exacerbation is needed to prevent and decrease the exacerbations. A better understanding of the pathogenesis of asthma exacerbation is an unmet need. Novel targeted therapies are required to prevent exacerbations in asthmatics.

Table 21.4: Pharmacological Management of Acute Severe Asthma

Medication	Dosing
Salbutamol	2.5 mg/2.5 ml (each dose), continuous nebulization for an hour and then re-assess for clinical response pMDI with spacer (recommended): up to 4–10 puffs every 20 minutes for the first hour, followed by 4–10 puffs every 3–4 hours, or more often
Ipratropium bromide	Nebulization of 0.5 mg/2.5 ml every 4–6 hours, along with salbutamol
Corticosteroids	OCS equivalent to 50 mg prednisolone or IV Hydrocortisone 200 mg in divided dose should be given for 5–7 days
Magnesium sulphate	Single intravenous infusion of 2 gm over 20 min
Methylxanthines	Not used routinely; potential harmful side effects and no added benefit
LTRAs	Not recommended in routine management
Heliox	Helium and oxygen combination in an 80:20 ratio
Epinephrine	0.3–0.5 mg (1 mg/ml, 1:1000) every 20 min, 3 doses if no response

REFERENCES

1. GINA-2020-report_20_06_04-1-wms.pdf [Internet]. [cited 2020 Dec 8]. Available from: https://ginasthma.org/wp-content/uploads/2020/06/GINA-2020-report_20_06_04-1-wms.pdf

2. O'Byrne PM, Inman MD. Airway hyperresponsiveness. Chest. 2003; 123:411S–416S.

3. An Official American Thoracic Society/European Respiratory Society Statement: Asthma Control and Exacerbations | Standardizing Endpoints for Clinical Asthma Trials and Clinical Practice | American Journal of Respiratory and Critical Care Medicine [Internet]. [cited 2020 Dec 8]. Available from: https://www.atsjournals.org/doi/full/10.1164/rccm.200801-060ST

4. Psychological, social and health behaviour risk factors for deaths certified as asthma: a national case-control study | Thorax [Internet]. [cited 2020 Dec 8]. Available from: https://thorax.bmj.com/content/57/12/1034.abstract

5. Skobeloff EM, Spivey WH, Clair SSS, Schoffstall JM. The influence of age and sex on asthma admissions. JAMA. 1992; 268:3437–4340.

6. Denlinger LC, Phillips BR, Ramratnam S, Ross K, Bhakta NR, Cardet JC, et al. Inflammatory and comorbid features of patients with severe asthma and frequent exacerbations. Am J Respir Crit Care Med. 2016; 195:302–313.

7. A Systematic Review of Risk Factors Associated with Near-Fatal and Fatal Asthma [Internet]. [cited 2020 Dec 8]. Available from: https://www.hindawi.com/journals/crj/2005/837645/

8. Trasande L, Thurston GD. The role of air pollution in asthma and other pediatric morbidities. J Allergy Clin Immunol. 2005; 115:689–699.

9. Community study of role of viral infections in exacerbations of asthma in 9–11-year- old children | BMJ. [Internet]. [cited 2020 Dec 8]. Available from: https://www.bmj.com/content/310/6989/1225

10. Jayasinghe H, Kopsaftis Z, Carson K. Asthma bronchiale and exercise-induced bronchoconstriction. Respiration. 2015; 89:505–512.

11. The impact of cold on the respiratory tract and its consequences to respiratory health. Clinical and Translational Allergy. | Full Text [Internet]. [cited 2020 Dec 8]. Available from: https://ctajournal.biomedcentral.com/articles/10.1186/s13601-018-0208-9

12. Berns SH, Halm EA, Sampson HA, Sicherer SH, Busse PJ, Wisnivesky JP. Food allergy as a risk factor for asthma morbidity in adults. J Asthma. 2007; 44:377–381.

13. Society BPGL and BT. Chapters 1-3. Thorax. 2003; 58:i1–16.

14. Kenyon N, Zeki AA, Albertson TE, Louie S. Definition of critical asthma syndromes. Clin Rev Allergy Immunol. 2015; 48:1–6.

15. Global, regional, and national deaths, prevalence, disability-adjusted life years, and years lived with disability for chronic obstructive pulmonary disease and asthma, 1990–2015: a systematic analysis for the Global Burden of Disease Study 2015 - Lancet Resp Medicine. [Internet]. [cited 2020 Dec 8]. Available from: https://www.thelancet.com/journals/lanres/article/PIIS2213-2600(17)30293-X/fulltext

16. Salvi SS, Apte KK, Dhar R, Shetty P, Faruqi RA, Thompson PJ, et al. Asthma insights and management in India: lessons learnt from the Asia Pacific—Asthma Insights and Management (AP-AIM) Study. J Assoc Physicians India. 2015; 63:36–43.

17. Medications that reduce emergency hospital admissions: an overview of systematic reviews and prioritisation of treatments | BMC Medicine. | Full Text [Internet]. [cited 2020 Dec 8]. Available from: https://bmcmedicine.biomedcentral.com/articles/10.1186/s12916-018-1104-9

18. Suissa S, Blais L, Ernst P. Patterns of increasing beta-agonist use and the risk of fatal or near-fatal asthma. Eur Respir J. 1994; 7:1602–1609.

19. Killian KJ, Watson R, Otis J, St. Amand TA, O'Byrne PM. Symptom perception during acute bronchoconstriction. Am J Respir Crit Care Med. 2000; 162:490–496.

20. Genetic risk factors for the development of allergic disease identified by genome-wide association - Portelli - 2015 - Clinical; Experimental Allergy - Wiley Online Library [Internet]. [cited 2020 Dec 8]. Available from: https://onlinelibrary.wiley.com/doi/10.1111/cea.12327

21. Du R, Litonjua AA, Tantisira KG, Lasky-Su J, Sunyaev SR, Klanderman BJ, et al. Genome-wide association study reveals class I MHC–restricted T cell–associated molecule gene (CRTAM) variants interact with vitamin D levels to affect asthma exacerbations. J Allergy Clin Immunol. 2012; 129:368-373.e5.

22. Tavendale R, Macgregor DF, Mukhopadhyay S, Palmer CNA. A polymorphism controlling ORMDL3 expression is associated with asthma that is poorly controlled by current medications. J Allergy Clin Immunol. 2008; 121:860–863.

23. Robroeks CMHHT, van Vliet D, Jöbsis Q, Braekers R, Rijkers GT, Wodzig WKWH, et al. Prediction of asthma exacerbations in children: results of a one-year prospective study. Clin Exp Allergy J Br Soc Allergy Clin Immunol. 2012; 42:792–798.

24. Rodriguez-Roisin R. Acute severe asthma: pathophysiology and pathobiology of gas exchange abnormalities. Eur Respir J. 1997; 10:1359–71.

25. Pepe PE, Marini JJ. Occult positive end-expiratory pressure in mechanically ventilated patients with airflow obstruction: the auto-PEEP effect. Am Rev Respir Dis. 1982; 126:166–170.

26. Differentiating vocal cord dysfunction from asthma | JAA [Internet]. [cited 2020 Dec 9]. Available from: https://www.dovepress.com/differentiating-vocal-cord-dysfunction-from-asthma-peer-reviewed-article-JAA

27. Carruthers DM, Harrison BD. Arterial blood gas analysis or oxygen saturation in the assessment of acute asthma? Thorax. 1995; 50:186–188.

28. White CS, Cole RP, Lubetsky HW, Austin JH. Acute asthma: admission chest radiography in hospitalized adult patients. Chest. 1991; 100:14–16.

29. Kirkland SW, Vandenberghe C, Voaklander B, Nikel T, Campbell S, Rowe BH. Combined inhaled beta-agonist and anticholinergic agents for emergency management in adults with asthma. Cochrane Database Syst Rev. 2017; 1:CD001284.

30. Newman KB, Milne S, Hamilton C, Hall K. A comparison of albuterol administered by metered-dose inhaler and spacer with albuterol by nebulizer in adults presenting to an urban emergency department with acute asthma. Chest. 2002; 121:1036–1041.

31. Peters JI, Shelledy DC, Jones AP, Lawson RW, Davis CP, LeGrand TS. A randomized, placebo-controlled study to evaluate the role of salmeterol in the in-hospital management of asthma. Chest. 2000; 118:313–320.

32. Corticosteroids for preventing relapse following acute exacerbations of asthma - Rowe, BH - 2007 | Cochrane Library [Internet]. [cited 2020 Dec 9]. Available from: https://www.cochranelibrary.com/cdsr/doi/10.1002/14651858.CD000195.pub2/full

33. Ratto D, Alfaro C, Sipsey J, Glovsky MM, Sharma OP. Are intravenous corticosteroids required in status asthmaticus? JAMA. 1988; 260:527–529.

34. Rowe BH, Vethanayagam D. The role of inhaled corticosteroids in the management of acute asthma. Eur Respir J. 2007; 30:1035–7.

35. Antibiotics for exacerbations of asthma - Normansell, R - 2018 | Cochrane Library [Internet]. [cited 2020 Dec 9]. Available from: https://www.cochranelibrary.com/cdsr/doi/10.1002/14651858.CD002741.pub2/full

36. Rowe B, Bretzlaff J, Bourdon C, Bota G, Camargo C. Magnesium sulfate is effective for severe acute asthma treated in the emergency department. West J Med. 2000; 172:96.

37. Lim WJ, Mohammed Akram R, Carson KV, Mysore S, Labiszewski NA, Wedzicha JA, et al. Non-invasive positive pressure ventilation for treatment of respiratory failure due to severe acute exacerbations of asthma. Cochrane Database Syst Rev. 2012; 12:CD004360.

38. Pallin M, Naughton MT. Noninvasive ventilation in acute asthma. J Crit Care. 2014; 29:586–593.

39. Davidson AC, Banham S, Elliott M, Kennedy D, Gelder C, Glossop A, et al. BTS/ICS guideline for the ventilatory management of acute hypercapnic respiratory failure in adults. Thorax. 2016; 71:ii1–35.

40. Risk Factors for Morbidity in Mechanically Ventilated Patients with Acute Severe Asthma | American Review of Respiratory Disease [Internet]. [cited 2020 Dec 9]. Available from: https://www.atsjournals.org/doi/abs/10.1164/ajrccm/146.3.607

41. Perrin K, Wijesinghe M, Healy B, Wadsworth K, Bowditch R, Bibby S, et al. Randomised controlled trial of high concentration versus titrated oxygen therapy in severe exacerbations of asthma. Thorax. 2011; 66:937–941.

42. Pilar J, Modesto i Alapont V, Lopez-Fernandez YM, Lopez-Macias O, Garcia-Urabayen D, Amores-Hernandez I. High-flow nasal cannula therapy versus non-invasive ventilation in children with severe acute asthma exacerbation: an observational cohort study. Med Intensiva. 2017; 41:418–424.

43. Mikkelsen ME, Woo YJ, Sager JS, Fuchs BD, Christie JD. Outcomes using extracorporeal life support for adult respiratory failure due to status asthmaticus. ASAIO J. 2009; 55:47–52.

44. Rodrigo GJ, Nannini LJ. Comparison between nebulized adrenaline and β2 agonists for the treatment of acute asthma. A meta-analysis of randomized trials. Am J Emerg Med. 2006; 24:217–222.

45. Nair P, Milan SJ, Rowe BH. Addition of intravenous aminophylline to inhaled beta(2)-agonists in adults with acute asthma. Cochrane Database Syst Rev. 2012; 12:CD002742.

46. Rodrigo GJ, Rodrigo C, Pollack CV, Rowe B. Use of helium-oxygen mixtures in the treatment of acute asthma: a systematic review. Chest. 2003; 123:891–896.

47. Camargo CA, Smithline HA, Malice M-P, Green SA, Reiss TF. A randomized controlled trial of intravenous montelukast in acute asthma. Am J Respir Crit Care Med. 2003; 167:528–533.

48. Vaschetto R, Bellotti E, Turucz E, Gregoretti C, Della Corte F, Navalesi P. Inhalational anesthetics in acute severe asthma [Internet]. Vol. 10(9), Current Drug Targets. 2009 [cited 2020 Dec 9]: p. 826–832. Available from: https://www.eurekaselect.com/70037/article

49. Nanchal R, Kumar G, Majumdar T, Taneja A, Patel J, Dagar G, et al. Utilization of mechanical ventilation for asthma exacerbations: analysis of a national database. Respir Care. 2014; 59:644–653.

22 Allergic Bronchopulmonary Aspergillosis (ABPA)

Venugopal Panicker and Arjun Suresh

CONTENTS

INTRODUCTION

Allergic bronchopulmonary aspergillosis (ABPA) is a pulmonary disorder caused by hypersensitivity to *Aspergillus fumigatus* (*A. fumigatus*) that complicates the course of patients with asthma and cystic fibrosis (CF).[1,2] Alhough ABPA was described first in 1952, awareness of the disease is low, with around one-third of patients in developing countries being misdiagnosed as having tuberculosis.[2] The disease occurs in patients with exposure to aspergillus spores, followed by their germination and colonization of the respiratory tract with a subsequent allergic response. Patients usually present with symptoms that are usually attributable to underlying diagnosis; this often results in a delay in diagnosis. Most cases are diagnosed in the third to fifth decade of life but can occur at any age. Treatment aims at reduction in inflammatory response either by steroids or reduction in antigen load. Focus must be on early diagnosis and treatment which may result in long-term remission and can prevent lung damage.

PATHOPHYSIOLOGY

The pathogenesis of ABPA is not completely understood, but is believed to be an exaggerated immunological response to chronic colonization of *Aspergillus* spp. Aspergillus is a ubiquitous fungi and grows optimally at body temperature.[4] In healthy individuals, fungal spores are usually cleared from the body. However in an allergic host, spores germinate in the lung with subsequent colonization, which results in an exaggerated Th2 response. The factors which influence colonization are poorly understood but are believed to be due to host factors which

DOI: 10.1201/9781003125785-22

Table 22.1: Genetic Factors That Increase the Risk of ABPA[6,7]

- CFTR mutations
- HLA-DR2/DR5 restriction
- IL-4Rα SNPs
- IL-10 promoter genotype
- Chitotriosidase 1 (CHIT1) exon 10 mutation
- Polymorphisms in the promoter region of the pathogen associated molecular pattern receptor, Toll-like receptor (TLR) 9
- Lung surfactant protein-A-2 gene polymorphisms
- Integrin β3 polymorphisms
- Disintegrin polymorphisms
- Metalloprotease gene polymorphisms
- Protocadherin 1 polymorphisms
- **MHC DQ2 allele may be protective**

(CFTR—Cystic fibrosis transmembrane conductance regulator, HLA-DR—Human Leukocyte Antigen-DR isotype, IL—interleukin, SNPs—single nucleotide polymorphisms.)

include genetic factors (Table 22.1), abnormalities in the airway mucosal defences of patients with asthma and cystic fibrosis, corticosteroid treatment or antibiotic misuse and the level of environmental exposure to the fungus.[5] ABPA develops only in a low percentage of asthmatics exposed constantly to the fungus, indicating a genetic predisposition.

Aspergillus proteolytic products can cause inflammation and increased antigen penetration into airway walls.[1,4] Aspergillus-derived proteases may stimulate proinflammatory cytokines, such as IL-8, and may also cause tissue damage and cell death as well as detachment, resulting in the development of bronchiectasis.[1,8]

Mycelial antigens are processed by dendritic cells, resulting in the release of cytokines and antigen presentation to T lymphocytes. In a normal host, this results in activation of nonallergic T helper (Th-1) and allergic (Th2) lymphocytes. The Th1 response results in macrophage and neutrophil cytotoxic action and the production of IgG and IgA antibodies, which may protect against aspergillus infection. Th2 response results in synthesis and secretion of IL-4, IL-5, IL-10, and IL-13 and immunoglobulin elaboration that mediate allergic inflammation.[1]

Th2 response predominates in allergic persons and this is greatest in ABPA. Th2 response also results in influx of macrophages and eosinophils. IL-10 down regulates Th1 CD4 + T cells, further skewing the responses to a Th2 pattern. IL-4 and IL-13 induce IgE isotype switching of B cells.[4,9]

Immunologic studies reveal the presence of a type I hypersensitivity reaction reflected by elevated serum levels of total IgE and *A. fumigatus*-specific IgE. An exaggerated Type III hypersensitivity reaction is indicated by the presence of *A. fumigatus*-specific IgG antibodies (classically called "precipitins" or precipitating antibodies) and circulating immune complexes during exacerbations. A type IV cell-mediated immune reaction may also play a role, as dual (immediate and delayed) cutaneous reactions and an in vitro lymphocyte transformation to *A. fumigatus* antigen stimulation have been noted in some patients.[10]

DIAGNOSIS

One of the earliest diagnostic criteria to have had widespread acceptance was Rosenberg–Patterson criteria (Table 22.2).[11] ISHAM proposed a modified diagnostic criterion, and this is now widely accepted (Table 22.3).

The criterion was refined in 2016 to include COPD and post tubercular fibrocavitary disease as predisposing factors and the presence of precipitating antibodies was replaced by *A. fumigatus*-specific IgE of more than 0.35 kU_A/l However, this needs validation.[2,12]

Features on HRCT chest and/or chest radiograph consistent with ABPA include transient abnormalities (i.e. nodules, consolidation, mucoid impaction, hyperattenuating mucus (HAM), fleeting opacities (toothpaste/gloved finger opacities, tram-track opacities), or permanent opacities (parallel lines, ring shadows, bronchiectasis and pleuropulmonary fibrosis).

ABPA is subdivided based on radiology into serological ABPA (ABPA-S), ABPA with

Table 22.2: Rosenberg-Patterson 1977 Criteria for Diagnosis of ABPA

Primary criteria (1–6 suggestive, +7 definite)

1. Episodic bronchial obstruction
2. Peripheral eosinophilia
3. Positive immediate skin test to Aspergillus
4. Positive precipitin test to Aspergillus
5. Increased total serum IgE
6. History of transient or fixed lung infiltrates
7. Proximal bronchiectasis

Secondary (supportive) criteria

1. Brown plugs/flecks in sputum
2. Positive late (6–12 h/Arthus) skin test to Aspergillus

Table 22.3: ABPA Working Group Criteria (ISHAM Criteria)

1. **Predisposing asthma or CF**
2. **Obligatory criteria**
   a. IgE > 1000 IU/mL and
   b. Positive immediate skin test or increased IgE antibody to Aspergillus
3. **Supportive criteria**
   a. Eosinophilia >500
   b. Precipitins or increased IgG antibody to Aspergillus
   c. Consistent radiographic opacities

bronchiectasis (ABPA-B), ABPA with high-attenuation mucus (ABPA-HAM), and ABPA with chronic pleuropulmonary fibrosis (ABPA-CPF)[2] (Table 22.4).

Patients with ABPA-CB, especially those with HAM, have a higher relapse rate, more immunologically severe disease, more severe clinical features, more serious small airway ventilatory dysfunction and more often associated with significantly higher peripheral eosinophil counts.[13]

Patients of ABPA have been reported rarely without asthma or CF. However, many such patients develop asthma along the course and may indicate a pre-clinical phase of disease.

ASPERGILLUS SKIN TEST

An immediate cutaneous hypersensitivity on skin testing of Aspergillus extract (commercial or in-house) done either by a skin prick test or intradermal injection can be used as surrogate marker for allergic sensitization to Aspergillus and usually represents IgE antibodies specific to *A. fumigatus*.[14] Intradermal tests are more sensitive.[15] The risk of anaphylaxis, the need for trained personnel and standardized antigen availability has led to a reduction in its role as a screening test.[12] SPT is preferred over intradermal testing because higher false positive results are seen with latter.[7] A negative prick skin

Table 22.4: Radiological Classification of ABPA Based on Computed Tomographic (CT) Chest Findings

ABPA-S (Serological ABPA)	All the diagnostic features of ABPA but no abnormality resulting from ABPA on HRCT chest
ABPA-B (ABPA with bronchiectasis)	All the diagnostic features of ABPA, including bronchiectasis on HRCT chest
ABPA-HAM (ABPA with high attenuation mucus)	All the diagnostic features of ABPA, including the presence of high-attenuation mucus

test followed by negative intradermal reactivity to Aspergillus virtually excludes ABPA.[7]

A. fumigatus-SPECIFIC IgE

Elevated IgE are considered hallmarks of ABPA however the cut-off value for diagnosis of ABPA is still widely debated. ISHAM working group proposed a cut-off value >0.35 kU_A/l which has a sensitivity of 100% and specificity of 66%. Hence the test can be used as an excellent screening test. Due to significant variability, it has no role in follow-up or assessing treatment.[12]

TOTAL IgE

Total IgE levels are elevated in patients with ABPA and do not usually return to normal levels despite treatment; the lowest value in the course of treatment is taken as the 'new' baseline.[16]

A latent class analysis showed that a cut-off of 1000 IU/ml has a sensitivity of 92% and specificity of 40% for the diagnosis of ABPA. A cut-off value 1000 IU/ml is recommended by the ISHAM group and appears appropriate, with an allowance for a lower value if all other criteria are met.[2,17]

The serum IgE is an important tool in follow-up of patients, and an increase in IgE levels may signify an impending exacerbation. An increasing level (>50% of the 'new' baseline) of total IgE, along with worsening respiratory symptoms and the appearance of consistent radiological findings, suggests an exacerbation of ABPA.[17]

TOTAL EOSINOPHIL COUNT

Peripheral eosinophilia is nonspecific and not always seen. Often, peripheral blood eosinophilia does not correlate with pulmonary eosinophilia. Patients on oral steroids can have lower or even normal eosinophil levels. Upon reflecting on the above-mentioned problems, the ISHAM working group has reduced the relevance of eosinophilia in the diagnosis of ABPA.[2]

PRECIPITATING ASPERGILLUS ANTIBODIES

Serum precipitins against *A. fumigatus* are seen in 69–90% of patients with ABPA and 10% of asthmatics with or without SAFS.[18,19] The *A. fumigatus*-specific IgG antibodies have traditionally been detected using the double diffusion technique of Ouchterlony (*Aspergillus precipitins*).[20] Newer immunoassays can be used to detect or confirm specific IgG antibodies against Aspergillus antigens and may be more sensitive than serum precipitins.[21] The sensitivity and specificity of *A. fumigatus*-specific IgG at a cutoff of 27 mgA/L was

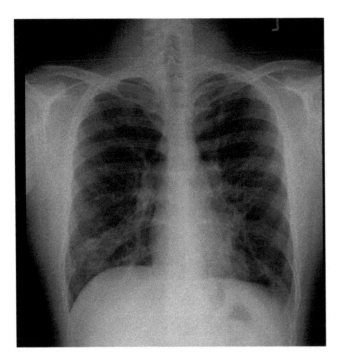

Figure 22.1   X-ray chest showing central bronchiectasis. (Picture courtesy of Dr Resmi Sekhar.)

around 89% and 100%, respectively in the diagnosis of ABPA, which makes it a good 'rule-in' test.[22] Aspergillus IgG is not specific for ABPA because high levels are often seen in other forms of aspergillosis, especially CPA.

SPUTUM CULTURE FOR
Aspergillus fumigatus

The vast majority of ABPA patients show the presence of Aspergillus on nucleic acid detection, but culture positivity is seen only in 40–60%.[23] As Aspergillus is ubiquitous, and colonization can occur without the development of ABPA, the diagnostic value is poor.

RADIOLOGY
Chest X-ray (Figure 22.1)

Chest X-ray may be normal in around 50% patients, making it a poor screening tool, but its utility is primarily as a follow-up tool.[13]

CXR findings are described in Table 22.5

HIGH-RESOLUTION CT SCAN (TABLE 22.6)

HRCT is the investigation of choice in suspected patient with ABPA. Radiological features can be either transient or permanent, based on the temporal manifestation of ABPA.[12] Nodules, consolidation, tram track opacities, finger in glove appearance and fleeting densities are the commonly seen transient abnormalities; while permanent

abnormalities described are ring shadows, bronchiectasis, and pleuropulmonary fibrosis, occasionally cavitation, localized emphysema and contracted upper lobe.[24] Fleeting shadows may be seen on CXR or HRCT and are seen in around 89% of patients with ABPA.[7]

The common HRCT findings are bronchiectasis with or without mucous impaction, consolidation, mosaic attenuation of lungs, centrilobular nodules with or without tree in bud appearance and chronic pleuropulmonary fibrotic changes. Bronchiectasis usually has an upper lobe

Table 22.5: X-ray Findings in ABPA

- "Tram line" shadows—due to thickened walls of nondilated bronchi
- "Parallel lines"—due to the presence of ectatic bronchi
- "Ring shadows"—due to bronchial wall thickening or saccular bronchiectasis
- "Toothpaste shadows"— due to mucoid impacted second- to fourth-order bronchi
- "Gloved finger shadows"—due to intrabronchial exudates with bronchial wall thickening, which appear as branched tubular radiodensities 2–3 cm long and 5–8 mm wide that extend from the hilum
- Perihilar opacities due to mucus plugging may mimic hilar adenopathy
- Fleeting infiltrates
- Fixed changes: Bronchiectatic cavities

Table 22.6: HRCT Findings in ABPA

Bronchial abnormalities

Bronchiectasis, usually central, as characterized by the "signet ring" and "string of pearls" appearances

Dilated bronchi with or without air–fluid levels

Totally occluded bronchi

Bronchial wall thickening

Parallel-line opacities extending to the periphery

High attenuation mucus plugs

Parenchymal changes

Consolidation

Non-homogeneous patchy opacities

Parenchymal scarring of varying extent

Segmental or lobar collapse

Cavitation

Emphysematous bullae

predilection with it being central in around two-third of patients.[13] Central bronchiectasis is an arbitrary definition which is used to describe bronchiectasis limited to the inner two-thirds or central half of the lungs[25] (Figure 22.2). Although CB is considered sine qua non for ABPA, peripheral bronchiectasis is seen in around 29–36% of involved lobes.[26]

Mucoid impaction (Figure 22.3) and atelectasis usually segmental or subsegmental are seen that rarely can involve the whole lung. Mucous plugs are often hypodense; however higher

attenuation is seen in around 20–30% of cases, described as 'high-attenuation mucus (HAM).'[27] HAM, defined as mucus visually denser than paraspinal skeletal muscle, is a pathognomonic finding of ABPA (Figure 22.4). Hyperattenuating mucoid impaction has a specificity of 100% (sensitivity 19–32%), which makes it an excellent 'rule-in' test.[28] Upper lobe pleural thickening, fibro cavitary disease and aspergilloma may indicate the development of CPA. HAM is believed to be due to the presence of calcium salts and metals (the ions of iron and manganese) or desiccated mucus.[29] The presence of HAM correlates with a poorly controlled course of ABPA.

Pleural findings may be seen in around 40% and include pleural effusions, spontaneous pneumothorax, bronchopleural fistula, and pleural thickening.[30]

MAGNETIC RESONANCE IMAGING

The role of MRI is usually limited to patients in whom radiation exposure may not be safe, especially in pregnancy. MRI can also detect HAM; however, this needs more evidence and validation.[12]

LUNG FUNCTION TESTING

Lung function usually varies with the stage of disease, exacerbation and therapy. An obstructive airflow pattern may be seen, especially during exacerbations. A normal PFT may be seen despite

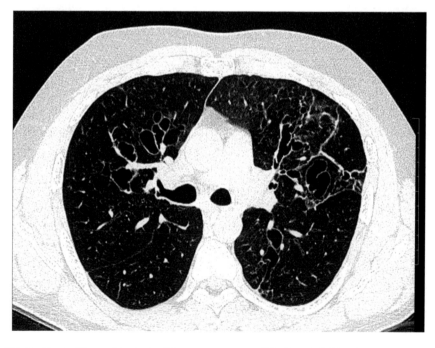

Figure 22.2   Central bronchiectasis. (Picture courtesy of Dr Resmi Sekhar.)

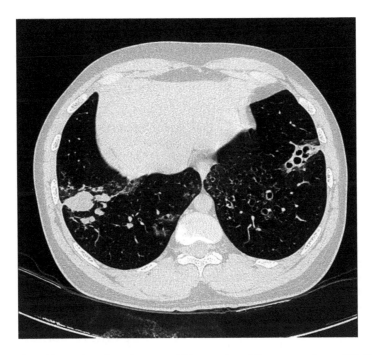

Figure 22.3 Dilated bronchus showing mucoid impaction. (Picture courtesy of Dr Resmi Sekhar.)

the presence of bronchiectasis, if asthma is well controlled. A restrictive pattern with impaired DLCO has also been reported and is seen more in patients with stage 5 disease. Further, a mixed pattern may also be seen.[31]

NEWER TESTS
Recombinant Aspergillus Antigens
Asp f1, Asp f2, Asp f3, Asp f4, Asp f6 are now available commercially for use in the clinical setting; however, their use needs further evidence and validation. Recombinant antigens may also play a role in differentiating ABPA from SAFS.[32]

Basophil Activation Tests
It detect upregulation of CD203c on the basophil surface after antigenic stimulation in sensitized patients, have shown promise in distinguishing ABPA from fungal colonization and CF related ABPA.[33]

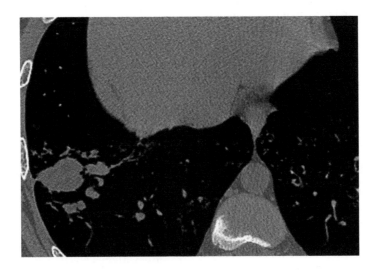

Figure 22.4 The high-attenuation mucus (HAM) with 111 HF density (usual value above 70 HF). (Picture courtesy of Dr Resmi Sekhar.)

CLINICAL FEATURES

ABPA can been seen among all ages (more in the 20- to 40-year age group) and sexes. Symptomatology can range from being asymptomatic or incidentally detected on a workup of asthma to a fatal destructive lung disease. Clinical presentation usually bears no correlation with duration of disease or its severity. Up to one-third of patients with significant lung damage may be relatively asymptomatic.[7]

Patients in exacerbation often present with fever, malaise, fatigue, cough with expectoration and haemoptysis. Clinical examination may show evidence of consolidation or atelectasis. The most common symptoms seen are breathlessness, cough, expectoration and pleuritic chest pain. Patients also can have non-specific complaints like anorexia, fatigue, generalized aches and pains, low-grade fever and loss of weight. Expectoration of brownish-black mucous plugs is specific but seen quite variably (in around 30–70%).[2] Features and examination findings of bronchiectasis and cor-pulmonale may be seen. Clubbing is uncommon and is seen in patients with long-standing bronchiectasis.

CLINICAL STAGES OF ABPA

ABPA conventionally was staged based on stages proposed by Patterson and Greenberg in 1982.[34] Based on clinicoradiological as well as immunological profile, 5 groups have been identified and described in Table 22.6.

The ISHAM working group has proposed a newer staging system to overcome the lack of precise definitions and to promote research into therapeutics (Table 22.7). It is important to understand that neither staging represents the natural evolution of the disease.[2,7]

It is important to note that seldom does the IgE level fall to normal after therapy; however, IgE levels do fall progressively with therapy and the nadir is considered new baseline. Further therapy does not aim to normalize IgE levels but to improve clinical and radiological features with a fall in IgE of 25–50% (Figure 22.5). Even in advanced stages, the disease can be clinically as well as immunologically active, thus requiring therapy.[2]

TREATMENT

The major goals of therapy are to attain symptom control whilst reducing pulmonary inflammation and exacerbation and to prevent lung damage.

Two approaches can summarize treatment options in ABPA:

1. Controlling the immune response
2. Decreasing the burden of organisms to decrease host exposure to the stimulus[31]

Control of the immune response is currently best achieved by steroids, which are the main stay in treatment of ABPA. Reduction in the antigen burden is established by antifungals which have been shown to be an effective add-on in patients with poor control despite steroid therapy, as well as being a safer alternative—though with slightly reduced efficacy.

Without treatment ABPA can result in significant lung damage; hence treatment is advised even in newly detected cases with controlled asthma. Treatment with either steroids or azoles are preferred.[35] Treatment of ABPA-S might prevent further lung damage and prevent progression of the disease. However, evidence is sparse. ABPA-S has been shown to progress to ABPA-CB if left untreated but the role of treatment in prevention of bronchiectasis requires further randomized controlled trials (RCTs).

Although steroids are the drug of choice, precise dosage and duration still needs validation. Available data suggest a low dose regimen to be as effective as medium dose regimens with lower side effects, but with a lower proportion of patients having initial response to treatment.[36] (See Figure 22.6 for treatment algorithm and Table 22.8 for various regimens practised.)

Patients who do not have an adequate response to steroids, or have a high risk of adverse effects, recurrent exacerbation on steroids or steroid dependence, may find azoles beneficial as either an add-on or as an alternative.

Pulsed methyl prednisolone (15 mg/kg max 1 gm) may be beneficial in patients who are non-responsive to steroids and azoles, especially in steroid dependent patients in exacerbation. However, this needs validation.[12]

The role of inhaled corticosteroids is limited to treatment of asthma and inhaled corticosteroids do not play a role in the treatment of ABPA. Although they can result in improvement in symptoms, ABPA remains immunologically active and progressive.

Oral itraconazole capsules are poorly absorbed. Liquid formulations are available. Voriconazole has better oral bioavailability but its use is limited by high rates of photosensitivity (20–40%), as well as risk of skin malignancy in long-term usage.[2,12] Posaconazole may be a valid alternative.

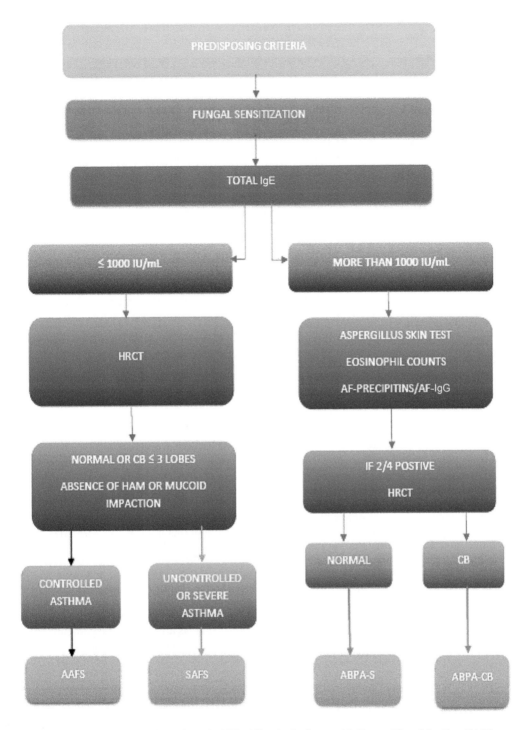

Figure 22.5 Diagnostic algorithm. (AAFS: Allergic Asthma with Fungal Sensitization; SAFS: Severe Asthma with Fungal Sensitization; ABPA-S: Allergic Bronchopulmonary Aspergillosis–Serology; ABPA-CB: Allergic Bronchopulmonary Aspergillosis–Central Bronchiectasis; HRCT: High-Resolution CT.)

Table 22.7: Newer Staging System by ISHAM Working Group

Stage	Definition	Features
0	Asymptomatic	• GINA definition of controlled asthma • Fulfils the diagnostic criteria of ABPA • Has not been previously diagnosed to have ABPA
1	Acute	• Patient has uncontrolled asthma/constitutional symptoms • Fulfils diagnostic criteria for ABPA • Not previously diagnosed to have ABPA
1a	With mucoid impaction	• Meets all the criteria • Documented mucoid impaction on CT or bronchoscopy
1b	Without mucoid impaction	• Meets all the criteria • No documented mucoid impaction on CT or bronchoscopy
2	Response	• Clinical improvement (resolution of constitutional symptoms, improvement in asthma control) • Major radiological improvement • IgE decline by ≥25% of baseline at 8 weeks
3	Exacerbation	• Clinical and/or radiological deterioration associated with an increase in IgE by ≥50%
4	Remission	• Sustained clinicoradiological improvement • IgE levels remaining at or below baseline (or increase by <50%) for ≥6 months on or off therapy *other than* systemic glucocorticoids
5a	Treatment-dependent ABPA	• Relapse on 2 or more consecutive occasions within 6 months of stopping treatment OR • Worsening of clinical, radiological, or immunological parameters on tapering oral steroids/azoles
5b	Glucocorticoid-dependent asthma	• Requires oral or parenteral glucocorticoids for control of asthma • ABPA is well controlled as reflected by IgE levels and chest radiograph
6	Advanced ABPA	• Type II respiratory failure and/or cor pulmonale • Radiological evidence of fibrotic findings consistent with ABPA on HRCT of the chest • Exclusion of reversible causes of acute respiratory failure

(CT, computed tomography; HRCT, high-resolution CT; GINA, Global Initiative for Asthma.)

Isavuconazole may also be effective. In cases that remain refractory, inhaled Amphotericin B may be attempted. A recent unblinded RCT did find voriconazole as effective as steroids in acute stages.[37] Other antifungal agents, including nystatin, miconazole, clotrimazole, and natamycin, are generally ineffective.

Bronchoscopy may be useful in patients with proximal bronchial obstruction unresponsive to medical therapy, even after 3–4 weeks, but otherwise is not recommended. Patients who have bronchiectasis should also be offered airway clearance techniques like hypertonic saline nebulization, percussion vests, airway clearance devices, long-term azithromycin, etc.

FOLLOW-UP AND MONITORING

Patients are followed up with a history and physical examination, chest radiograph, total IgE levels and a quality of life questionnaire every 8 weeks.

A ≥25% decline in IgE levels, along with clinicoradiological improvement signifies a satisfactory response to therapy. If the patient cannot be tapered off prednisolone/azole, it implies that the disease has evolved into stage 4.

Management should be attempted with alternate-day prednisone/azole in the least possible dose.

The aim of therapy is not to normalize IgE levels, but to decrease the IgE levels by 25–50%, which in most cases leads to clinical and radiographic improvement. Further, it is important to identify the new baseline.[2]

ROLE OF BIOLOGICS IN ABPA

Omalizumab is an anti-IgE recombinant humanized monoclonal antibody that prevents binding of IgE to receptor on mast cells and basophils and has been approved for use in uncontrolled asthma. Current evidence is limited but suggests that omalizumab can reduce the number of exacerbations, eosinophil levels, corticosteroid requirements and IgE levels, as well as the basophil sensitivity to *A. fumigatus* during the treatment period.[38] Further, ideal dosages are unknown, with IgE levels often going well beyond the routine prescribing limits.[39] The optimal duration of therapy is also unknown. Omalizumab can be considered in the case of patient intolerance or non-responsiveness to conventional therapy, or

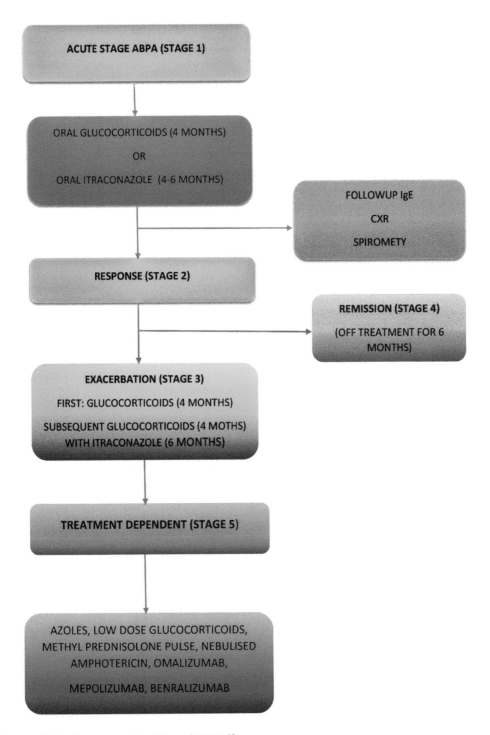

Figure 22.6 Treatment algorithm of ABPA.[35]

in the case of steroid dependence, in an attempt to reduce dependence.[31]

Mepolizumab, benralizumab and dupilumab have also been reported to be effective, but more evidence is required before use in clinical practice.

COMPLICATIONS

Complications occur, especially in inadequately treated patients or patients with a delay in diagnosis or initiation of therapy. The development of bronchiectasis is the most

171

Table 22.8: Dosage Regimens of Steroids and Itraconazole for ABPA[2]

Oral Glucocorticoids

Regimen 1

Prednisolone 0.5 mg/kg/day for 1–2 weeks, then on alternate days for 6–8 weeks, then taper by 5–10 mg every 2 weeks and discontinue

Regimen 2

Prednisolone, 0.75 mg/kg for 6 weeks, 0.5 mg/kg for 6 weeks, then taper by 5 mg every 6 weeks to continue for a total duration of at least 6–12 months

Oral Itraconazole

Dose: 200 mg twice a day, with therapeutic drug monitoring for at least 16 weeks

Response often takes longer than 16 weeks

Recurrent short courses or long-term therapy

Table 22.9: Diagnostic Criteria of SAFS

Severe Asthma

Evidence of fungal sensitization	Total serum IgE <1000 IU/mL Positive immediate skin test reactivity to *Aspergillus fumigatus* OR Elevated specific serum IgE to *A. fumigatus*
Exclusion of ABPA	Absence of serum precipitins (by gel diffusion) and elevated specific serum IgG to *A. fumigatus*
Normal radiology	No bronchiectasis or infiltrates

dreaded complication, as this alone can predispose to recurrent exacerbations and also brings in a plethora of associated complications like recurrent infections, haemoptysis, etc.

Aspergillus can continue to grow and may result in formations of aspergilloma or the development of invasive pulmonary aspergillosis. Chronic necrotising aspergillosis can occur and cause upper lobe fibrosis and cavitation. Chronic or recurrent atelectasis can also occur. Pulmonary fibrosis, localized emphysema and honeycombing may occur. In progressive disease, patients may develop type 2 failure with cor pulmonale.[2]

ALLERGIC BRONCHOPULMONARY MYCOSIS (ABPM)

Some patients with asthma have clinical and radiological presentation similar to ABPA but lack serological evidence and have a negative skin test to *Aspergillus fumigatus*. However, total IgE remains elevated and these patients show sensitivity to fungi other than aspergillus. The common fungi causing ABPM are *Candida albicans, Bipolaris, Schizophyllum commune, Curvularia lunata, Penicillium, Dreschlera hawaiiensis, Pseudoallescheria boydii, Alternaria alternata, Fusarium vasinfectum, Rhizopus oryzae, Geotrichum candidum,* and *Stemphylium lanuginosum*.[3] ABPM can cause progressive lung damage. Treatment is similar to ABPA and is responsive to steroids.[7]

SEVERE ASTHMA WITH FUNGAL SENSITIZATION (SAFS)

Severe asthma with fungal sensitization (SAFS) was first described by Denning et al. in 2006. It can be considered to be part of

spectrum of allergic disorders, with asthma and asthma with fungal sensitization at one end, and ABPA-CB at another. It may even represent a natural progression in some. It is characterized by severe asthma with fungal sensitization and exclusion of ABPA and is described in Table 22.9.[40]

SAFS should be treated like asthma. If unresponsive, additional antifungals or anti-IgE therapy or a combination may be considered. Itraconazole has been shown to be effective.

Omalizumab may improve FEV_1; however, even in studies which did show improvement, FEV_1 did not return to normal levels as observed with itraconazole therapy.[40]

ABPA IN CYSTIC FIBROSIS

Cystic fibrosis is characterized by impaired mucociliary clearance, increased mucus viscosity, reduced antimicrobial activity of airway secretions, recurrent antibiotic use and altered airway microbiome, all of which predispose to fungal colonization and ABPA in a subset of these patients.[41–43] Further aggressive long-term azithromycin and chronic inhaled antibiotics at an early age may have decreased the prevalence of *S. aureus* and *Pseudomonas aeruginosa* but increased Aspergillus airway colonization.[44] Low BMI in cystic fibrosis has been associated with an increased risk of ABPA.[45]

Diagnosis of ABPA in CF is challenging because bronchiectasis and recurrent exacerbations are part of the natural course of the disease. Ideal cut-off values for serological markers remain unclear. A diagnosis can be made from criteria proposed by the ISHAM working group or Cystic Fibrosis Foundation Consensus Conference[46] (Table 22.10).

Annual screening is recommended with total serum IgE; if more than 500 IU/ml, this should be followed by an immediate skin test or RAST.

Table 22.10: Diagnostic Criteria of Cystic Fibrosis Associated ABPA[47]

Cystic Fibrosis Foundation Consensus Conference Diagnostic Criteria

Cystic fibrosis with acute or subacute clinical deterioration

Serum total IgE concentration >1000 IU/mL unless the patient is receiving systemic corticosteroids

Positive serum-specific IgE (>0.35 kUA/L) or immediate skin test

Precipitating antibodies to *A. fumigatus* or serum IgG antibodies to *A. fumigatus* by an in vitro test

New or recent infiltrates (or mucus plugging) on chest radiography or CT that do not respond to antibiotics and standard physiotherapy

More recently, Denning et al. proposed a newer classification for Aspergillosis based on additional evidence from sputum galactomannan and real-time Aspergillus PCR with Aspergillus serum-specific IgE and IgG[48] (Table 22.11).

Treatment is similar to ABPA in asthmatics.

A fall in IgE of 35% is considered a good response. However, levels often fall by 25% in the first month, and by 60% by 2 months.[49]

Omalizumab and mepolizumab have shown promise and can bring down steroid requirements while stabilising lung function.[49] Vitamin D levels were found to be lower among CF patients with ABPA, and there is evidence that vitamin D supplementation can reduce Th2 inflammation and reduce Aspergillus-specific IgE.[2,50]

ABPA IN SPECIAL CIRCUMSTANCES

Management of ABPA in children is similar to adults with extra care taken to reduce the corticosteroid dose to the least possible, as these drugs can cause growth retardation. Once remissions are achieved, it may be optimal to switch to an antifungal azole.[12]

Table 22.12: Differential Diagnosis[1,4]

- Refractory asthma
- Newly diagnosed cystic fibrosis
- Tuberculosis
- Sarcoidosis
- Infectious pneumonia
- Eosinophilic pneumonia
- Aspergillus-sensitive asthma
- Churg–Strauss syndrome
- Bronchocentric granulomatosis
- Allergic bronchopulmonary mycosis
- Severe asthma with fungal sensitization

Pregnant and lactating patients should be treated with corticosteroids. ABPA exacerbations are increased in pregnancy.[51] Itraconazole has been associated with higher miscarriage rates. Newer azoles are also contraindicated; however, they may be used in the case of life-threatening diseases, especially when therapeutic options are limited. Omalizumab is better avoided.[12]

There are certain clinical conditions that resemble ABPA clinically or radiologically (Table 22.12).

CONCLUSION

ABPA can lead to significant lung damage, which can be prevented by early therapy. Diagnosis is hindered by the lack of availability of a single diagnostic test and a lack of adequate awareness. Currently, IgE appears to be the best screening test, and ISHAM working group criteria is simple, cost effective and practical. Despite the difficult course, lung damage can be prevented in most patients while maintaining a good quality of life. ABPA should be suspected and evaluated in all asthmatics and treated promptly. Steroids with or without azoles are effective in controlling the disease in most patients. Adverse effects to medications must be actively sought and treated. The urgent need for newer, less toxic therapies cannot be overstated.

Table 22.11: Novel Immunologic Classification of Aspergillosis in Adult CF[48]

Class	PCR	Serology	Galactomannan
Aspergillus bronchitis	PCR positive	*A. fumigatus* IgG elevated	Sputum galactomannan positive
Aspergillus sensitized	PCR negative or positive	*A. fumigatus* IgE (not IgG) elevated	Sputum galactomannan negative
ABPA	PCR positive	Total and specific *A. fumigatus* IgE/IgG elevated	Sputum galactomannan positive

Abbreviation: PCR—Polymerase chain reaction.

REFERENCES

1. Agarwal R. Allergic Bronchopulmonary Aspergillosis. *CHEST* 2009; **135**: 805–826.

2. Agarwal R, Chakrabarti A, Shah A, Gupta D, Meis JF, Guleria R et al. Allergic bronchopulmonary aspergillosis: review of literature and proposal of new diagnostic and classification criteria. *Clin Exp Allergy* 2013; **43**: 850–873.

3. Chowdhary A, Agarwal K, Kathuria S, Gaur SN, Randhawa HS, Meis JF. Allergic bronchopulmonary mycosis due to fungi other than Aspergillus: a global overview. *Crit Rev Microbiol* 2014; **40**: 30–48.

4. Patterson K, Strek ME. Allergic Bronchopulmonary Aspergillosis. *Proc Am Thorac Soc* 2010; **7**: 237–244.

5. Gago S, Overton NLD, Ben-Ghazzi N, Novak-Frazer L, Read ND, Denning DW et al. Lung colonization by *Aspergillus fumigatus* is controlled by ZNF77. *Nat Commun* 2018; **9**. https://doi.org/10.1038/s41467-018-06148-7.

6. Jat KR, Vaidya PC, Mathew JL, Jondhale S, Singh M. Childhood allergic bronchopulmonary aspergillosis. *Lung India* 2018; **35**: 499–507.

7. Shah A, Panjabi C. Allergic aspergillosis of the respiratory tract. *Eur Respir Rev* 2014; **23**: 8–29.

8. Tomee JF, Kauffman HF, Klimp AH, de Monchy JG, Köeter GH, Dubois AE. Immunologic significance of a collagen-derived culture filtrate containing proteolytic activity in Aspergillus-related diseases. *J Allergy Clin Immunol* 1994; **93**: 768–778.

9. Knutsen AP, Chauhan B, Slavin RG. Cell-mediated immunity in allergic bronchopulmonary Aspergillosis. *Immunology and Allergy Clinics of North America* 1998; **18**: 575–599.

10. Slavin RG, Hutcheson PS, Chauhan B, Bellone CJ. An overview of allergic bronchopulmonary Aspergillosis with some new insights. *Allergy Asthma Proc* 2004; **25**: 395–399.

11. Rosenberg M, Patterson R, Mintzer R, Cooper BJ, Roberts M, Harris KE. Clinical and immunologic criteria for the diagnosis of allergic bronchopulmonary Aspergillosis. *Ann Intern Med* 1977; **86**: 405–414.

12. Agarwal R, Sehgal IS, Dhooria S, Aggarwal AN. Developments in the diagnosis and treatment of allergic bronchopulmonary Aspergillosis. *Expert Rev Respir Med* 2016; **10**: 1317–1334.

13. Agarwal R. Allergic bronchopulmonary Aspergillosis: Lessons for the busy radiologist. *World J Radiol* 2011; **3**: 178–181.

14. Pastorello EA. 3. Skin tests for diagnosis of IgE-mediated allergy. *Allergy* 1993; **48**: 57–62.

15. Agarwal R, Aggarwal AN, Gupta D, Jindal SK. Aspergillus hypersensitivity and allergic bronchopulmonary aspergillosis in patients with bronchial asthma: systematic review and meta-analysis. *Int J Tuberc Lung Dis* 2009; **13**: 936–944.

16. Agarwal R, Gupta D, Aggarwal AN, Saxena AK, Saikia B, Chakrabarti A et al. Clinical significance of decline in serum IgE levels in allergic bronchopulmonary Aspergillosis. *Respir Med* 2010; **104**: 204–210.

17. Agarwal R, Maskey D, Aggarwal AN, Saikia B, Garg M, Gupta D et al. Diagnostic performance of various tests and criteria employed in allergic bronchopulmonary Aspergillosis: A latent class analysis. *PLoS One* 2013; **8**. https://doi.org/10.1371/journal.pone.0061105.

18. McCarthy DS, Pepys J. Allergic broncho-pulmonary Aspergillosis: Clinical immunology. 2. Skin, nasal and bronchial tests. *Clin Allergy* 1971; **1**: 415–432.

19. Agarwal R, Gupta D, Aggarwal AN, Saxena AK, Chakrabarti A, Jindal SK. Clinical significance of hyperattenuating mucoid impaction in allergic bronchopulmonary Aspergillosis: an analysis of 155 patients. *Chest* 2007; **132**: 1183–1190.

20. Ouchterlony O. Diffusion-in-gel methods for immunological analysis. *Prog Allergy* 1958; **5**: 1–78.

21. Dhooria S, Agarwal R. Diagnosis of allergic bronchopulmonary Aspergillosis: a case-based approach. *Future Microbiol* 2014; **9**: 1195–1208.

22. Agarwal R, Dua D, Choudhary H, Aggarwal AN, Sehgal IS, Dhooria S et al. Role of *Aspergillus fumigatus*-specific IgG in diagnosis and monitoring treatment response in allergic bronchopulmonary Aspergillosis. *Mycoses* 2017; **60**: 33–39.

23. Chakrabarti A, Sethi S, Raman DSV, Behera D. Eight-year study of allergic bronchopulmonary Aspergillosis in an Indian teaching hospital. *Mycoses* 2002; **45**: 295–299.

24. Shah A. Allergic bronchopulmonary and sinus Aspergillosis: the roentgenologic spectrum. *Front Biosci* 2003; **8**: e138–e146.

25. Hansell DM, Strickland B. High-resolution computed tomography in pulmonary cystic fibrosis. *Br J Radiol* 1989; **62**: 1–5.

26. Greenberger PA, Patterson R. Allergic bronchopulmonary Aspergillosis: model of bronchopulmonary disease with defined serologic, radiologic, pathologic and clinical findings from asthma to fatal destructive lung disease. *Chest* 1987; **91**: 165S–171S.

27. Agarwal R, Gupta D, Aggarwal AN, Behera D, Jindal SK. Allergic bronchopulmonary Aspergillosis: lessons from 126 patients attending a chest clinic in north India. *Chest* 2006; **130**: 442–448.

28. Agarwal R, Khan A, Gupta D, Aggarwal AN, Saxena AK, Chakrabarti A. An alternate method of classifying allergic bronchopulmonary Aspergillosis based on high-attenuation mucus. *PLOS ONE* 2010; **5**: e15346.

29. Kaur M, Sudan DS. Allergic bronchopulmonary Aspergillosis (ABPA)—The high resolution computed tomography (HRCT) chest imaging scenario. *J Clin Diagn Res* 2014; **8**: RC05–RC07.

30. Panchal N, Bhagat R, Pant C, Shah A. Allergic bronchopulmonary Aspergillosis: the spectrum of computed tomography appearances. *Respir Med* 1997; **91**: 213–219.

31. Agarwal R, Sehgal IS, Dhooria S, Muthu V, Prasad KT, Bal A *et al*. Allergic bronchopulmonary Aspergillosis. *Indian J Med Res* 2020; **151**: 529–549.

32. Muthu V, Singh P, Choudhary H, Dhooria S, Sehgal IS, Prasad KT *et al*. Role of recombinant *Aspergillus fumigatus* antigens in diagnosing Aspergillus sensitisation among asthmatics. *Mycoses* 2020; **63**: 928–936.

33. Gernez Y, Waters J, Mirković B, Lavelle GM, Dunn CE, Davies ZA *et al*. Blood basophil activation is a reliable biomarker of allergic bronchopulmonary Aspergillosis in cystic fibrosis. *Eur Respir J* 2016; **47**: 177–185.

34. Allergic Bronchopulmonary Aspergillosis: Staging as an Aid to Management | Annals of Internal Medicine. https://www.acpjournals.org/doi/10.7326/0003-4819-96-3-286?url_ver=Z39.88-2003&rfr_id=ori:rid:crossref.org&rfr_dat=cr_pub%20 200pubmed (accessed 23 Sep2020).

35. Dhooria S, Sehgal IS, Muthu V, Agarwal R. Treatment of allergic bronchopulmonary Aspergillosis: from evidence to practice. *Future Microbiol* 2020; **15**: 365–376.

36. Agarwal R, Aggarwal AN, Dhooria S, Sehgal IS, Garg M, Saikia B *et al*. A randomised trial of glucocorticoids in acute-stage allergic bronchopulmonary Aspergillosis complicating asthma. *Eur Respir J* 2016; **47**: 490–498.

37. Agarwal R, Dhooria S, Sehgal IS, Aggarwal AN, Garg M, Saikia B *et al*. A randomised trial of voriconazole and prednisolone monotherapy in acute-stage allergic bronchopulmonary Aspergillosis complicating asthma. *Eur Respir J* 2018; **52**:1801159. https://doi.org/10.1183/13993003.01159-2018.

38. Li J-X, Fan L-C, Li M-H, Cao W-J, Xu J-F. Beneficial effects of Omalizumab therapy in allergic bronchopulmonary Aspergillosis: A synthesis review of published literature. *Respir Med* 2017; **122**: 33–42.

39. Hochhaus G, Brookman L, Fox H, Johnson C, Matthews J, Ren S *et al*. Pharmacodynamics of omalizumab: implications for optimised dosing strategies and clinical efficacy in the treatment of allergic asthma. *Curr Med Res Opin* 2003; **19**: 491–498.

40. Mirsadraee M, Dehghan S, Ghaffari S, Mirsadraee N. Long-term effect of antifungal therapy for the treatment of severe resistant asthma: an active comparator clinical trial. *Curr Med Mycol* 2019; **5**: 1–7.

41. Tracy MC, Moss RB. The myriad challenges of respiratory fungal infection in cystic fibrosis. *Pediatr Pulmonol* 2018; **53**: S75–S85.

42. Kolwijck E, van de Veerdonk FL. The potential impact of the pulmonary microbiome on immunopathogenesis of Aspergillus-related lung disease. *Eur J Immunol* 2014; **44**: 3156–3165.

43. Role of Antibiotics and Fungal Microbiota in Driving Pulmonary Allergic Responses | Infection and Immunity. https://iai.asm.org/content/72/9/4996.short (accessed 9 Oct 2020).

44. Breuer O, Schultz A, Turkovic L, de Klerk N, Keil AD, Brennan S *et al*. Changing prevalence of lower airway infections in young children with cystic fibrosis. *Am J Respir Crit Care Med* 2019; **200**: 590–599.

45. Risk Factors for Aspergillus Colonization and Allergic Bronchopulmonary Aspergillosis in Children With Cystic Fibrosis - Jubin - 2010 - Pediatric Pulmonology - Wiley Online Library. https://onlinelibrary.wiley.com/doi/abs/10.1002/ppul.21240 (accessed 9 Oct 2020).

46. Maleki M, Mortezaee V, Hassanzad M, Mahdaviani SA, Poorabdollah M, Mehrian P *et al*. Prevalence of allergic bronchopulmonary Aspergillosis in cystic fibrosis patients using two different diagnostic criteria. *Eur Ann Allergy Clin Immunol* 2019; **52**: 104–111.

47. Stevens DA, Moss RB, Kurup VP, Knutsen AP, Greenberger P, Judson MA *et al*. Allergic bronchopulmonary Aspergillosis in cystic fibrosis— State of the art: cystic fibrosis foundation consensus conference. *Clin Infect Dis* 2003; **37**: S225–S264.

48. Baxter CG, Dunn G, Jones AM, Webb K, Gore R, Richardson MD *et al*. Novel immunologic classification of Aspergillosis in adult cystic fibrosis. *J Allergy Clin Immunol* 2013; **132**: 560–566.e10.

49. Lattanzi C, Messina G, Fainardi V, Tripodi MC, Pisi G, Esposito S. Allergic bronchopulmonary Aspergillosis in children with cystic fibrosis: An update on the newest diagnostic tools and therapeutic approaches. *Pathogens* 2020; **9**: 716.

50. Vitamin D supplementation decreases *Aspergillus fumigatus* specific Th2 responses in CF patients with aspergillus sensitization: a phase one open-label study | SpringerLink. https://link.springer.com/article/10.1186/s40733-015-0003-5 (accessed 9 Oct2020).

51. Sehgal IS, Dhooria S, Prasad KT, Muthu V, Aggarwal AN, Chakrabarti A *et al*. Pregnancy complicated by allergic bronchopulmonary Aspergillosis: A case-control study. *Mycoses*; **n/a**. doi:10.1111/myc.13180.

23 Pulmonary Eosinophilia

Kiran Vishnu Narayan

CONTENTS

INTRODUCTION

Eosinophils were first discovered by Paul Ehrlich in 1879[2]. The association between pulmonary infiltrates and eosinophilia was first reported by Loeffler in 1932, and the term "Pulmonary Infiltrates with Eosinophilia" was coined by Reeder and Goodrich in 1952[3,4,5]. Eosinophils are a subset of white blood cells involved in host response to infection, immune response and tumour surveillance. Eosinophils are derived from a clonal population of CD 34+ myeloid progenitor cells in the bone marrow.

The precursor being the same for both basophils and eosinophils, differentiation into the eosinophilic lineage is under the influence of cytokines IL-3, IL-5 and GM-CSF. They then migrate along the vascular endothelium (rolling) and into interstitium of organs through diapedesis. The migration into specific organs is decided by eotaxins, which are chemokines that attract eosinophils. Eotaxins bind to the eosinophil chemokine receptor CCR3. As such, the eosinophils are several hundred-fold more abundant in tissues than in

DOI: 10.1201/9781003125785-23

the blood. The survival of eosinophil in tissues will depend on the presence of cytokines that regulate its apoptosis.

Pulmonary eosinophilia is considered when there is the following:[6-8]

1. Absolute eosinophil count in blood >500/ul with lung imaging showing infiltrates

2. BAL eosinophil >10%

3. Transbronchial/open lung biopsy shows evidence of eosinophilic infiltration.

Peripheral eosinophilia is not mandatory, e.g, acute eosinophilic pneumonia may have no eosinophils in the early phase. Lung imaging, especially if a conventional chest X-ray, may miss the infiltrates.[9,10]

AETIOLOGY

Pulmonary eosinophilia may develop due to a known cause, as in parasitic transit through the lung, or due to an unknown cause or other association as described in Table 23.1.

PULMONARY EOSINOPHILIA DUE TO A KNOWN CAUSE

Simple Pulmonary Eosinophilia (Loeffler's Syndrome)

This was named after Loeffler who identified transpulmonary migration of Ascaris. Loeffler's syndrome can be applied to Ascaris species (*Ascaris lumbricoides* and *Ascaris suum*) Hookworm species (*Ancylostoma duodenale*,

Table 23.1: Classification of Pulmonary Eosinophilia

Due to a Known Cause

- Parasitic infestation-transpulmonary migration (Loefflers)/direct pulmonary invasion/heavy seedling
- Tropical pulmonary eosinophilia
- Infections
- ABPA
- Drug-/toxin-induced/post-radiation

Due to an Undetermined Cause

- Eosinophilic pneumonias-idiopathic, acute, chronic
- EGPA (Churg–Strauss syndrome)
- Idiopathic hypereosinophilic syndromes
- Idiopathic hypereosinophilic obliterative bronchiolitis

Lung Diseases with Associated Eosinophilia

- Allergic rhinitis
- Asthma
- Non-asthmatic eosinophilic bronchitis
- Organising pneumonia/Sarcoidosis/ Hypersensitivity pneumonitis
- Connective tissue disease related ILD
- Langerhans cell histiocytosis
- Post-lung transplantation
- Solid organ tumours

Necator americanus, Necator brasilensis) and *Strongyloides* species[11]. All these three species have a stage of larval migration through blood stream into pulmonary capillaries and then pass through the stages of alveolar penetration, maturation and migration upwards into airways and move into digestive tract. The pulmonary manifestations are believed to result from an immune hypersensitivity reaction to the parasite larvae most commonly due to Ascariasis. Pulmonary symptoms begin approximately 9–14 days following ingestion of parasitic ova and occur during the migration of larvae through the lung. It is characterized clinically by low-grade fever, an irritating non-productive cough, dyspnea, a burning substernal discomfort which is aggravated on deep breathing and coughing, and occasional haemoptysis. Symptoms are usually self-limiting, and typically resolve in 1–2 weeks. Peripheral blood examination reveals moderate-to-severe eosinophilia, which is at its peak as respiratory symptoms resolve. Chest X-ray shows non segmental, bilateral, interstitial, and peripheral/pleural based alveolar infiltrates (often fleeting). Infiltrates typically clear spontaneously after several weeks. Stool examinations for ova and parasites are generally negative when pulmonary symptoms predominate and become positive only after 8 weeks. Pulmonary function evaluation typically reveals a mild-to-moderate restrictive ventilator defect with a reduced diffusing capacity for carbon monoxide (DLCO). Symptomatic management includes bronchodilators and rarely steroids. To prevent the late digestive tract manifestations of Ascariasis, patients may be treated with antihelminthics. Oral mebendazole (100 mg twice a day for 3 days) or a single dose of Albendazole 400 mg can be given.

Direct Pulmonary Invasion Due to Parasite

Parasitic larvae can invade lung parenchyma rather than simply migrating through it. eg Paragonimia and Cestodes (*Echinococcus, Taenia solium*).[12]

Paragonimiasis/Lung Flukes

Can invade the lungs and produce haemoptysis, pneumothorax and an eosinophil rich pleural effusion. Peripheral eosinophilia is most marked in the initial stages and reduces as days progress irrespective of treatment. Chest X-ray shows a peripheral subpleural nodular lesion with halo or a cavity in the mid-lower zones of lung. CT scan shows round low-attenuation cystic lesions filled with fluid or air, which is seen within an area of consolidation.

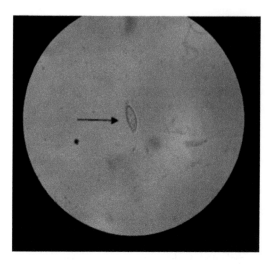

Figure 23.1 A wet smear from BAL showing *Paragonimus ova.*

Peripheral linear opacities seen on chest X-rays are actually worm migration tracks and can be seen on CT scans. Induced sputum or BAL will show eosinophilia and can demonstrate ova and eggs (see Figure 23.1). Medical treatment is usually with Praziquantel at a dose of 75 mg/kg/day for 3–5 days. Some patients may require surgery for persistent pneumothorax, pleural effusion or empyema[12].

Echinococcal Cyst/Hydatid Cyst

Common species include *Echinococcus granulosus* and *Echinococcus multilocularis*. They can present with lung and liver cysts. Leakage or accidental/iatrogenic rupture of pulmonary cysts of echinococcosis can cause pulmonary eosinophilia, secondary bacterial infection and rarely anaphylaxis. Chest imaging will show cystic lesions, which may be intact or ruptured. IgM antibodies to echinococcus can be detected by enzyme-linked immunosorbent assay (ELISA)

Heavy Haematogenous Seedling

This occurs due to helminth larvae and eggs being deposited in the lungs from a heavy haematogenous load especially in immunosuppression. Unlike transpulmonary migration described above this form of spread is not part of the parasitic life cycle. Eg. visceral larva migrans.[13]

Visceral Larva migrans

This is caused by Ascarid species (*Toxocara canis, Toxocara cati, Ascaris suum*). It presents predominantly in children, the majority of whom remain asymptomatic and undiagnosed. Patients can manifest with fever, fatigue, cough, wheezing, dyspnoea seizures, hepatomegaly and leucocytosis with eosinophilia. Chest imaging shows poorly defined, diffuse nodular alveolar infiltrates in almost half the patients with pulmonary symptoms. Diagnosis of Toxocariasis is difficult. Cutaneous *Larva migrans* produced by *Ancylostoma brasiliense* (creeping eruption) may also produce simple pulmonary eosinophilia in 50% of cases. Treatment is symptomatic and role of antihelminthics is controversial. Steroids are useful in severe lung involvement.[14]

Strongyloides stercoralis

Strongyloides stercoralis is an intestinal nematode that can produce lung involvement in different ways. In addition to the transpulmonary migration through lungs as mentioned above, it can produce disseminated infection and autoinfection. These are usually seen in immunocompromised patients. Severe COPD and poorly controlled asthma patients on systemic steroids are at risk of hyperinfection syndrome. Peripheral blood eosinophilia, in association with pneumonia, bronchospasm and abdominal pain or diarrhoea suggests strongyloidiasis in patients living or having travelled in endemic areas. Diagnosis of strongyloidiasis depends on the demonstration of eggs or larvae in BAL fluid. Eosinophilia is usually present in recently infected patients, but it is often absent in disseminated disease. Serologic testing by ELISA for IgG antibodies to *Strongyloides* is often positive, while stool examination is often negative. Because of the risk of hyperinfection syndrome that persists for years, all infected patients are treated when diagnosed (Ivermectin 200 µg/kg daily for 2 days and repeated 2 weeks later).[15]

Schistosomiasis

They can present with pulmonary involvement in two ways. In early acute Schistosomiasis (*S. hematobium or S. mansoni*) 3–6 weeks after infection, patients may develop cough, dyspnoea wheezing and eosinophilia. Chest imaging shows transient multiple small pulmonary nodules and ground glassing. An alternate phase is seen following antihelminthic treatment in patients with portal hypertension. Adult worms travel to the lungs via portosystemic collaterals, which is known as Lung shift/verminous pneumonia or reactionary Loffler like Pneumonitis. Chronic schistosomiasis may result in pulmonary hypertension. Diagnosis is clinical in persons coming from the endemic zones. Serology and stool examination is negative during the acute stages.[16]

Eosinophilic Pneumonias of Other Infectious Causes

Pulmonary infection with eosinophilia has been reported with the fungi *Coccidioides immitis* (most commonly), *Cryptococcus neoformans*, *Aspergillus niger* and *Mucormyces*[17-19] Bacterial or viral pulmonary infection (e.g., tuberculosis [TB], brucellosis, respiratory syncytial virus, influenza infection) may occasionally be a cause of eosinophilic pneumonia. TB can produce an undulating pattern of eosinophilia. It has been noted that eosinophilia correlates with a good prognosis, and eosinopenia was noted in miliary or fulminant TB disease.[20,21]

Tropical Pulmonary Eosinophilia

Tropical eosinophilia, one of the most common causes of chronic cough in tropical areas (Indian subcontinent, South East Asia, Africa, South America) with endemic filariasis, is caused by the nematodes *Wuchereria bancrofti* and *Brugia malayi*. It is an immune response to the blood borne microfilarial stages of these parasites spread by mosquitoes. Those affected usually present with severe spasmodic nocturnal cough (wake up coughing at 1–5 a.m.), breathlessness, wheeze, fever, leucocytosis and marked peripheral eosinophilia (AEC>3000/uL).[22,23] The circulating microfilariae are trapped in the lung vasculature where they release their antigenic contents, further triggering the inflammatory pulmonary reaction. Blood eosinophilia (2 weeks) is followed by pneumonia (1–3 months), with the formation of eosinophilic abscesses and granulomatous lesions. Untreated disease may lead to pulmonary fibrosis.[24] There are elevated serum IgE (>1000 units/mL) and markedly elevated antifilarial IgG antibodies. BAL shows intense alveolitis with a mean percentage of 54% of eosinophils with marked degranulation. Chest X-rays typically show diffuse opacities or miliary nodules, and approximately 20% of affected patients have a normal chest radiograph. CT scans are more sensitive than chest radiography, and typical findings include reticulonodular opacities, bronchiectasis, air trapping, calcification, and mediastinal adenopathy.[25]

The diagnostic criteria of tropical pulmonary eosinophilia includes[26]

- Residence in a filarial endemic area

- Nocturnal spasmodic cough

- Eosinophil count greater than 3000/μL; and

- Clinical and hematologic response to diethylcarbamazine (DEC)

The standard treatment recommended by the World Health Organization is DEC at 6 mg/kg in divided doses for 3 weeks. Steroids in addition to DEC may be beneficial for eosinophilic apoptosis and preventing end organ damage due to the high eosinphil load. Most patients improve within 3 weeks. However, a sizeable proportion do not have complete resolution and may have a mild form of interstitial lung disease, which can relapse also. Therefore, it is recommended to give a repeat monthly course of DEC at 3 month-intervals for 1–2 years, especially in endemic areas[27-29].

Drugs, Toxic Agents and Radiation-Induced Eosinophilic Pneumonias

Drugs

Many drugs have been reported to cause pulmonary opacities and especially acute eosinophilic pneumonia. Drugs causing eosinophilic pneumonia are mainly non-steroidal anti-inflammatory drugs and antibiotics.[5]

A list of common drugs causing eosinophilic pneumonia is shown in Table 23.2.

It can occur with any drug, including non-prescription drugs, herbal preparations, dietary supplements, street drugs, and environmental exposures. They can have an acute or subacute

Table 23.2: Drugs That May Cause Acute Eosinophilic Pneumonia

Antimicrobials

- Nitrofurantoin
- Penicillins
- Sulphonamides
- Tetracycline
- Isoniazid
- Ethambutol
- Streptomycin

Antineoplastic/Immunosuppressive

- Bleomycin
- Methotrexate
- Azathioprine

NSAID

- Aspirin
- Naproxen
- Piroxicam

Cardiovascular/Antidiabetic

- Amiodarone
- ACE inhibitors
- Beta-blockers

Miscellaneous

- Carbamazepine
- Phenytoin
- Iodinated contrast agents
- Progesterone

Toxins

- Rubber manufacturing chemicals inhalation
- Dust/smoke/fireworks/tobacco smoke inhalation

onset and are not always related to either the cumulative dose of drug used or the duration of treatment. Respiratory symptoms vary widely in severity, from being asymptomatic with pulmonary infiltration and eosinophilia (Loeffler-like illness), chronic cough with or without dyspnoea and fever, acute eosinophilic pneumonia, drug reaction with eosinophilia and systemic symptoms (DRESS) to severe fulminant respiratory failure. Chest X-ray typically shows interstitial or alveolar infiltrates, and common HRCT findings include bilateral peripherally located consolidation and ground-glass opacities. A diagnosis of drug or toxin-induced eosinophilic pneumonia is based upon a careful review of all drugs and other exposures and resolution of symptoms on elimination of the offending agent. Withdrawing the agent usually leads to disappearance of eosinophilia, pulmonary infiltrates, and normalization of lung function within a month. Supplemental therapy with corticosteroids can hasten recovery in patients who are severely ill.

Radiation Therapy

Chronic eosinophilic pneumonia may develop after radiation therapy for cancer. It usually occurs in women with a history of asthma or allergy, at a median time of 3.5 months and up to 10 months after completion of radiotherapy for breast cancer. Chest radiograph shows unilateral (involving the irradiated lung) or even contralateral to irradiated chest, bilateral and possibly migratory opacities. All patients have blood eosinophilia of 1.0×10^9/L (1000/μL) or greater and/or eosinophilia greater than 40% on the BAL differential cell count. Patients rapidly improve with oral corticosteroids without sequelae, but relapse can occur.[5]

EOSINOPHILIC LUNG DISEASES OF UNDETERMINED CAUSE

Idiopathic Chronic Eosinophilic Pneumonia

Idiopathic chronic eosinophilic pneumonia (ICEP) was first described in detail by Carrington and colleagues in 1969. It is seen predominantly in women (with a 2:1 female-to-male ratio). The incidence of ICEP peaks in the fourth decade, with a mean age of 45 years at diagnosis. A vast majority of patients with ICEP are non-smokers. A prior history of atopy is found in about half of the patients, with allergic rhinitis in 12–24%. Asthma is usually late onset and may also develop concomitantly with the diagnosis of ICEP in 15% of patients, or develop after ICEP in 13%.[6] Cases have been reported wherein patients initially diagnosed with CEP later developed Eosinophilic Granulomatosis with Polyangitis.

Clinical Features

The most common respiratory symptoms are cough, dyspnea, wheeze and chest pain. Haemoptysis may occur rarely. Systemic symptoms and signs are often prominent, with fever, weight loss (>10 kg in about 10%), fatigue, anorexia, weakness and night sweats.

Diagnosis

The diagnosis of ICEP is based on the presence of compatible clinical, radiographic, and BAL findings, in absence of an obvious infection or other known causes of eosinophilic lung disease. Routine blood investigations show peripheral blood eosinophilia with a mean percentage of blood eosinophils at a differential count of 26%. A lack of peripheral blood eosinophilia does not rule out the diagnosis, since eosinophilia may be absent in 10–30% of cases.[30] ESR and CRP levels are increased. Total blood IgE level is increased in about half of the cases and is greater than 1000 IU/mL in 15%. Antinuclear antibodies may occasionally be present.

Radiology

Peripheral opacities in the upper and mid zones of lungs are present in almost all cases and are fleeting or migratory in a quarter of cases. The alveolar opacities have ill-defined margins, with a density varying from ground-glass to consolidation. The classic pattern of "photographic negative of pulmonary oedema or reversal of the shadows" described in ICEP, is seen in only one-fourth of patients. The reverse halo or atoll sign is rare.[31] Follow up imaging, months after the onset of symptoms, may also show linear band-like opacities parallel to the pleural surface or lobar atelectasis. The band shadows in fact cross the fissures also. A pleural effusion may be observed in <10% of cases, as compared to acute eosinophilic pneumonia.[32]

PFT

Obstructive pattern may be seen in those without a history of asthma, and the restrictive pattern occurs due to eosinophilic infiltration into the interstitium. Diffusing capacity may be reduced and the alveolar–arterial oxygen gradient may be mildly elevated. BAL has replaced lung biopsy for the diagnosis of ICEP, and eosinophilia ranging from 12–95% is a characteristic and constant feature. Lung biopsy is usually not necessary to make a confident diagnosis of CEP.

Treatment

Treatment with steroids should be initiated as soon as a diagnosis of CEP is made, as fewer than 10% of cases spontaneously improve or recover, and untreated CEP can lead to irreversible fibrosis.[33] In fact, if a patient does not improve with glucocorticoid treatment, alternative diagnoses should be considered. Therapy is started with 0.5 mg/kg/day of prednisone and continued in the same dosage for 2 weeks after a complete resolution of symptoms and plain chest radiographic abnormalities (usually 4–6 weeks). Slow tapering is done over 6–12 months based on clinicoradiological evaluation and blood eosinophil count. Most patients require prolonged treatment beyond 6–9 months because of relapse while decreasing below a daily dose of 10–15 mg/day of prednisone, or after stopping the corticosteroid treatment. Relapses occur on restarting smoking.[30] Newer monoclonal antibodies have also been tried in those with steroid dependence, e.g. omalizumab, anti-IL5 monoclonal antibody mepolizumab, and antibody against alpha-chain of the interleukin-5 receptor benralizumab. Paradoxically, the dual monoclonal antibody against IL-5 and 13 dupilumab has caused the development of CEP in a patient with asthma.[34–37]

Acute Eosinophilic Pneumonia (AEP)

This is an acute onset pneumonia associated with the rapid development of acute respiratory failure in a previously healthy patient. AEP tends to occur in patients between the age of 20 and 40 and is more common in men. The majority of patients with AEP have a history of smoking (up to 70%). It has also been reported among persons who have been involved in activities with unusual exposures (including exposure to dust from the World Trade Center collapse in New York City, after military deployment in Iraq, cave exploration, gasoline tank cleaning, plant repotting, woodpile moving, cocaine inhalation, indoor renovations, etc.).

Diagnostic Criteria for Idiopathic Acute Eosinophilic Pneumonia

1. Acute onset of febrile respiratory manifestations (≤1 *month* before consultation)

2. Bilateral diffuse opacities on chest radiography

3. Low oxygen levels as assessed by SpO_2 on room air <90% and/or PaO_2 on room air <60 mm Hg and/or $PaO_2/FiO_2 \leq 300$ mm Hg,

4. BAL showing >25% eosinophils (or eosinophilic pneumonia on lung biopsy)

5. Absence of an evident infection, drugs or of other known causes of eosinophilic lung disease.

Clinical Features

Most patients present with an acute febrile illness of a week with myalgia, nonproductive cough, dyspnea and pleuritic chest pain which rapidly progress to Acute Respiratory Distress syndrome (ARDS) in 2–3 days. A characteristic feature unlike acute viral pneumonias like SARS-CoV-2 would be absence of any multisystem involvement despite severe respiratory failure. Hypoxemia may be severe and refractory to breathing 100% oxygen.

Investigations

When performed in less severe cases, lung function tests show a mild restrictive ventilatory defect with normal FEV_1/FVC ratio and reduced diffusing capacity. There is leucocytosis but peripheral eosinophilia is rare at presentation and may increase during the course of the disease. Sputum and pleural fluid eosinophilia is also present. The chest radiograph shows bilateral opacities, with mixed alveolar or interstitial opacities and bilateral pleural effusion. HRCT chest shows ground-glass opacities and air space consolidation. Poorly defined nodules and interlobular septal thickening are also seen. Bilateral pleural effusion and interlobular septal thickening with preserved cardiac left ventricular function on Echocardiography are highly suggestive of IAEP in a patient with eosinophilic pneumonia. BAL is the key to the diagnosis of IAEP, showing an average percentage of 37–54% eosinophils on the differential cell count, with sterile bacterial cultures.

Treatment and Prognosis

When a diagnosis of IAEP is made, steroids are usually started as intravenous methylprednisolone pulses of 15–20 mg/kg for 3 days and later changed to oral therapy that can be tapered over 2–4 weeks. They respond well to corticosteroids within 3 days. Recovery is rapid with no significant clinical or imaging sequelae and no relapse after stopping corticosteroid treatment.

Hypereosinophilic Syndrome

Idiopathic HES is a rare disorder first described in 1968 by Hardy and Anderson. It is also called Loefflers Endocarditis and Eosinophilic Leukaemia.[5] Hypereosinophilic syndromes (HES) are a heterogeneous group of rare disorders defined by the presence of marked peripheral or tissue eosinophilia resulting in end-organ damage and variable presentations in terms of severity. Organ damage occurs due to Eosinophilic infiltration and/or thromboembolic phenomena. Current consensus defines **hypereosinophilia** as blood eosinophils $>1.5 \times 10^9$/L on two examinations separated by ≥ 1 month and/or tissue eosinophilia (defined as $>20\%$ of cells in a bone marrow specimen, tissue infiltration, and/or marked deposition of EDGP in tissue).[38,39]

HES can be of different forms.

- *Lymphocytic variant* of HES—A monoclonal proliferation of T lymphocytes producing eosinophilopoietic chemokines and eosinophilia.

- *Myeloproliferative variant* of HES (Chronic Eosinophilic Leukaemia)—A clonal proliferation of the eosinophil cell lineage itself

- *Familial HE/HES*—an extremely rare autosomal dominant condition, likely due to dysregulation of IL-5 expression.

- *Idiopathic HES*—HES not fitting into any of the above categories.

Lymphocytic Variant HES

It accounts for about 30% of patients with HES. It results from the production of eosinophilopoietic chemokines (especially IL-5) by clonal Th2 lymphocytes. Serum levels of IgE are elevated as a consequence of IL-4 and IL-13 production by these Th2 lymphocytes. Most reported patients are atopic and have skin manifestations like papules or urticarial plaques infiltrated by lymphocytes and eosinophils (and in some of them, a cutaneous T-cell lymphoma or the Sezary syndrome was ultimately present). In such cases, the HES may be considered a premalignant T-cell disorder. They respond to steroids.

Myeloproliferative Variant HES (Chronic Eosinophilic Leukaemia)

It accounts for 20–30% of cases and is caused by a interstitial chromosomal deletion of a region in the long arm of chromosome 4q12 resulting in the fusion of FIP1L1–PDGFRA (Fip1-like 1 (*FIP1L1*)-platelet-derived growth factor receptor alpha). Depending on the stage of the disease and the organ involved, patients may have few or no clinical manifestations or be acutely ill. Anaemia, hepatosplenomegaly, mucosal ulcerations, severe cardiac manifestations resistant to corticosteroid treatment and thrombocytopenia are common and suggestive of the diagnosis. Here, cutaneous manifestations are infrequent. The presence of the FIP1L1–PDGFRA rearrangement is sufficient for the diagnosis of myeloproliferative HES.

Clinical Features of Hypereosinophilic Syndrome

HES is more common in men than in women (9:1) and appears between 20 and 50 years. The onset is generally insidious, with eosinophilia discovered incidentally in 12% of the patients. Extremely high values of eosinophilia, in excess of 100×10^9/L (100,000/µL), are found in some patients. The main presenting symptoms are fever, weakness, fatigue, weight loss, cough and dyspnoea. The dominant organs involved include heart, nervous system, lungs, skin, GIT, eye and joints. 25–40% of the patients may have asthmatic symptoms, including nocturnal cough, wheezing and dyspnoea which may progress to ARDS. Pleural effusion, thromboembolism and pulmonary hypertension may develop over time. Cardiovascular involvement is a major cause of morbidity and mortality with restrictive cardiomyopathy, frequent congestive heart failure, mitral regurgitation and intramural thrombus formation. Peripheral arterial and venous thromboses can also occur. Neurological manifestations include cerebrovascular accidents due to thromboemboli, central nervous system dysfunction and peripheral neuropathies. Cutaneous manifestations include erythematous pruritic papules and nodules, urticaria and angioedema. There can be diarrhoea, ascites, colitis, pancreatitis and Budd Chiari syndrome. Arthralgia and polyarthritis are also associated with HES.[40,41]

Investigations

Chest CT findings consist of focal areas of ground-glass attenuation mainly in the lung periphery and small nodules with or without a halo sign. Only mild eosinophilia at BAL contrasting with high levels of eosinophilia in the blood has been reported in patients with the HES. Treatment depends on the underlying variety of HES and the organ involvement.

Treatment

In clonal and idiopathic forms, the aim is to limit or reverse the end organ damage, provide symptomatic improvement and keep the AEC<1500/uL. Emergency management is needed if the AEC>100,000 cells/uL, there is evidence of leukostasis (e.g. pulmonary or neurologic dysfunction with AEC>50,000/uL) or there is evidence of life-threatening complications like pulmonary emboli and acute heart failure. In asymptomatic patients with peripheral eosinophilia alone, follow-up can be done every 3–6 months to assess any evidence of end organ damage. Imatinib is the first-line therapy in patients with the myeloproliferative variant of HES, especially (but not exclusively) when the FIP1L1–PDGFRA fusion protein is present. Initial dosage is 400 mg/day for rapid cytogenic response. Rapid improvement of symptoms with normalisation of eosinophil counts occur within 1–2 weeks. If there is no response in 2–4 weeks, it should be discontinued and other treatment considered. In Imatinib resistance, other agents with PDGFR-like activity in HES like dasatinib, sorafenib, and nilotinib, are available.[42–44] Steroids are given in the lymphocytic variety and idiopathic variety of HES. Prednisolone is given in a range of 20–60 mg daily, depending on the severity of the disease manifestations and the degree of eosinophilia at presentation. Other treatments include chemotherapeutic agents (hydroxyurea, vincristine, etoposide); cyclosporin A; interferon-α; anti-IL-5 antibody mepolizumab and anti-IL-5 α receptor antibody benralizumab.[45]

Idiopathic Hypereosinophilic Obliterative Bronchiolitis

A distinct entity coined hypereosinophilic obliterative bronchiolitis has been recently identified and is defined by the following provisional working criteria:[45,46]

- A peripheral eosinophil cell count greater than 1×10^9/L (>1000/μL) and/or bronchoalveolar lavage eosinophil count greater than 25%

- Persistent airflow obstruction with FEV_1/FVC<70% and post bronchodilator FEV_1<80% predicted despite 4–6 weeks of high-dose inhaled corticosteroids and bronchodilators

- Lung biopsy showing an Eosinophilic bronchiolitis and/or HRCT evidence of bronchiolitis (centrilobular nodules and branching opacities)

The blood eosinophil cell count is elevated (with a mean of 2.7×10^9/L (2700/μL), and the mean eosinophil differential percentage at BAL is 63%. Whitish tracheal and bronchial granulations or bronchial ulcerative lesions can be present with prominent eosinophilia at bronchial biopsy. They respond well to oral prednisolone at an initial dose of 0.5–1 mg/kg/day and tapered to a maintenance dose of approximately 10 mg/day. Other important eosinophilic lung diseases like ABPA are discussed elsewhere in this textbook.

Eosinophilic Granulomatosis with Polyangitis (EGPA)/Churg–Strauss Syndrome

It was first described in the early 1950s and is an uncommon disease, with the diagnosis often missed or delayed. It usually affects those from 30–50 years of age, without any sex predilection.[47]

EGPA/Churg–Strauss syndrome classically progresses in 3 stages:

1. Prodromal stage—Patient presents with late onset allergic rhinitis, nasal polyposis and asthma, in the absence of a family history. This stage can last from months to years.

2. Eosinophilic stage—There is eosinophilic infiltration into multiple organs like lungs, skin and GIT.

3. Vasculitic stage—It is characterised by the onset of vasculitic manifestations such as-constitutional symptoms, eosinophilic vasculitis and granulomas.

Diagnosis is based on criteria from the American College of Rheumatology in 1990. At least 4 out of the 6 criteria are needed, with a sensitivity of 85% and specificity of 99.7%:[48]

1. Asthma

2. Paranasal sinusitis

3. Migratory or transient pulmonary infiltrates

4. Mono- or polyathropathy

5. Peripheral Eosinophilia >10%

6. Extravascular eosinophils in a blood vessel

Clinical Features

Systemic manifestations include fever, weight loss, arthralgia/arthritis, lymphadenopathy and ocular manifestations, and they herald the onset of vasculitis. Respiratory manifestations include upper respiratory tract involvement (75–85%), asthma, Loefflers like syndrome, pleurisy, thromboembolism and pleural effusion. Compared to granulomatosis with polyangitis (Wegners), no necrosis is seen in the upper respiratory tract. Asthma is predominant in the prodromal and eosinophilic stages. Asthma may be there for a long time and usually subsides with the onset of the vasculitic phase. A short interval between asthma onset and vasculitis depicts an increased severity of CSS. Cardiovascular involvement is the leading cause of mortality. Coronary vasculitis can lead to myocardial infarction, Ischemic cardiomyopathy and congestive cardiac failure. Neurological changes are seen in two-thirds of patients. They consist of mononeuritis multiplex, polyneuropathy, seizures, CVA and subarachnoid haemorrhage. Eosinophilic gastroenteritis develops characterised by abdominal pain, bleeding, diarrhoea, intestinal

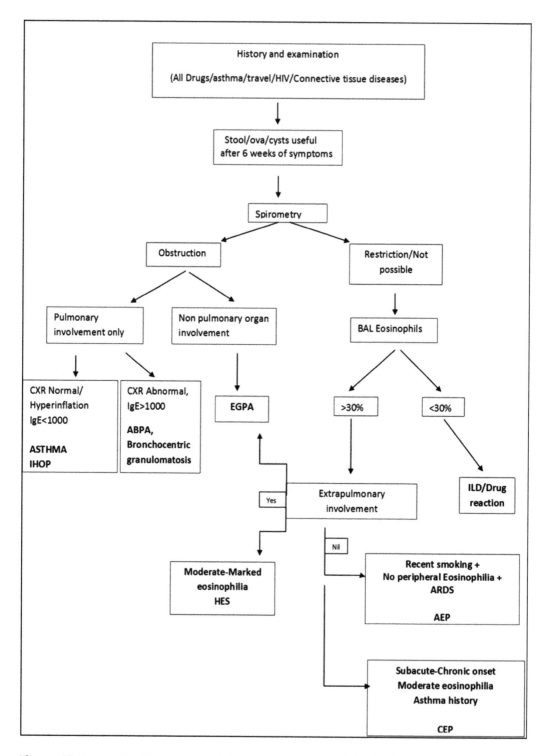

Figure 23.2 An algorithmic approach to pulmonary eosinophilia. (AEP: Acute Eosinophilic Pneumonia; CEP: Chronic Eosinophilic Pneumonia; HES: Hypereosinophilic Syndrome; IHOP: Idiopathic hypereosinophilic obliterative bronchiolitis; ABPA: Allergic bronchopulmonary aspergillosis; EGPA: *Eosinophilic granulomatosis* with polyangitis.)

obstruction, ulcers and perforation. Palpable purpura, maculopapular rash, nodules and ulcers can occur. Renal involvement includes haematuria, hypertension following renal infarction, interstitial nephritis and focal segmental glomerulosclerosis.

Investigations

There is leucocytosis with eosinophilia and a high ESR. IgE levels are elevated and parallel the disease activity. A positive p-ANCA is seen in only 30–60% of patients, and the majority of patients have antibodies against Myeloperoxidase. p-ANCA can be used only for an initial diagnosis because the follow-up levels do not have use as a marker. Pleural fluid is eosinophilic with low glucose levels. Loeffler-like infiltrates can be seen in 40% of patients and pleural effusions in 30% of cases. Other findings include ground glassing, consolidation, non cavitating nodules, peribronchial thickening and pulmonary artery enlargement. PFT shows an obstructive pattern. BAL reveals eosinophilia. A histopathology of biopsied organs may show intravascular and extravascular non caseating granulomas, eosinophilic infiltration and vasculitis of small and medium sized vessels, thus drawing the new terminology of allergic granulomatosis with angitis.

Treatment

Steroids form the backbone of treatment. Prednisolone in doses of 60–100 mg/day should be given for good control and tapered slowly to a maintenance dose that will prevent relapse. Maintenance may be needed for 12–18 months or more to prevent relapse. Disease activity is assessed clinically by the disappearance of constitutional symptoms, normalisation of blood pressure and improvement in organ functions. If there is an inadequate response to high dose steroids and severe life-threatening organ involvement, immunomodulators like Pulse cyclophosphamide are the treatment of choice. Other alternatives include mycofenolate, azathioprine and methotrexate. The Anti-IL-5 monoclonal antibody mepolizumab at a dose of 300 mg every 4 weeks has been approved by the FDA for EGPA.[49,50] Beta-blockers should not be used to control BP because they may produce bronchospasm and precipitate congestive cardiac failure. Prognosis is assessed by using the five factor score (FFS) with cardiac involvement, gastrointestinal disease and age ≥65 being the strongest indicators of a poor prognosis.[51,52]

An algorithmic approach to diagnosis of pulmonary eosinophilia is shown in Figure 23.2.

CONCLUSION

In clinical practice, the diagnosis of eosinophilic pneumonia is suspected in patients presenting with respiratory symptoms, pulmonary opacities on imaging and demonstration of eosinophilia in the peripheral blood or, preferably, in the lung. Eosinophilia can occur as an incidental finding during evaluation or as a clue to the clinical condition. Work up of eosinophilia is based on the severity of clinical condition, eg sick patients would require urgent treatment, eosinophilic count e.g., very high counts would need intervention, evidence of end organ involvement/damage and possibility of a neoplastic aetiology. A detailed history with physical examination to identify pattern of organ involvement is needed[53,54]. Patient presenting with persistent eosinophilia with no improvement to a therapeutic trial of antifilarials (Diethyl carbamazine) and steroids should always be worked up for an underlying haematological disorder.

REFERENCES

1. Vincet C, Jean Francois C. Eosinophilic Lung diseases. In: Broaddus VC, Mason RJ, Ernst JD, King TE Jr, Lazarus SC, Murray JF, Nadel JA, Slutsky A, Gotway MB. Murray and Nadels Textbook of Respiratory Medicine. 6th edition: Elsevier; 2016. pp 1221–42.

2. Hirsch JJ, Hirsch BI. Paul Ehrlich and the discovery of the Eosinophil. In: Mahmoud AAF, Austen KF. The Eosinophils in Health and Disease. New York: Grune and Stratton; 1980. pp 3–13.

3. Löffler, W. Zur Differential-Diagnose der Lungeninfiltrierungen. Beiträgezur Klinik der Tuberkulose 1932; 79:368–82.

4. Reeder WH, Goodrich BE. Pulmonary infiltration with eosinophilia (PIE syndrome). Ann Intern Med. 1952; 36(5):1217–40.

5. S Varma, A Jindal. Pulmonary eosinophilic disorders. In: SK Jindal, PS Shankar, S Raoof, D Gupta, AN Aggarwal, R Agarwal. Textbook of Pulmonary and Critical Care Medicine. India. 1st edition: Jaypee; 2012. pp 1217–28.

6. Allen JN, Davis WB. Eosinophilic lung diseases. Am J Respir Crit Care Med 1994; 150:1423.

7. Bain GA, Flower CD. Pulmonary eosinophilia. Eur J Radiol 1996; 23:3.

8. Umeki S. Reevaluation of eosinophilic pneumonia and its diagnostic criteria. Arch Intern Med 1992; 152:1913.

9. Hayakawa H, Sato A, Toyoshima M, et al. A clinical study of idiopathic eosinophilic pneumonia. Chest 1994; 105:1462.

10. Dejaegher P, Derveaux L, Dubois P, Demedts M. Eosinophilic pneumonia without radiographic pulmonary infiltrates. Chest 1983; 84:637.

11. Loffler W. Transient lung infiltrations with blood eosinophilia. Int Arch Allergy Appl Immunol 1956; 8:54.

12. Wilson ME, Weller PF. Eosinophilia. In: Guerrant RL, Walker DH, Weller PF. Tropical Infectious Diseases: Principles, Pathogens and Practice. Philadelphia: 2nd edition: Elsevier; 2006. pp 1478.

13. Phills JA, Harrold AJ, Whiteman GV, Perelmutter L. Pulmonary infiltrates, asthma and eosinophilia due to Ascaris suum infestation in man. N Engl J Med. 1972; 286:965–970.

14. Fillaux J, Magnaval JF: Laboratory diagnosis of human toxocariasis. Vet Parasitol 2013; 193:327–336.

15. Igra-Siegman Y, Kapila R, Sen P, et al: Syndrome of hyperinfection with Strongyloides stercoralis. Rev Infect Dis 1981; 3:397–407.

16. Schwartz E, Rozenman J, Perelman M. Pulmonary manifestations of early schistosome infection among nonimmune travelers. Am J Med 2000; 109:718.

17. Lombard CM, Tazelaar HD, Krasne DL. Pulmonary eosinophilia in coccidioidal infections. Chest 1987; 91:734.

18. Yamaguchi H, Komase Y, Ikehara M, et al. Disseminated cryptococcal infection with eosinophilia in a healthy person. J Infect Chemother 2008; 14:319.

19. Hirano T, Yamada M, Sato K, et al. Invasive pulmonary mucormycosis: rare presentation with pulmonary eosinophilia. BMC Pulm Med 2017; 17:76.

20. Elsom KA, Ingelfinger FJ. Eosinophilia and pneumonitis in Chronic Brucellosis:report of 2 cases. Ann Intern Med 1942;16:995–1002

21. Vijayan VK, Reetha AM, Jawahar MS, et al. Pulmonary eosinophilia in pulmonary tuberculosis. Chest 1992; 101:1708.

22. Boggild AK, Keystone JS, Kain KC. Tropical pulmonary eosinophilia: a case series in a setting of nonendemicity. Clin Infect Dis 2004; 39:1123.

23. Ottesen EA, Nutman TB. Tropical pulmonary eosinophilia. Annu Rev Med 1992; 43:417.

24. Mullerpattan JB, Udwadia ZF, Udwadia FE. Tropical pulmonary eosinophilia–a review. Indian J Med Res 2013; 138:295.

25. Sandhu M, Mukhopadhyay S, Sharma SK. Tropical pulmonary eosinophilia: a comparative evaluation of plain chest radiography and computed tomography. Australas Radiol 1996; 40:32.

26. Cooray JH, Ismail MM: Re-examination of the diagnostic criteria of tropical pulmonary eosinophilia. Respir Med 1999; 93:655–59.

27. Ganatra RD, Sheth UK, Lewis RA. Diethylcarbamazine (hetrazan) in tropical eosinophilia. IJMR 1958; 46(2) 205–22.

28. Ray D. Lung functions in tropical eosinophilia. Indian J Chest Dis 1974; 16:368–73.

29. Vijayan VK. Tropical pulmonary eosinophilia. CurrOpinPulm Med 2007; 13:428–33.

30. Marchand E, Reynaud-Gaubert M, Lauque D, et al. Idiopathic chronic eosinophilic pneumonia. A clinical and follow-up study of 62 cases. The Grouped'Etudeset de Recherchesur les Maladies "Orphelines" Pulmonaires (GERM"O"P). Medicine (Baltimore) 1998; 77:299.

31. Gholamnejad M, Rezaie N. Unusual presentation of chronic eosinophilic pneumonia with "reversed halo sign": a case report. Iran J Radiol 2014;11(2):e7891.

32. Ebara H, Ikezoe J, Johkoh T, Kohno N, Takeuchi N, Kozuka T, et al. Chronic eosinophilic pneumonia: evolution of chest radiograms and CT features. J Comput Assist Tomogr 1994; 18(5):737–44.

33. Yoshida K, Shijubo N, Koba H, et al. Chronic eosinophilic pneumonia progressing to lung fibrosis. EurRespir J 1994; 7:1541.

34. Kaya H, Gümüş S, Uçar E, et al. Omalizumab as a steroid-sparing agent in chronic eosinophilic pneumonia. Chest 2012; 142:513.

35. Brenard E, Pilette C, Dahlqvist C, et al. Real-Life Study of Mepolizumab in Idiopathic Chronic Eosinophilic Pneumonia. Lung 2020; 198:355.

36. Isomoto K, Baba T, Sekine A, et al. Promising Effects of Benralizumab on Chronic Eosinophilic Pneumonia. Intern Med 2020; 59:1195.

37. Menzella F, Montanari G, Patricelli G, et al. A case of chronic eosinophilic pneumonia in a patient treated with dupilumab. TherClin Risk Manag 2019; 15:869.

38. Weller PF, Bubley GJ. The idiopathic hypereosinophilic syndrome. Blood 1994; 83:2759.

39. Simon HU, Rothenberg ME, Bochner BS, et al. Refining the definition of hypereosinophilic syndrome. J Allergy ClinImmunol 2010; 126:45.

40. Dulohery MM, Patel RR, Schneider F, Ryu JH. Lung involvement in hypereosinophilic syndromes. Respir Med 2011; 105:114.

41. Fauci AS, Harley JB, Roberts WC, et al. NIH conference. The idiopathic hypereosinophilic syndrome. Clinical, pathophysiologic, and therapeutic considerations. Ann Intern Med 1982; 97:78.

42. Cools J, DeAngelo DJ, Gotlib J, et al. A tyrosine kinase created by fusion of the PDGFRA and FIP1L1

genes as a therapeutic target of imatinib in idiopathic hypereosinophilic syndrome. N Engl J Med 2003; 348:1201.

43. Baumgartner C, Gleixner KV, Peter B, et al. Dasatinib inhibits the growth and survival of neoplastic human eosinophils (EOL-1) through targeting of FIP1L1-PDGFRalpha. Exp Hematol 2008; 36:1244.

44. Lierman E, Folens C, Stover EH, et al. Sorafenib is a potent inhibitor of FIP1L1-PDGFRalpha and the imatinib-resistant FIP1L1-PDGFRalpha T674I mutant. Blood 2006; 108:1374.

45. Cordier JF, Cottin V, Khouatra C, et al. Hypereosinophilic obliterative bronchiolitis: a distinct, unrecognised syndrome. Eur Respir J 2013; 41:1126.

46. Takayanagi N, Kanazawa M, Kawabata Y, Colby TV. Chronic bronchiolitis with associated eosinophilic lung disease (eosinophilic bronchiolitis). Respiration 2001; 68:319.

47. Sinico RA, Bottero P. Churg-Strauss angiitis. Best Pract Res Clin Rheumatol 2009; 23:355.

48. Pagnoux C, Guilpain P, Guillevin L. Churg-Strauss syndrome. Curr Opin Rheumatol 2007; 19:25.

49. Wechsler ME, Akuthota P, Jayne D, et al. Mepolizumab or Placebo for EosinophilicGranulomatosis with Polyangiitis. N Engl J Med 2017; 376:1921.

50. Kim S, Marigowda G, Oren E, et al. Mepolizumab as a steroid-sparing treatment option in patients with Churg-Strauss syndrome. J Allergy Clin Immunol 2010; 125:1336.

51. Samson M, Puéchal X, Devilliers H, et al. Long-term outcomes of 118 patients with eosinophilicgranulomatosis with polyangiitis (Churg-Strauss syndrome) enrolled in two prospective trials. J Autoimmun 2013; 43:60.

52. Guillevin L, Cohen P, Gayraud M, et al. Churg-Strauss syndrome. Clinical study and long-term follow-up of 96 patients. Medicine (Baltimore) 1999; 78:26.

53. Tefferi A. Blood eosinophilia: a new paradigm in disease classification, diagnosis, and treatment. Mayo Clin Proc 2005; 80:75.

54. Roufosse F, Weller PF. Practical approach to the patient with hypereosinophilia. J Allergy Clin Immunol 2010; 126:39.

PART III

MANAGEMENT OF ALLERGY AND ASTHMA IN ADOLESCENTS AND YOUNG ADULTS

24 Patient Education and Lifestyle Modification in Asthma Management

Alpa Dalal, Tarang Kulkarni and Manas Mengar

CONTENTS

INTRODUCTION

Asthma is known to be a heterogeneous disease. This heterogeneity is based not only on the presentation of the disease, but also on the comorbidities and triggers leading to possible flare-ups/exacerbations. This phenomenon has led to the development of asthma phenotyping and biological therapy. Whether or not this phenotype-based approach may be used in prescribing non-pharmacological treatment is something that remains to be seen.

In recent years, there has been an increased emphasis on pharmacotherapy like inhaled corticosteroids with the long-acting beta agonist (ICS+LABA) being the mainstay of asthma treatment. However, patient education, lifestyle modification and other non-pharmacological methods of asthma management, although much needed, have not received the same level of attention. Over reliance on pharmacotherapy has also increased the overall cost of the management of asthma. The annual cost of the management of asthma in India is estimated to be $261, whereas severe asthma is managed at an even greater cost of $334 per year (1). These costs impart a significant economic burden, especially in middle- to low-income countries like India. Lifestyle modification in asthma patients may be a relatively inexpensive modality that may lead to a significant improvement in control of symptoms, resulting in an increased asthma related quality of life. As noted in a review by Clark et al, including lifestyle modifications in a routine asthma treatment plan was associated with

significantly fewer symptoms and decreased asthma health care utilization (2).

Patient Education and Training

Patient education is generally defined as 'a systematic learning experience in which a combination of methods (Table 24.1) is generally used, such as the provision of information and advice and behaviour modification techniques, which influence the patient experiences and/or their knowledge and health behaviour aimed at improving or maintaining health or learning to cope with a condition, usually a chronic one' (3).

Addressing Stigma and Perception of Control

Patient education is important in understanding the nature of the disease, perception of symptom control, and importance of taking inhalers. In the Indian context, based on a questionnaire study on 1012 patients (testing perception of asthma), it was found there are many barriers in the way of optimal asthma treatment (4). Inability to recognize warning signals, belief in a permanent cure for asthma, preference for seeking treatment only at the time of an asthma attack, aversion to inhaled therapy and inclination towards complementary therapies (saintly therapy, fish therapy, etc.) are some of the barriers to optimal asthma management in India. These lead to under-treatment with resulting moderate airflow obstruction in the majority of subjects. An understanding of the disease among the Indian population was low—only 15.3% of the patients understood that asthma is not curable but can be controlled (4).

DOI: 10.1201/9781003125785-24

Table 24.1: Components of Patient Education in Asthma

No.	Components	Problems	Strategies to Overcome
1.	Nature of asthma as a disease	Poor perception of asthma symptoms	Detailed explanation in local language about asthma symptoms and monitoring
2.	Stigma of asthma	Impairs diagnosis and leads to non-adherence	Patient education, awareness and strategies for behavioural change Asthma support groups and counselling sessions.
3.	Monitoring asthma control	Easy access to health care	Asthma self-guided management approach in mild cases Understanding symptoms and need to seek help
4.	Inhaler technique	Not following 7-step technique	Checking and training inhaler technique at each visit Switching inhaler devices in certain cases Device maintenance
5.	Compliance with therapy	Stopping inhalers once symptoms reduced Concerns about inhalers being 'addictive' Cost of inhaler	Checking for compliance at each visit Education about need and benefit of inhalers Partnership between physician and patient regarding choosing inhaler in terms of cost, side effects, device, frequency and ease of use
6.	Trigger avoidance	Continued trigger exposure leading to poor asthma control	Identification of and, ideally, the complete avoidance of trigger Meditation/Yoga to address triggers like anxiety and stress
7.	Smoking cessation	Lack of motivation Withdrawal symptoms	Cessation counselling Nicotine replacement therapies

In India, social stigma, due to the reasons mentioned above, is a significant barrier to treatment. In a study conducted in rural Punjab, 58.6% of patients refused inhaled treatment for asthma due to the associated social stigma (5). On the bright side, in more recent studies that number has dropped to only 6.7% (6).

The GINA guidelines provides a comprehensive algorithmic approach towards management of asthma (7). Patient education and a self-guided asthma action plan are important aspects of the GINA approach. Patient training starts with education related to the nature of the disease, prescriptions, inhaler techniques and—most importantly—control of possible triggers.

Physician and Patient Partnership

In the Indian context, the physician and patient relationship has been an important topic of discussion in recent times. Possible causes hampering the physician–patient relationship include time constraints, language barrier, poor social support, cultural conditioning, educational level and patient intellectual capacity, etc. Asthma management begins at the point where the physician conveys the diagnosis to the patient. Expectedly, this is an important moment for the patient because every diagnosis is met with anxiety, questions about the prognosis and the nature of the illness. This is where the physician needs to be compassionate and attentive to the patient's emotional and spiritual needs. It is important that the patient undergoes counselling and rapport building with attention, care and humor to build a strong physician-patient relationship (8). Even in terms of pharmacotherapy, the decision of choosing the right treatment, the side effects and a further follow up plan need to be discussed with the patient and any concerns need to be addressed. Measures to improve communication skills have been listed in Table 24.2.

Self-Management

Patients are also trained regarding the use of asthma diaries and peak flow meters for

Table 24.2: Measures to Improve Physician–Patient Communication in Asthma

1. Offer reassurance and alleviate fears regarding disease and treatment.
2. Use interactive dialogue (open-ended questions).
3. Take a personalized approach to lifestyle modifications.
4. Adopt responsible non-verbal engagement and communication.
5. Address the emotional and spiritual concerns regarding long-term management.
6. Share decision-making regarding treatment related goals.
7. Provide a written action plan.
8. Appreciate when the patient has followed correct management strategies.

monitoring their asthma symptoms. Newer smartphone applications and online asthma control test score calculators also seem to help patients monitor their asthma symptoms. Factors like low literacy and socio-economic status are identified as important barriers for the implementation of self-management programs for asthma patients.

Patients also need to be educated regarding avoidance of possible triggers. Asthma triggers are agents that on exposure can lead to the worsening of asthma symptoms. These triggers can range from respiratory viral infections to a host of factors like change in temperature, tobacco smoke, dust, cold air, etc. In the Indian population, almost half of the asthmatics considered air-pollution to be a trigger for their asthma. Other reported triggers were strong odours, biomass fuel fumes, incense sticks and tobacco smoke (9). Sensitisation to house dust mite and aspergillus have also been reported in Asian asthmatics.

Avoidance of Triggers

Identification of triggers causing worsening of asthma symptoms is the first step towards evaluation. Such assessment should take into consideration the intensity, duration, sensitivity and clinical significance of the allergen in the context of the patient's medical history. Diagnostic tests such as allergic skin prick testing or in vitro IgE assays could be useful in this regard. This is particularly useful since immunotherapy for patients sensitized to house dust mite allergy is now approved for use in severe asthma (7). Details of occupational exposures, indoor/outdoor air pollutants, exercise, etc., need to be sought. However allergen exposure cannot be completely avoided in certain cases (e.g. changing the department or environment in case of occupational asthma). In cases where an exposure to allergen is unavoidable (e.g. exercise-induced bronchospasm), the authors suggest an extra dose of the patient's inhaler prior to exposure. This approach is generally advised when the first two approaches are not possible or have failed.

Respiratory viral infections have also been identified as a potential trigger for worsening asthma control in Indian population (10). In such cases strategies for prevention of viral infections like attention to hand hygiene and avoidance of contact with infected individual may be undertaken. Annual influenza and pneumococcal vaccination could be useful to prevent worsening of asthma symptoms (11).

A few patients experienced worsening of asthma symptoms after having episodes of anxiety, chronic stress and depression (12). Vocal cord dysfunction is an important differential here that needs to be excluded by the treating physician. Counselling techniques like cognitive behavioural therapy have proved to be useful to alleviate depression and stress. Cognitive behavioural therapy assists asthma patients in recognizing and altering negative thought patterns, thereby blocking negative emotions.

Meditation in this cohort of patients has been associated with better asthma related outcomes. In a systematic review consisting of over 200 patients, meditation techniques were associated with a significant improvement in asthma associated quality of life (13). Even in the author's experience, meditation has been shown to consistently reduce anxiety levels, ultimately leading to improved asthma control.

The ultimate purpose of patient education is to bring about sustainable health promoting behaviour change to improve long-term outcomes. It has been observed that in many patients mere knowledge sharing, information and skills training (inhaler techniques, self-monitoring) does not translate into a change in their beliefs, habits and behaviours. For this subset of patients, we need to develop interventions and strategies that help us to break through their barriers of strong conditioning and beliefs and empower them to change their mindset, habits, behaviour and bring about health supportive lifestyle change on long-term basis (Table 24.3).

Table 24.3: Physician's Checklist for Asthma Education Advice

1. Have I informed the patient about the nature of asthma as a disease?

2. Have I focussed on building a healthy physician-patient relationship?

3. Have I addressed the patient's concerns and asthma stigma related issues?

4. Have I advised the patient on monitoring asthma symptoms with tools like asthma diaries, Home PEFR monitoring, etc?

5. Have I demonstrated and confirmed the proper technique to take inhalers?

6. Have I explained to the patient the benefit of inhalers and the need of adherence to inhalers?

7. Have I checked the intellectual and social competency of either the patient or the caregiver?

8. Have I explained to the patient the importance of trigger identification and avoidance?

9. Have I counselled my patient to adopt a healthy lifestyle? (diet and exercise)

10. Have I informed the patient regarding the next follow up schedule and need of PFTs at regular intervals?

Lifestyle Modifications in Asthma
Obesity and Asthma

The relationship between obesity and asthma derives from a complex interplay of biologic, physiologic and environmental factors. Mass loading of the chest wall and abdomen with adipose tissue decreases the functional residual capacity (the lung volume at the end of normal tidal exhalation); breathing at lower functional residual capacity may increase airway reactivity (14, 15). In asthma, evidence supports weight loss interventions that incorporate diet and exercise, with multiple trials showing improvements in lung function, asthma control, quality of life and exacerbation frequency (16).

It is still unknown if eosinophil function is altered by obesity. While submucosal eosinophils are increased in obese patients with asthma relative to overweight and lean subjects, eosinophils in induced sputum and peripheral blood are not increased with obesity.

Weight loss interventions range from liquid-diet replacement to diet and exercise to bariatric surgery. In general, studies of weight loss interventions show improvements in asthma control, asthma related quality of life, and lung function if a sufficient amount of weight loss (at least 5%) is attained (17). This is generally associated with increased PEFR, lung function and expiratory reserve volume. Most improvement in asthma control was seen in patients experiencing the maximum weight loss. For obese patients with asthma, bariatric surgery is typically reserved for those with a BMI ≥35 kg/m who have not been able to lose sufficient weight by other methods. As bariatric surgery carries the risk of peri- and post-operative morbidity that may be exacerbated by severe asthma, it requires lifelong lifestyle changes and a careful evaluation of the risks and benefits of surgery should be discussed in detail with each patient.

Diet and Asthma

Diet is an important modifiable risk factor in chronic conditions like asthma. Moreover, it is an important aspect of the patient's life which is closely associated with habit patterns, significant cultural and emotional conditioning. Several studies have evaluated the benefit of an anti-inflammatory diet in asthma. In a recent systematic review, it was observed that adherence to a Mediterranean diet (rich in fruits, vegetables, dietary fibres and omega-3 fatty acids) was associated with fewer asthma symptoms (18). Similarly, in a study involving adult asthma patients, the Dietary Approaches to Stop Hypertension (DASH) diet was associated with clinically important improvements in quality of life and asthma control (19). Antioxidants have also been investigated in asthma in recent times (20). Vitamic C is the most commonly used antioxidant. Despite its wide usage, the evidence supporting its routine use is scarce. Given the recent data demonstrating the positive impact of fruits, vegetables and a high fibre diet on asthma control, vitamin C should be consumed as a part of one's whole food intake rather than as supplements.

Omega-3 polyunsaturated fatty acids (PUFA), probiotics and synbiotics have been studied in various randomized controlled trials for their anti-inflammatory effect on asthma control in adults and children with inconsistent results. Based on this, it is not possible to recommend probiotic/synbiotic supplements and omega-3 PUFA use for their benefits in asthma. Vitamin D is hypothesized to be useful in asthma, owing to its impact on the immune function and asthma susceptibility genes (21). Deficiency of vitamin D in adults has been linked to persistent airway inflammation leading to a poorer lung function and increased symptom burden. In a recent systematic review involving 9 trials, vitamin D supplement was associated with a significant reduction in exacerbation rates and need of oral corticosteroids. In the author's opinion, vitamin D may be useful in asthma for its anti-inflammatory effect, but more research particularly regarding dose based on geographical area, environmental exposures, age and gender is needed.

Gastroesophageal reflux is a comorbidity associated with severe or difficult-to-treat asthma. Micro-aspiration of gastric contents into the upper airway, increased vagal tone and heightened bronchial reactivity produce bronchoconstriction and therefore exacerbate airflow obstruction in asthmatics. GE reflux was a frequent comorbidity (46%) in patients with severe or difficult-to-treat asthma in 341 patients enrolled in The Epidemiology and Natural History of Asthma: Outcomes and Treatment Regimens (TENOR) II study (22).

Asthma improvement during a three-month empiric trial of twice daily PPI therapy, in combination with appropriate lifestyle modifications for GERD, is considered diagnostic of GE reflux-triggered asthma.

Exercise and Asthma

Patients with asthma are less likely to exercise than their non-asthmatics counterparts (23). The primary reason for this is thought to be fear of increased shortness of breath

Table 24.4: Components of Pulmonary Rehabilitation (27)

1. Education	Education involves teaching patients about respiratory diseases and supporting them through self-management training.
2. Exercise	Exercise is the cornerstone of rehabilitation—it consists of strength and endurance training.
3. Physical activity	Physical activity, coupled with conventional pharmacotherapy, has been shown to reduce exacerbation rates and asthma related emergency room visits.
4. Breath retraining	Breath retraining techniques reduce respiratory rate, improve ventilation and gas exchange in order to reduce air trapping.
5. Weight loss counselling	Weight loss interventions show improvements in asthma control, asthma related quality of life and lung function if a sufficient amount of weight loss (at least 5%) is attained.
6. Psychological counselling	Counselling should be offered either individually or in small groups to adults with persistent asthma because discussion will enable patients to feel more comfortable with their disease and make them more inclined to participate in social activities.

and, in a few cases, exercise-induced bronchoconstriction. This leads to a vicious cycle of exercise avoidance, resulting in asthma related morbidity and invalidity. Therefore, it is strongly recommended for asthma patients to participate in 20–60 minutes of physical activity, at least 3 times/week (24). When coupled with conventional pharmacotherapy, exercise has shown to reduce exacerbation rates and asthma related emergency room visits. However, the impact of exercise training on airway and systemic inflammation is still unclear, and more evidence is currently needed in this regard.

In the author's practice, many patients with moderate to severe asthma are enrolled in a pulmonary rehabilitation program or yoga meditation program (see Table 24.4.). The evidence in this regard is also strong, as it has shown significant short-term and long-term improvement in asthma control and health related quality of life. While pulmonary rehabilitation in asthmatics is effective, it should be used with caution in patients with exercise-induced bronchoconstriction (EIB). Exercise-induced asthma is defined as episodic bronchoconstriction during or immediately post-exercise. Such patients should be counselled regarding prevention of EIB with regular inhaled corticosteroids (ICS) and leukotriene receptor antagonist therapy. Warm up exercises and a low dose ICS-formoterol before exercise is also recommended in these patients (25). Traditional approaches recommend swimming over other land based exercises for patients with asthma. Swimming was thought to be free of cold air and pollen exposure. However, in a meta-analysis, including randomized control trials comparing water based exercises with other methods, no significant differences were observed between water based and land based exercises (26). Given the current evidence in this regard, it is

not possible to recommend one form of physical activity over the other.

Yoga and Asthma

The ancient practice of Yoga which includes physical postures, breathing techniques and meditation has been widely used for physical, mental and spiritual rehabilitation for many chronic disease conditions. Yoga is culturally accepted and widely available across the country.

Yoga was systemized and standardized by Rishi Patanjali in the Yoga Sutras (300–200 BC). Yoga is popularly understood to be a program of physical exercises (asana) and breathing exercises (pranayama). But its real purpose is to bring about Integration, Balance, Self-Awareness and Mind Management through the eight components of Rishi Patanjali's classical yoga, known as Ashtang Yoga.

The first four parts are called external limbs and the next four parts are called internal limbs.

All of these eight components are interconnected and can be used comprehensively for patient education and lifestyle modification.

We can draw parallels from the Eight Limbs of Yoga and integrate them with medical science to create a Comprehensive Patient Empowerment Programme based on yoga philosophy. The first two limbs, Yama and Niyama, are about 'dos and don'ts' that we address in Patient Education and Awareness Programme (trigger avoidance, regular inhaler use, techniques, diet, etc). The third limb is Asana, physical postures,which are equivalent to physical exercises. This component helps to improve muscle tone, strength, stamina and improve flexibility and recruitment of respiratory muscles. The fourth limb, Pranayam, can be compared to breath retraining and breathing exercises that helps asthma patients to improve their breathing patterns and allow good control over thoughts and emotions.

The next 4 components are called Internal Limbs: Pratyahar, (directing one's attention and energy inwards), Dharana (single focus; for example, focussing on breathing), Dhyan (meditation) and Samadhi (blissful deep meditation). This internal aspect of yoga is less known and under-utilized. These practices help one move across the barriers of strong thought emotion patterns and perceptions to bring about changes in mindset and attitudes. We have been running the Yoga and Meditation Programme in our setup for the past 8 years. Many of our asthma patients having triggers like anxiety and stress, and comorbidities like GERD and rhinitis, developed significant changes in their attitudes and lifestyle, which translated into better compliance with treatment and symptom control and a significant reduction in exacerbations (unpublished work).

The author's study, conducted in 53 healthy subjects using Kriya Yoga (sequential breathing practices followed by Six Step Meditation) for 48 days, demonstrated a significant reduction in mean Anxiety and Depression score of HADS, and WHO QoLBREF scores increased significantly over 48 days (28). In 32 subjects there was statistically significant cortical activity in area 23 demonstrated on EEG after 48 days of practice. Broadman area 23 is associated with better self-awareness, judgement, memory, sense of well-being and happiness.

Based on the findings of this study, we conducted a controlled study in COPD patients (more than half of these patients were Asthma COPD overlap). The intervention used involved 8 types of breathing exercises, six step meditation and sound therapy for 12 weeks.

QoL as measured by SGRQ showed a statistically significant improvement in the intervention group compared to the control group. 6MWD decreased in the control group but remained stable in the yoga group (29).

There are many learning points in this case study (Table 24.5) that can help us develop interventions for larger patient groups. This well-educated, working professional, living in urban area suffered from three decades of faulty treatment, lack of guidance and her own misconceptions. A treatable reversible airway obstruction deteriorated into an irreversible airway obstruction with profound physical and psychological impact on her life.

Although the last 7 years of evidence-based medical management with patient education, counselling, yoga exercises and lifestyle

Table 24.5: Case Study Showing the Effect of Lifestyle Modification in Asthma

- 64-year-old woman
- Employed as a bank manager
- Diagnosed as asthmatic in 1983
- For 31 years, received only oral and inhaled sos Salbutamol
- In 2014, after a routine PFT picked up moderate airflow obstruction, she was referred to a chest physician
- ICS+LABA was initiated for this patient.
- Had frequent anxiety about dependence of inhalers and had a deeply rooted steroid phobia, leading to frequent non-compliance and worsening of asthma control
- Patient was subjected to thorough counselling and asthma education and lifestyle modification. Yoga and 'pranayama' programs were implemented
- Dissatisfaction and anxiety about her long-term inhaler dependence, however, still persisted!
- She was later enrolled in asthma support group therapy—a breathing exercise and meditation program—in 2019, which led to a significantly improved psychological state and better acceptance of her disease symptoms and therapy, which led to improved asthma control
- In turn, we could also 'step-down' her inhaled corticosteroid dose, which made her pleasantly surprised!

modifications brought about significant symptom relief, she still remained anxious and dissatisfied with inhaler dependence, leading to brief periods of non-adherence to inhalers and missing follow-ups.

The last 2 years of being part of group therapy based on breathing exercises, meditation and counselling has resulted in a change in her mindset, physical and psychological benefits and sustained behavioural change. It is unfortunate and unacceptable that in today's era of advanced therapeutics and evidence based medicine we continue to hear and see such stories. We need to conduct more research into this area and develop comprehensive strategies incorporating patient education, lifestyle counselling and interventions to empower our patients to bring about sustained behavioural change to deal with this chronic condition. In India, the question of whether or not we can explore the role of yoga in this context needs to be addressed!

CONCLUSION

Understanding our patient's needs, addressing their concerns and empowering them with knowledge and skills for self-care is most crucial component of asthma management. The core purpose of patient education is to establish a partnership based on knowledge and mutual trust. Lifestyle modification is a cost effective patient management intervention. Diet and nutrition, physical exercise, weight reduction and addressing comorbidities like GERD, obesity, anxiety, etc., are emerging as effective measures to improve patient outcomes in various studies. Yoga and meditation are emerging as very effective interventions for improving physical and psychological health and proving to be very useful tools to help patients change their attitudes to adopt healthy behaviours and lifestyles. In India, yoga is culturally accepted and widely available across the country. Future research should focus on standardization of yoga intervention and its impact on various components of asthma management. In countries like India, clinicians need to focus on developing different tools to educate their patients who are from different cultural, educational and socioeconomic backgrounds and speak diverse languages. Patient education and lifestyle modification should become part of our undergraduate and postgraduate training so that it may become an integral part of our clinical practice.

REFERENCES

1. Koul PA, Dhar R. Economic burden of asthma in India. Lung India 2018;35(4):281–283.

2. Clark NM, Griffiths C, Keteyian SR, Partridge MR. Educational and behavioral interventions for asthma: who achieves which outcomes? A systematic review. J Asthma Allergy. 2010 Dec 10;3:187–97.

3. van den Borne HW. The patient from receiver of information to informed decision-maker. Patient Educ Couns. 1998 Jun 1;34(2):89–102.

4. Singh V, Sinha HV, Gupta R. Barriers in the management of asthma and attitudes towards complementary medicine. Respir Med. 2002 Oct;96(10):835–840.

5. Prasad R, Gupta R, Verma S. A study on perception of patients about bronchial asthma. Indian J Allergy Asthma Immunol. 2003;17(2):85–87.

6. Prasad R, Kushwaha RAS, Verma S, Kumar S, Verma A, Prakash V, et al. A study to know the knowledge, attitude, and practices of patients of bronchial asthma. Int J Med Public Health. 2013;3(3):159.

7. Global Initiative for Asthma. Global Strategy for Asthma Management and Prevention, 2019. Available from: www.ginasthma.org.

8. Partridge MR, Hill SR. Enhancing care for people with asthma: the role of communication, education, training and self-management. 1998 World Asthma Meeting Education and Delivery of Care Working Group. Eur Respir J. 2000 Aug 1;16(2):333–48.

9. Thompson PJ, Salvi S, Lin J, Cho YJ, Eng P, Abdul Manap R, et al. Insights, attitudes and perceptions about asthma and its treatment: findings from a multinational survey of patients from 8 Asia-Pacific countries and Hong Kong. Respirol Carlton Vic. 2013 Aug;18(6):957–967.

10. Chhabra SK, Dash DJ. Acute exacerbations of chronic obstructive pulmonary disease: causes and impacts. Indian J Chest Dis Allied Sci. 2014 Jun;56(2):93–104.

11. Dhar R, Ghoshal AG, Guleria R, Sharma S, Kulkarni T, Swarnakar R, et al. Clinical practice guidelines 2019: Indian consensus-based recommendations on influenza vaccination in adults. Lung India Off Organ Indian Chest Soc. 2020 Aug;37(Supplement):S4–18.

12. Kewalramani A, Bollinger ME, Postolache TT. Asthma and mood disorders. Int J Child Health Hum Dev IJCHD. 2008;1(2):115–123.

13. Paudyal P, Jones C, Grindey C, Dawood R, Smith H. Meditation for asthma: Systematic review and meta-analysis. J Asthma Off J Assoc Care Asthma. 2018;55(7):771–778.

14. Peters U, Dixon AE, Forno E. Obesity and asthma. J Allergy Clin Immunol. 2018;141(4):1169–1179.

15. Barros R, Moreira P, Padrão P, Teixeira VH, Carvalho P, Delgado L, et al. Obesity increases the prevalence and the incidence of asthma and worsens asthma severity. Clin Nutr Edinb Scotl. 2017;36(4):1068–74.

16. Alwarith J, Kahleova H, Crosby L, Brooks A, Brandon L, Levin SM, et al. The role of nutrition in asthma prevention and treatment. Nutr Rev. 2020 Nov 1;78(11):928–938.

17. Adeniyi FB, Young T. Weight loss interventions for chronic asthma. Cochrane Database Syst Rev. 2012 Jul 11;(7):CD009339.

18. Papamichael MM, Itsiopoulos C, Susanto NH, Erbas B. Does adherence to the Mediterranean dietary pattern reduce asthma symptoms in children? A systematic review of observational studies. Public Health Nutr. 2017 Oct;20(15):2722–2734.

19. Ma X, Cui J, Wang J, Chang Y, Fang Q, Bai C, et al. Multicentre investigation of pathogenic bacteria and antibiotic resistance genes in Chinese patients with acute exacerbation of chronic obstructive pulmonary disease. J Int Med Res. 2015 Oct;43(5):699–710.

20. Stoodley RG, Aaron SD, Dales RE. The role of ipratropium bromide in the emergency management of acute asthma exacerbation: a metaanalysis of randomized clinical trials. Ann Emerg Med. 1999 Jul;34(1):8–18.

21. Riverin BD, Maguire JL, Li P. Vitamin D supplementation for childhood asthma: A systematic review and meta-analysis. PLOS ONE. 2015 Aug 31;10(8):e0136841.

22. Chipps BE, Haselkorn T, Paknis B, Ortiz B, Bleecker ER, Kianifard F, et al. More than a decade follow-up in patients with severe or difficult-to-treat asthma: The epidemiology and natural history of asthma: Outcomes and treatment regimens (TENOR) II. J Allergy Clin Immunol. 2018;141(5):1590–1597.e9.

23. Panagiotou M, Koulouris NG, Rovina N. Physical activity: A missing link in asthma care. J Clin Med [Internet]. 2020 Mar 5 [cited 2020 Dec 14];9(3). Available from: https://www.ncbi.nlm.nih.gov/pmc/articles/PMC7141291/

24. Guidelines for the Diagnosis and Management of Asthma (EPR-3) | NHLBI, NIH [Internet]. [cited 2020 Dec 14]. Available from: https://www.nhlbi.nih.gov/health-topics/guidelines-for-diagnosis-management-of-asthma

25. Parsons JP, Hallstrand TS, Mastronarde JG, Kaminsky DA, Rundell KW, Hull JH, et al. An official American Thoracic Society clinical practice guideline: exercise-induced bronchoconstriction. Am J Respir Crit Care Med. 2013 May 1;187(9):1016–1027.

26. Grande AJ, Silva V, Andriolo BNG, Riera R, Parra SA, Peccin MS. Water-based exercise for adults with asthma. Cochrane Database Syst Rev. 2014 Jul 17;(7):CD010456.

27. Zampogna E, Zappa M, Spanevello A, Visca D. Pulmonary rehabilitation and asthma. Front Pharmacol [Internet]. 2020 [cited 2020 Dec 14];11. Available from: https://www.frontiersin.org/articles/10.3389/fphar.2020.00542/full

28. Dalal A, Deshpande A, Gandhi M, Pawaskar A. A prospective, single arm intervention study to evaluate the effect of kriya yoga on neuro-cardiac physiology and quality of life. Int J Public Ment Health Neurosci. 2018; 5(2):15–23. https://doi.org/10.13140/RG.2.2.20790.96328

29. Rasam S, Vanjare N, Katkar S, Nirmal P, Das V, Kale N, et al. Yoga and meditation improve quality of life in subjects with moderate-to-very severe COPD without any effect on lung function. Eur Respir J [Internet]. 2019 Sep 28 [cited 2020 Dec 14];54(suppl 63). Available from: https://erj.ersjournals.com/content/54/suppl_63/PA769

25 Role of Antihistamines, Antileukotrienes and Mast Cell Stabilizers in Allergy and Asthma

Paramez Ayyappath

CONTENTS

INTRODUCTION

Initial manifestations of allergic diseases like asthma and rhinitis usually appear during childhood and early adolescence. The timely diagnosis and appropriate management of these diseases is important during childhood and adolescence because an uncontrolled disease may affect their cognitive and academic performance. Although topical corticosteroids remain the main controller therapy for these diseases, the compliance to the same remains a major concern, leading to inappropriate and undesirable outcomes. Antihistamines, antileukotrienes, and mast cell stabilizers play an important role in the management of allergic diseases. Antihistamines are primarily rapid relievers of allergic symptoms—especially in allergic rhinitis (AR) and urticaria—while the other two are primarily controller medicines to prevent the allergic cascade. Most of these drugs are administered orally (some antihistamines like azelastine and mast cell stabilizers are used topically), providing rapid symptom relief with minimal side effects as compared to systemic corticosteroids.

PATHOGENESIS OF ALLERGIC DISEASES

The term *atopy* implies a tendency to manifest asthma, rhinitis, urticaria, and atopic dermatitis alone or in combination, in association with the presence of allergen-specific IgE. Mast cells are key effector cells in allergic rhinitis and asthma, and the dominant effector in urticaria, and anaphylaxis. The binding of IgE to human mast cells and basophils, a process termed *sensitization*, prepares these cells for subsequent antigen-specific activation. IgE mediated cell activation of mast cells initiate two pathways for the production of lipid mediators and cytokines.[1,2] The biosynthesis of leukotrienes

and their action on cysteinyl leukotriene receptors is elucidated in Figure 25.1.

IgE-mediated immune responses can be classified chronologically according to 3 reaction patterns. The early-phase response is the immediate response after allergen is introduced into target organs. This response is characterized by mast cell degranulation and release of preformed mediators including histamine, occurring within an immediate time frame of 1–30 minutes after allergen exposure and resolving within 1–3 hours. Acute reactions are associated with increased local vascular permeability, which leads to leakage of plasma proteins, tissue swelling, and increased blood flow, as well as itching, sneezing, and wheezing.

A second, late-phase response can occur within hours of allergen exposure, reaching a maximum at 6–12 hours and resolving by 24 hours. Late-phase responses are characterized in the skin by edema, redness, and induration; in the nose by sustained nasal blockage; and in the lung by airway obstruction and persistent wheezing. Late-phase responses are associated with early infiltration of neutrophils and eosinophils, followed by basophils, monocytes, macrophages, and Th2-type cells. TNF-α released by activated mast cells induces the vascular endothelial expression of cell adhesion molecules, and leads to transendothelial migration of various inflammatory cells especially accumulation of eosinophils.

In the third reaction pattern, chronic allergic disease, tissue inflammation can persist for days to years. Several factors contribute to persistent tissue inflammation, including recurrent exposure to allergens and microbial agents.

The repeated stimulation of allergic effector cells such as mast cells, basophils, eosinophils,

DOI: 10.1201/9781003125785-25

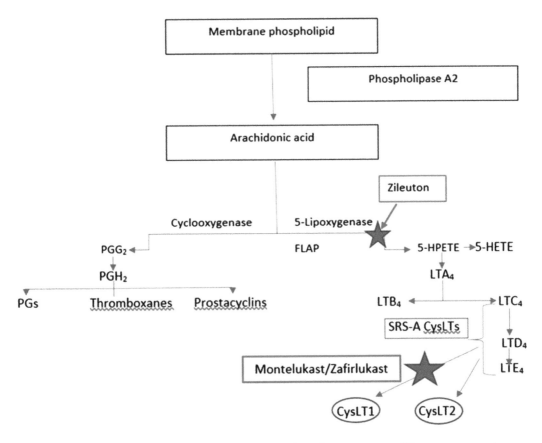

Figure 25.1 Metabolism of arachidonic acid through cyclooxygenase and lipoxygenase pathways. (HPETE—hydroperoxy ecosatetraenoic acid, HETE—hydroxyl tetraenoic acid, SRS-A—slow-reacting substance of anaphylaxis, CystLT—cysteinyl leukotriene, CystLT 1—cysteinyl leukotriene receptor 1, CystLT 2—cysteinyl leukotriene receptor 2.)

and Th2 cells contribute to unresolved inflammatory conditions.[2]

ANTIHISTAMINES[4,5]

Antihistamines typically reduce itching, sneezing, and rhinorrhea but are less effective for nasal congestion compared with glucocorticoid sprays. H1-antihistamines are classified as first-generation (relatively sedating) or second-generation (relatively non-sedating). Antihistamines usually are administered by mouth but are also available for topical ophthalmic and intranasal use. Second-generation antihistamines are preferred because they cause less sedation. These lipophobic agents were developed primarily to avoid the unwanted anticholinergic and central nervous system effects of the first-generation drugs.[6]

Mechanism of action: H1 antihistamines are not actually receptor antagonists, but rather inverse agonists. They bind the H1 receptor and

downregulate its constitutive activity, shifting the equilibrium from the active form of the H1 receptor to the inactive form.[7]

In experimental models, second- and third-generation antihistamines also have a variety of anti-inflammatory properties, including decreased mast cell mediator release and down regulation of adhesion molecule expression. Inhibition of interleukin 4 (IL-4) and interleukin 13 (IL-13) production may explain reports of their dose-dependent beneficial effect in asthma.[8]

Diphenhydramine, chlorpheniramine, hydroxyzine, brompheniramine, and triprolidine are first-generation antihistamines and are infrequently used due to their side effects.

Second-generation agents include cetirizine, terfenadine and loratadine. Metabolites of second-generation agents, such as fexofenadine (metabolite of terfenadine), desloratadine (metabolite of loratadine), and levocetirizine (purified isomer of cetirizine) were designed to have fewer central nervous system effects than their parent compounds.[9]

COMMONLY USED ANTIHISTAMINES (SECOND GENERATION)

Cetirizine: The standard dose of 10 mg once daily is appropriate for adults and children ages ≥6 years. The usual dose for children ages 2–5 years is 5 mg once daily. Smaller children ages 6 months to 2 years may be given 2.5 mg once daily. The maintenance dose is halved for patients with significant renal and/or hepatic insufficiency

Levocetirizine: Levocetirizine is an active enantiomer of cetirizine and produces effects equivalent to cetirizine at about one-half of the dose. For adults and children ≥12 years, the standard dose is 5 mg once daily. For children ages 6–11 years, the standard dose is 2.5 mg once daily in the evening. Levocetirizine is unlikely to be effective as an alternative for patients who do not respond adequately to cetirizine. Significant dose alteration is necessary in renal insufficiency.

Loratadine: Loratadine is a long-acting selective H1 antihistamine and has a standard dose of 10 mg once daily for age ≥6 years. For children ages 2–5 years, the usual dose is 5 mg once daily. For patients with significant renal and/or hepatic insufficiency, the usual dose is administered every other day. Its chemically distinct from cetirizine

Desloratadine: Desloratadine is the active metabolite of loratadine and produces effects equivalent to loratadine at about one-half of the dose. For adults and children ≥12 years, the standard dose is 5 mg once daily. For children ages 6–11 years, the dose is 2.5 mg once daily; for those ages 1–5 years, the dose is 1.25 mg once daily and 1 mg once daily for small children ages 6 months to 1 year. For patients with significant renal and/or hepatic insufficiency, the usual dose is administered every other day.

Fexofenadine: The dose of fexofenadine is 180 mg daily for ages ≥12 years or 30 mg twice daily for children ages 2–11 years. A lower dose of 15 mg twice daily is approved in the United States for small children ages 6 months to 2 years. It is best taken without food and specifically not with fruit juices.

Other new-generation orally active antihistamines are **Ebastine** (10–20 mg/day), **Mizolastine** (10 mg/day), **Rupatadine** (2.5–10 mg/day) and **Bilastine** (20 mg/day).

Antihistamine nasal sprays: Azelastine and olopatadine are available as nasal sprays and are similarly effective.

Azelastine: This is available in two strengths, 0.1% or 0.15%. Only the lower strength should be used in children 6 months to 6 years of age. The dose is 1 spray per nostril twice daily. Children 6–12 years can use either strength at a dose of 1 spray per nostril twice daily. In older children and adults, the dosing of both strengths is the same: 1 or 2 sprays per nostril once or twice daily.[10]

Olopatadine: This may be obtained without a prescription and is available in one strength. The dose for children 6–11 years is 1 spray per nostril twice daily. The dose for children ≥12 years and adults is 2 sprays per nostril twice daily.

Antihistamine nasal sprays have some anti-inflammatory effect and improve nasal congestion. They have a rapid onset of action (in 10–15 minutes) and can be administered for rapid relief on demand. The onset of action is faster than that of intranasal corticosteroid sprays. They can be used in combination with topical corticosteroids for patients with uncontrolled symptoms.

Adverse effects and safety: First-generation antihistamines cause significant sedation because they are lipophilic and easily cross the blood-brain barrier. Adverse effects on intellectual and motor function, even in the absence of subjective awareness of sedation are well documented. In school-aged children, sedating antihistamines are associated with impaired school performance. In infants and toddlers, first-generation antihistamines can cause paradoxical agitation, and have been linked to a small number of deaths in children <2 years of age. Anticholinergic effects, including dry mouth and eyes, urinary hesitancy, and confusion are more prominent in adults.[11,12]

ANTILEUKOTRIENE AGENTS

The leukotrienes are proinflammatory mediators produced from arachidonic acid via the 5-lipoxygenase (5-LO) pathway. Resident leukocytes produce leukotrienes rapidly and the binding of LTs to leukotriene receptors is a key in pathogenesis of asthma and allergic rhinitis. LTD_4, acting at $CysLT_1$ receptors, is a potent bronchoconstrictor, whereas LTE_4 induces a vascular leak and induces recruitment of eosinophils to bronchial mucosa. CysLT1 receptor has a preference for LTD4 and is blocked by the receptor antagonists in clinical use, while the CysLT2 receptor is equally responsive to LTD4 and LTC4, is unaffected by these antagonists, and is a negative regulator of the function of the CysLT1 receptor.[13]

Table 25.1: Commonly Used Antileukotrienes and Their Doses

Medication	Preparations	Infant and Small Child	Paediatric	Adolescent and Adult
Montelukast	Granules: 4 mg per packet Chewable tablets: 4 mg, 5 mg Tablet: 10 mg	12 months* to 5 years: 4 mg granules or chewable tablet, once daily in evening	6 to 14 years: 5 mg chewable tablet, once daily in evening	≥15 years and adult: 10 mg tablet, once daily in evening
Zafirlukast	Tablets: 10 mg, 20 mg	(Not used)	5–11 years: 10 mg, twice per day	≥12 years and adult: 20 mg, twice per day
Zileuton	Immediate-release tablet: 600 mg Extended-release tablet: 600 mg	(Not used)	(Not used)	≥12 years and adult: Immediate release: 600 mg, four times per day Extended release: 1200 mg, twice per day
Pranlukast	Capsule: 112.5 mg, 225 mg Granules: 50 mg, 70 mg, 100 mg per packet	24 months to 5 years: 7 to 10 mg/kg granules per day in two divided doses	6 to 11 years: 7 to 10 mg/kg per day granules in two divided doses (maximum 225 mg twice per day)	≥12 years and adult: 225 mg, twice per day

* US Food and Drug Administration approved prescribing information. Available at https://dailymed.nlm. nih.gov/dailymed/.

Two approaches to interrupting the leukotriene pathway are inhibition of 5-lipoxygenase, thereby preventing leukotriene synthesis; and inhibition of the binding of LTD4 to its receptor on target tissues, thereby preventing its action (Figure 25.1). Efficacy in blocking airway responses to antigen challenge has been shown for drugs in both categories. Montelukast zafirlukast and pranlukast are cysteinyl leukotriene receptor antagonists (LTRA) which blocks LTD4 receptors, while zileuton inhibits formation of both CysLTs and LTB4 by inhibiting 5-lipooxygenase[14] (Table 25.1). Montelukast is used extensively in clinical practice as compared to other drugs of this class.

Montelukast: This is an orally active, highly selective cysteinyl leukotriene type-1 receptor antagonist of LTD4, with affinities approximately 2-fold greater than the natural ligand. It is rapidly absorbed achieving peak plasma concentration (Cmax) in 3–4 hours and with a mean bioavailability of 64% following a 10 mg oral administration.

More than 99% is bound to plasma proteins with minimal distribution across the blood–brain barrier. Metabolism occurs via liver P450 (CYP) 3A4 and 2CP microsomes, with potent inhibition of P450 2C8. Excretion occurs almost exclusively in bile with a half-life from 2.7 to 5.5 hours in healthy adults.[15]

The pharmacokinetic profile is similar in females and males, young and elderly. 10 mg is recommended for ages 15 and older, 5 mg chewable tablets for patients 6–14 years of age, 4 mg chewable in patients 2–5 years of age, and 4 mg oral granule formulation in pediatrics for asthma in 12–23 months and AR in 6–23 months of age.

In patients with mild to moderate hepatic insufficiency, no dosage adjustment is required but data are lacking regarding severe hepatic impairment. Dose adjustment in severe renal failure is not well known as the drug is almost exclusively excreted through the biliary system.

Tolerability: Montelukast is well tolerated and has a similar safety profile in pediatric and adult populations. Side effects most commonly reported above placebo included headache, otitis media, upper respiratory infection, and pharyngitis. Neuropsychiatric changes have been reported in association with montelukast, including dream abnormalities, insomnia, anxiety, depression, suicidal thinking, and in rare cases, suicide. A boxed warning was added to the product insert in 2020 with a recommendation from the US Food and Drug Administration (FDA) to avoid the use of montelukast in patients with allergic rhinitis or mild asthma, in favor of other treatments.

Efficacy and quality of life: The efficacy of montelukast in the treatment of seasonal AR has been studied quite extensively over the past few years as monotherapy, combined with a second-generation antihistamine, and with or without intranasal corticosteroids.

Night time symptoms (difficulty falling asleep, night time awakenings, and congestion upon awakening) appeared to have a better response with montelukast compared with antihistamines.[15]

Although various studies reinforce the greater efficacy of intranasal corticosteroids when compared to montelukast monotherapy, montelukast in combination with antihistamines was found to be as effective as intranasal corticosteroids in controlling daytime symptoms in seasonal allergic rhinitis. When montelukast is added for uncontrolled symptoms of AR, effective symptom control is achieved in patients already treated with intranasal corticosteroids and antihistamines.[16]

Montelukast is routinely used as the controller drug in steps 2, 3 and 4 in the management for asthma in children and adults, though it is considered less effective than an inhalational corticosteroid.[17] Monotherapy with montelukast as first-line controller medicine has shown benefit in certain subset of mild to moderate persistent asthma resulting in improvement in FEV_1, decreased exacerbation rates, improved quality of life and less requirement for rescue medications. Although not considered first-line therapy, the leukotriene-modifying agents are sometimes given instead of inhaled corticosteroids for mild asthma when prescription of an ICS meets patient resistance. Montelukast exert anti-inflammatory effects, such as reducing the numbers of circulating and sputum eosinophils, exhaled nitric oxide, and nonspecific bronchial hyperresponsiveness, in addition to their bronchodilator actions. Both in children and adults, the adherence to therapy—which is a key aspect in asthma control—with a once daily montelukast was seen to be higher than in inhaled corticosteroids.[18]

Zileuton: This inhibits the formation of leukotrienes by inhibiting 5 lipoxygenase-activating protein (FLAP). It is available in 2 preparations: immediate release (600 mg, four times daily) and controlled release (1200 mg, twice daily). This agent is only available in the United States and is approved for use in children 12 years and older. Regular monitoring of serum alanine aminotransferase is recommended and the drug is not recommended in pregnancy.

MAST CELL STABILIZERS

Cromolyn sodium: Cromolyn sodium is a mast cell stabilizer. It inhibits mast cell release of histamine and other inflammatory mediators by inhibiting the intermediate conductance chloride channel pathways of mast cells, eosinophils, epithelial and endothelial cells, fibroblasts, and sensory neurons

Cromolyn sodium is more effective than placebo in the treatment of seasonal allergic rhinitis. It also has no serious side effects and is available over-the-counter as a nasal spray. However, most studies show it to be less effective than glucocorticoid nasal sprays or second-generation antihistamines.[19]

Cromolyn blocks symptoms associated with the immediate- and late-phase nasal allergen challenge and is effective in doing so, even when used shortly before allergen inhalation. This makes cromolyn particularly useful for individuals who experience episodic symptoms to allergens, where it may be used 30 minutes prior to exposure. For seasonal allergic rhinitis, it is most effective when initiated just prior to the pollen season, rather than after symptoms have begun. Frequent dosing is required to attain a good effect in seasonal allergic rhinitis. The dose is 1–2 sprays, 3–4 times daily. Dose frequency can be reduced after the first 2–3 weeks of treatment. Though not frequently used for asthma, cromolyn preparations are available as nebulizer solutions, MDI or DPI.

Nedocromil generally is more potent in protecting patients against nonimmunologic stimuli and has better steroid sparing effect compared to cromolyn without much side effects. It is available as pMDI as 2 mg per puff and used as 2 puffs, 4 times a day. It may be tried if other agents are not well-tolerated or if patients are not keen on using inhaled glucocorticoids.

CONCLUSION

Antihistamines are the mainstay of treatment for allergic rhinitis and urticaria. Antileukotrienes, by virtue of their ease of administration, tolerability, lack of significant side effects and good compliance are extensively used as controller medicines for the management of allergic conditions, especially asthma. Currently, mast cell stabilizers are rarely used, due to the availability of more effective topical agents like inhalational corticosteroids. These agents have a role in appropriate clinical settings in carefully selected individuals.

REFERENCES

1. Jameson JL, Fauci AS, Kasper, DL, Hauser SL, Longo DL, Loscalzo J. *Harrison's Principles of Internal Medicine.* 20th ed. New York: McGraw-Hill; 2018.

2. Kleigman RM, St Geme J. *Nelson Textbook of Pediatrics.* 21st ed. New York: Elsevier: 2019.

3. Brunton LL, Chabner BA, Knollmann BC. *Goodman & Gilman's: The Pharmacological Basis of Therapeutics.* 12th ed. New York: McGraw-Hill; 2011.

4. Tripathi KD. *Essentials of Medical Pharmacolog.* 6th ed. New Delhi: Jaypee Brothers; 2008.

5. Katzung BG. *Basic & Clinical Pharmacology.* 14th ed. New York: McGraw-Hill Lange; 2018.

6. Borish L. Allergic rhinitis: systemic inflammation and implications for management. *J Allergy Clin Immunol* 2003; 112:1021.

7. Church MK. H(1)-antihistamines and inflammation. *Clin Exp Allergy* 2001; 31:1341.

8. Watts AM, Cripps AW, West NP, Cox AJ. Modulation of allergic inflammation in the nasal mucosa of allergic rhinitis sufferers with topical pharmaceutical agents. *Front Pharmacol* 2019 Mar 29;10:294.

9. Verster JC, Volkerts ER. Antihistamines and driving ability: evidence from on-the-road driving studies during normal traffic. *Ann Allergy Asthma Immunol* 2004; 92:294.

10. Lee TA, Pickard AS. Meta-analysis of azelastine nasal spray for the treatment of allergic rhinitis. *Pharmacotherapy* 2007; 27:852.

11. Simons FE, Simons KJ. Clinical pharmacology of new histamine H1 receptor antagonists. *Clin Pharmacokinet* 1999; 36:329.

12. O'Byrne PM, Israel E, Drazen JM. Antileukotrienes in the treatment of asthma. *Ann Intern Med* 1997; 127:472.

13. Bender BG, Berning S, Dudden R, et al. Sedation and performance impairment of diphenhydramine and second-generation antihistamines: a meta-analysis. *J Allergy Clin Immunol* 2003; 111:770.

14. Lagos JA, Marshall GD. Montelukast in the management of allergic rhinitis. *Ther Clin Risk Manag* 2007:3(2) 327–332.

15. Philip G, Nayak A, Berger W, et al. The effect of montelukast on rhinitis symptoms in patients with asthma and seasonal allergic rhinitis. *Curr Med Res Opin* 2004; 10:1549–1558.

16. Pullerits T, Praks L, Ristioja V, et al. Comparison of a nasal glucocorticoid, antileukotriene, and a combination of antileukotriene and antihistamine in the treatment of seasonal allergic rhinitis. *J Allergy Clin Immunol* 2002; 109:949–955.

17. Global Initiative for Asthma. Global strategy for asthma management and prevention, 2020, www.ginaasthma.org

18. Malmstrom K, Rodriguez-Gomez G, Guerra J, et al. Oral montelukast, inhaled beclomethasone, and placebo for chronic asthma. A randomized, controlled trial. Montelukast/Beclomethasone Study Group. *Ann Intern Med* 1999; 130:487.

19. Norris AA, Alton EW. Chloride transport and the action of sodium cromoglycate and nedocromil sodium in asthma. *Clin Exp Allergy* 1996; 26:250.

26 Role of Bronchodilators in Asthma

Vishnu Sharma

CONTENTS

INTRODUCTION

Asthma is characterized by recurrent episodes of breathlessness due to bronchial smooth muscle spasm, airway oedema and increased airway secretions. There will be narrowing of the airway lumen leading to symptoms in asthma. Bronchodilators are medications which relieve bronchospasm and give immediate relief to breathlessness. Bronchodilators are used as and when required, for relief of symptoms in asthma. A spasm of bronchial smooth muscle is readily relieved by beta-2 agonists. Hence, beta-2 agonists are the preferred bronchodilators in asthma for the relief of symptoms. The bronchodilator reversibility test is useful to differentiate bronchial asthma from COPD by spirometry.

CLASSIFICATION OF BRONCHODILATORS (TABLE 26.1)

Bronchodilators consist of beta agonist, anticholinergic and xanthine.

Beta-2 Agonists

According to the duration of action, beta agonists are grouped into the following:

- Short acting with duration of action of 3–6 hours: e.g. Salbutamol, levosalbutamol and terbutaline.

- Long acting with duration of action of 12 hours: e.g. Salmeterol and formoterol.

- Ultra long acting with duration of action of 24 hours: e.g. Indacaterol and velanterol.

Mechanism of Action of Beta-2 Agonists

Beta-2 agonists act mainly on the smooth muscle of the airway, uterus, intestine and systemic vasculature, which are rich in beta-2 adrenergic receptors. Activation of the receptors initiates a transmembrane signal cascade, involving the heterotrimeric G protein and the effector, adenylyl cyclase[1]. Adenylyl cyclase increases intracellular cAMP by hydrolysis of ATP. The elevated cAMP concentration activates cAMP-dependent protein kinase A (PKA). PKA phosphorylates intracellular substrates, which modulate various effects within the cell. In airway smooth muscle, PKA acts to phosphorylate Gq-coupled receptors, leading to a cascade of intracellular signals which have been proposed to reduce intracellular calcium ion or decrease the sensitivity of calcium ion. The change in calcium ion results in the inhibition of myosin light chain phosphorylation, preventing airway smooth muscle contraction. This action is the underlying mechanism behind beta-2 agonists, which leads to the bronchodilatory

DOI: 10.1201/9781003125785-26

Table 26.1: Bronchodilators

Drug	Group	Formulations
Salbutamol	Short-acting beta-2 agonist	DPI MDI Nebulizing solution Respule Tablet Syrup
Levosalbutamol	Short-acting beta-2 agonist	DPI MDI Respule Tablet Syrup
Formoterol	Long-acting beta-2 agonist	DPI MDI Alone or in combination with GCS, Respule for nebulization
Salmeterol	Long-acting beta-2 agonist	DPI MDI Alone or in combination with GCS
Ipratropium	Short-acting anticholinergic	Nebulizing solution and Respule, DPI, MDI–alone or in combination with SABA
Tiotropium	Long-acting anticholinergic	DPI, MDI–alone or in combination with LABA and GCS
Glycopyrronium	Long-acting anticholinergic	DPI, MDI–alone or in combination with LABA and GCS, Respule for nebulization
Methyl xanthines	Theophylline	Tablet and Injection IV/IM

effects. Beta-2 agonists also provide anti-inflammatory effects within the airway smooth muscle through the reduction of intercellular adhesion molecule-1, reduction of granulocyte-macrophage colony-stimulating factors, stabilization of mast cell degranulation and inhibition of multiple inflammatory pathways.

SALBUTAMOL

Salbutamol was the first selective B-2-receptor agonist to be marketed in 1968. It is available as oral tablet, syrup, intravenous preparation, metered dose inhalers (MDI), dry powder inhalers (DPI) and nebulising solution.

Onset of action by inhalation is 5–15 minutes and by oral route, 30 minutes. Duration of action when inhaled is 3–6 hours and by oral administration, 6–8 hours. Modified-release oral preparations are available with a duration of action of 12 hours.

It is readily absorbed from the GI tract, and metabolism is hepatic and in the gut wall.

Excretion is through urine as metabolites and the unchanged drug. A small portion is excreted through the faeces.

Adverse Reactions

Common side effects are fine skeletal muscle tremor, especially in the hands, tachycardia, palpitations, muscle cramps, headache and paradoxical bronchospasm. Rarely, it causes angioedema, urticaria, hypotension and collapse. Potentially serious hypokalaemia may occur after large doses. Over dosage may lead to tachycardia, tremor, CNS stimulation, hypokalaemia and hyperglycaemia. Symptomatic treatment is recommended.

Special Precautions

These drugs should be administered with caution in pregnancy with mild to moderate pre-eclampsia, arrhythmias, hyperthyroidism, hypertension, diabetes mellitus and myocardial insufficiency. Serum potassium levels should be monitored when administered to avoid untoward effects. In women treated for premature labour, hydration status, cardiac and respiratory function should be monitored. The volume of infusion fluid should be minimized. Treatment should be discontinued if the patient develops signs of pulmonary oedema.

DRUG INTERACTIONS

Concurrent administration of diuretics, corticosteroids and xanthines may augment hypokalaemia. Cardiovascular side effects are potentiated by concomitant administration of monoamine oxidase inhibitors (MAOIs), Tricyclic antidepressants (TCAs) and sympathomimetics. When used together. absorption of sulfamethoxazole is increased. Salbutamol can reduce serum levels of digoxin. Hypokalaemia induced by salbutamol increases the risk of digitalis toxicity. Blood pressure should be closely monitored if linezolid is used concurrently with salbutamol.

Salbutamol is contraindicated in situations like eclampsia, severe pre-eclampsia, intra-uterine infection, intra-uterine fetal death, antepartum haemorrhage, placenta previa, cord compression, threatened abortion and cardiac diseases.

Other short-acting beta-2 agonists being used are levosalbutamol and terbutaline.

Long-acting beta agonists being used are salmeterol, formoterol, indacaterol and velanterol.

The beta-2 agonist group of drugs are the most commonly used and preferred bronchodilators of choice in bronchial asthma. In acute exacerbation nebulized short-acting beta-2 agonist is preferred, as the onset of action is rapid[2]. In emergency situations when nebulizer is not available, short-acting beta-2 agonist metered dose inhaler can be used during acute exacerbation.

Long-acting beta-2 agonists are preferred in patients who require regular medications to control their symptoms[2]. It should be remembered that long-acting beta-2 agonists should never be used as monotherapy in an asthmatics. Increased number of asthma exacerbations, and increased deaths due to asthma have been reported in patients who used long-acting beta-2 agonists as monotherapy[3]. This is because, when only bronchodilators are administered in an asthmatic, airway inflammation worsens over a period of time. The long-acting beta-2 agonist should always be combined with an inhaled glucocorticosteroid which is a controller medication in asthma. A controller medication in bronchial asthma is one that reduces airway inflammation. Glucocorticosteroids are the most potent controller medications in asthma. The combination of long-acting beta-2 agonist with a glucocorticosteroid is more effective than doubling the dose of steroids in an asthmatic[4]. Steroids up regulate the receptors of the beta-2 agonist. This combination has the advantage of positive drug to drug interaction, where one drug potentiates the action of the other.

For patients who require regular medications to control their symptoms, the combination of long-acting beta-2 agonist with inhaled glucocorticosteroid should be used[4]. Combination preparations avoid monotherapy with beta-2 agonists and are more potent than using individual drugs for the reasons cited earlier.

Smart therapy (Single inhaler maintenance and reliever therapy) is ideal in asthmatic patients who require regular medications for symptom control[5]. Formoterol has a faster onset of action, its bronchodilator action increases with an increase in dose without an increase in the side effect profile, it does not lead to cumulative side effects, and adverse effects—if any—are shorter in duration in comparison to Salmeterol. Hence, formoterol is the preferred bronchodilator over salmeterol in SMART therapy.

The majority of asthmatic patients who come with exacerbations start experiencing the first symptom of exacerbation 24–48 hours prior to the development of severe symptoms. In these patients, if the dose of inhaled steroid and bronchodilator is increased at the onset of the first symptom of exacerbation, the chance of progression into severe symptoms is much less[5]. SMART therapy contains inhaled glucocorticosteroid and formoterol combination, the dose of which can be conveniently increased without any significant increase in side effects. SMART therapy reduces severity of exacerbations, reduces the number of emergency hospital visits and admissions, reduces systemic steroid requirement and leads to better control of asthma. It is simple and easy for the patient to understand and use, as the same medication is used for exacerbation and during steady state. Dosage can be stepped up and stepped down by the patient, depending upon the symptoms.

Indacaterol is not preferred in the treatment of asthma. Terbutalin has an increased side effect profile, especially tremor and cardiac side effects. Hence, it is not preferred in asthma. Salmeterol should not be used in acute exacerbation because the onset of action is slow, and its side effects increase with increase in dose[6].

The most frequent and common adverse effects due to beta-2 agonists include tremors, nervousness, palpitation and muscle cramps. They can increase underlying anxiety, particularly among those in the younger age group[2]. Serious adverse effects of bronchodilators include paradoxical bronchospasm, hypersensitivity reactions, hypertension, hypotension, cardiac arrhythmias, hypokalaemia and hyperglycaemia[2]. A bronchospasm caused by a bronchodilator is known as a paradoxical bronchospasm. The exact mechanism of a paradoxical bronchospasm is not known but it is thought to be due to a hypersensitivity reaction to the other components in the medication. Patients with underlying cardiac diseases, mitral valve prolapse and hypoxia are more prone to develop cardiac side effects due to beta-2 agonists. All the adverse reactions increase with age, increase in dose and in frequency of administration. Patients with hypoxia, severe bronchospasm, ischemic heart disease, arrhythmias or hypokalaemia should be monitored for adverse reactions.

Anticholinergic Drugs

There are two groups of anticholinergic drugs:

- Short acting with duration of action of 4–6 hours: e.g. Ipratropium bromide.

- Long acting with duration of action of 24 hours: e.g. Tiotropium bromide and glycopyrronium bromide.

Mechanisms of Action

Acetylcholine leads to the stimulation of the airway smooth muscle and increases secretion of mucous from bronchial mucosa in the medium-to-large airways. M1 receptors, present on the cholinergic ganglia, facilitate neural transmission. M2 receptors, located on the post ganglionic endings of the cholinergic fibres, lead to further acetylcholine release from the post ganglionic endings. M3 receptors, located on the smooth muscle cells, mucosal glands and vascular endothelium in the airway wall, induce bronchoconstriction, mucus hypersecretion and airway wall oedema. All these pathophysiologic features are present in asthma, and hence, anticholinergic drugs have been considered to be useful in the treatment of asthma.

Patients with bronchial asthma have increased resting airway smooth muscle tone due to cholinergic activity. Increased cholinergic activity and elevated smooth muscle tone in bronchial asthma leads to airway hyper responsiveness and airway remodelling. This can be reduced with anticholinergic drugs[7]. Anticholinergic drugs reduce non-neuronal inflammatory mediators of airways and reduce airway secretions in bronchial asthma[7]. Anticholinergic drugs can lead to adverse effects like dry mouth, urinary retention, tachycardia, constipation, delirium and gastric upset. These adverse reactions are more common in the elderly and in males.

When to Use Anticholinergics in Asthma

Anticholinergics are used as an add-on medication in asthma, in addition to inhaled beta-2 agonists and glucocorticosteroids. Short-acting anticholinergic (Ipratropium) can be used, along with short-acting beta-2 agonists, to treat acute severe asthma or status asthmaticus, severe asthma that does not respond to standard treatment, asthma in a smoker and asthma COPD overlap[7]. Long-acting anticholinergic drugs may be used in patients with difficult to control asthma, those with inadequate response to ICS–LABA, asthma in smokers and asthma COPD overlap[7].

METHYLXANTHINES

Theophylline and Aminophylline are the most commonly used drugs in this group. Methylxanthines act by inhibiting phosphodiesterase enzymes[8]. They also antagonize adenosine receptors, thus reducing the bronchoconstrictor action of adenosine. Phosphodiesterase (PDE) is an enzyme which breaks a phosphodiester bond. The cyclic nucleotide phosphodiesterases comprise a group of enzymes which degrade the phosphodiester bond in the second messenger molecules, namely cAMP and cGMP. Inhibition of phosphodiesterase enzyme will prolong or enhance the physiological processes mediated by cAMP or cGMP. Methylxanthines lead to bronchial smooth muscle relaxation, increase diaphragmatic contraction, accelerate mucociliary transport in the airways, reduce the release of inflammatory mediators from mast cells, lower pulmonary artery pressure and augment hypoxic respiratory drive[8].

Duration of action of Theophylline is 8 hours. This is shortened by cytochrome P450 inducers (e.g. polycyclic hydrocarbons in smokers, alcohol consumers with normal hepatic function, carbamazepine, phenytoin, barbiturates, and rifampicin)[9]. Duration of action of theophylline increases (up to 20 hours) in hepatic failure, left ventricular failure, increasing age and in patients who take medications that are metabolized by the cytochrome P450 system (e.g. cimetidine, erythromycin, ciprofloxacin, propranolol, oral contraceptives)[9]. Approximately 55% of serum theophylline is protein bound. The bronchodilator effect is proportional to the log of the serum concentration over the range of 3–45 mg/L (i.e. 17–248 µmol/L). Toxic effects of theophylline increase when the serum concentration exceeds 20 mg/L (110 µmol/L). Theophylline can be administered orally or intravenously.

Intravenous administration of aminophylline, to maintain plasma levels between 10–20 mg/L (55–110 µmol/L), in addition to nebulized salbutamol and intravenous methylprednisolone, has shown to produce more rapid and sustained improvement in airflow rates in acute exacerbation of asthma.

In adults with acute severe and resistant asthma (i.e. status asthmaticus), aminophylline (2 mg/kg i.v) should be given before mechanical ventilation is considered, followed by a further 4 mg/kg over 30 minutes to raise the serum level to 10 mg/L (55 µmol/L)[9]. Usually 1 mg of aminophylline per kg of body weight raises the plasma theophylline level by about 2 mg/L (11 µmol/L). Thereafter, a continuous infusion of 0.5 mg/kg/h of aminophylline (i.e. 0.4 mg/kg/h theophylline) is administered to keep the plasma theophylline level between 10–20 mg/L (55–110 µmol/L). If theophylline has been previously administered, a plasma level should be checked before treatment. Again, serum levels should be checked 1 hour after the intravenous loading dose to allow the maintenance dose to be changed if required[8]. To review the maintenance dose, a further plasma level should be taken 12 hours later and thereafter, as required. When changing from intravenous aminophylline to oral theophylline therapy, the 24-hour oral dose should be 80% of the intravenous aminophylline dose.

The side effects of theophylline include insomnia, headache, anorexia, nausea, vomiting, agitation, seizures, tachycardia, hypotension (due to peripheral vasodilatation), arrhythmias, diuresis (due to renal vasodilatation) and hypoxia (due to a worsening of the ventilation perfusion mismatch)[8]. Aminophylline can rarely lead to rashes, urticaria, angio-oedema, exfoliative dermatitis, fever and even bronchospasm[8]. This is due to a hypersensitivity reaction to ethylenediamine. Theophylline can also reduce the bactericidal activity of alveolar macrophages, which may have an adverse effect in patients who have pulmonary infections. However, this does not seem to be clinically significant.

Theophylline is also a potent inhibitor of pyridoxal kinase (the enzyme responsible for converting vitamin B6 to its active form pyridoxal 5-phosphate)[8]. Hence, it can lead to vitamin B6 deficiency, which may be responsible for some of the central nervous system excitatory effects associated with theophylline toxicity. This can be reversed by pyridoxine supplementation.

When to Use Methylxanthines in Asthma

Methylxanthines are used along with short-acting beta-2 agonists to treat acute severe asthma or status asthmaticus, severe asthma which does not respond to standard treatment, asthma in a smoker and asthma COPD overlap[8]. It can also be used as a convenient oral drug in the elderly and in patients who refuse to use inhaled medications and as an add-on therapy in asthma in addition to standard inhaled medications.

ADRENALINE

Adrenalin is the drug of choice for acute bronchospasm, due to hypersensitivity reaction and anaphylaxis. The subcutaneous administration of 0.3–0.5 mg of adrenaline repeated every 15–30 minutes, if required, is often used to treat an acute severe attack of asthma[10]. It has the advantage of rapid onset of action with immediate improvement in symptoms. It is a vasoconstrictor and hence reduces bronchial mucosal oedema and has bronchodilator action more than selective β^2 adrenergic agonists. For acute severe asthma, adrenaline (20–200 µg as an intravenous bolus followed by an infusion of 1–10 µg/min) is used, particularly when bradycardia and hypotension are present. In patients with acute severe asthma where breathing is laboured, inhaled medications may not reach the lower respiratory tract. Adrenalin gives rapid relief and may be life saving in such patients.

Because of the potentially serious cardiovascular side effects, use of adrenalin in asthma has been reduced since the 1980s. It can lead to angina, arrhythmias, hypertension and cerebral haemorrhage. These side effects are more in elderly patients with underlying cardiovascular diseases, hypertension and hyperthyroidism. Sometimes it can worsen breathlessness due to the development of cardiogenic pulmonary edema[10]. This is more common in elderly with underlying cardiovascular disease. Minor side effects of adrenalin include anxiety, apprehensiveness, restlessness, tremor, weakness, dizziness, sweating, palpitations, pallor, nausea and vomiting and headache.

NEWER AGENTS

Available bronchodilators do not inhibit/ antagonize all the pathways involved in airway narrowing in asthma. In some patients, responses to currently available bronchodilators are suboptimal. Patients require rapid response to medications during acute exacerbation of symptoms. Once daily medications become more convenient, patient compliance and adherence is much improved. Hence, the search is on to find newer bronchodilators with these properties.

At least nine potential new classes of bronchodilators have been identified[11].

1. Selective phosphodiesterase inhibitors

2. Bitter-taste receptor agonists

3. E-prostanoid receptor 4 agonists

4. Rho kinase inhibitors

5. Calcilytics

6. Agonists of peroxisome proliferator-activated receptor-γ

7. Agonists of relaxin receptor 1

8. Soluble guanylyl cyclase activators

9. Pepducins

These drugs are in preclinical phase. We still do not know which classes will actually be available for clinical use. If developed, these new drugs may be a useful addition to, rather than a substitution for, the bronchodilator therapy currently used, in order to achieve further optimization of bronchodilation.

ROUTE OF ADMINISTRATION

As far as possible, it is preferable to use the inhalation route for administration of medications. Advantages include rapid onset of action and less side effects. Disadvantages include (if the patient does not use the inhalation device properly) the medication may be ineffective and some patients may be reluctant to use inhaled medications.

How does the younger generation differ from adults?

Response to medications is more rapid in the young. Hence, the dose required may be less and should be proportional to the clinical response and symptom relief. In the younger age group, comorbidities are much less compared to adults. Hence, the side effects, especially cardiac side effects due to drugs, are much less compared to those for the elderly. Drug adverse reactions like tremors, anxiety, paradoxical bronchospasm, hypersensitivity reactions, ventilation perfusion mismatch leading to worsening of hypoxia are more common in the younger age group. The elderly may tolerate bronchodilators better, even at a higher dose.

Key Points

- Bronchodilators are the mainstays of treatment for relief of symptoms in bronchial asthma

- Short-acting beta-2 agonists should be used in acute exacerbation of asthma

- Inhaled long-acting beta-2 agonists in combination with glucocorticosteroid is preferred in asthmatics who require regular medication

- SMART therapy (inhaled formoterol with glucocorticosteroid) is ideal in asthmatics who require regular medication

- Beta-2 agonists should not be used as monotherapy in asthma—they should always be combined with glucocorticosteroid

- Bronchodilators should be used by the inhalation route

- Anticholinergics and Methylxanthines can be used as add-on medications in a select group of patients who do not respond adequately to beta-2 agonists

- Adrenalin is the drug of choice for bronchospasm due to hypersensitivity reaction

- Adrenalin can be used in patients with acute severe asthma who fail to respond to standard therapy

- Cardiac side effects due to bronchodilators is less in younger age group

- Compared to the elderly population, cardiac side effects due to bronchodilators is less in the younger age group

- Hypoxia, hypokalaemia and underlying cardiac conditions increase the risk of side effects

GINA 2020 GUIDELINES ON BRONCHODILATORS (FIGURE 26.1)

Regular or frequent use of SABA is associated with adverse effects. Higher use of SABA is associated with adverse clinical outcomes. For safety, GINA no longer recommends SABA-only treatment for Step 1. GINA now recommends that all adults and adolescents with asthma should receive ICS-containing controller treatment to reduce the risk of serious exacerbations. ICS can be delivered by regular daily treatment or, in mild asthma, by as-needed low-dose ICS-formoterol.

CONCLUSION

Inhaled beta-2 agonists are the bronchodilators of choice for the relief of symptoms in asthma. Anticholinergics, theophylline and adrenalin

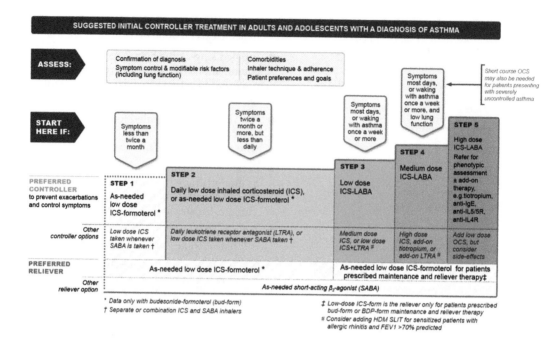

Figure 26.1 The role of beta-2 agonists in the management of asthma. (From GINA 2018.)

may be used in a select group of patients who fail to respond adequately to beta-2 agonists, along with other standard therapy. Bronchodilators should never be used as monotherapy in asthma but should always be combined with inhaled glucocorticosteroids. Serious side effects due to bronchodilators are found to be less in younger age groups.

REFERENCES

1. Walker JK, Penn RB, Hanania NA, Dickey BF, Bond RA. New perspectives regarding beta-2 adrenoceptor ligands in the treatment of asthma. Br J Pharmacol 2011; 163:18–28.

2. Billington CK, Penn RB, Hall IP. β₂ Agonists. Handb Exp Pharmacol 2017; 237:23–40. https://doi.org/10.1007/164_2016_64

3. Wijesinghe M, Perrin K, Harwood M, Weatherall M, Beasley R. The risk of asthma mortality with inhaled long acting beta-agonists. Postgrad Med J 2008; 84(995):467–472. https://doi.org/10.1136/pgmj.2007.067165. PMID: 18940948.

4. Hiroyuki Ohbayashi, Sahori Kudo, Mitsue Ariga. Evaluation of ICS/LABA combination therapy on respiratory function in patients with asthma: Open-label, randomized, cross-over trial, Eur Respir J 2018; 52 (suppl 62): PA1024;. https://doi.org/10.1183/13993003.

5. Chapman KR, Barnes NC, Greening AP, et al, Single maintenance and reliever therapy (SMART) of asthma: a critical appraisal, Thorax 2010; 65:747–752.

6. Chapman KR, Reality-based medicine. Chest 2000; 118:281–283.

7. Reinoud Gosens, Nicholas Gross, The mode of action of anticholinergics in asthma, Eur Respir J 2018; 52 (4): 1701247;. https://doi.org/10.1183/13993003.01247-2017.

8. Tilley SL. Methylxanthines in asthma. Handb Exp Pharmacol 2011; (200):439–456. https://doi.org/10.1007/978-3-642-13443-2_17. PMID: 20859807.

9. Makino S, Fueki M, Fueki N. Efficacy and safety of methylxanthines in the treatment of asthma. Allergol Int 2004; 53(1):13–22.

10. Pancorbo S, Fifield G, Davies S, Fraser G, Helmink R, Heissler J. Subcutaneous epinephrine versus nebulized terbutaline in the emergency treatment of asthma. Clin Pharm 1983; 2(1):45–48.

11. Cazzola M, Rogliani P, Gabriella Matera M. The future of bronchodilation: looking for new classes of bronchodilators, Eur Respir Rev 2019; 28 (154):190095;. https://doi.org/10.1183/16000617.0095-2019

27 Role of Corticosteroids in Allergic Disorders in Adolescents and Young Adults

Abha Mahashur and Ashok Mahashur

CONTENTS

INTRODUCTION

Allergic disorders are very common and rising all over the world. They affect the physical as well as the psychological health of those afflicted and are known to impair quality of life due to the morbidity associated with them. The prevalence of diseases associated with atopy has increased in many parts of the world over the past 20–30 years. Common allergic diseases include allergic asthma, allergic rhinitis, atopic dermatitis, food allergy, insect venom allergy and drug allergy. *Adolescents and young adults* are patients ages 11–25 years. This age group poses a challenge in management of allergic disorders for various reasons. This may be due to rapidity of changes in lifestyle habits and inability to sense the responsibility of perceiving symptoms for self-management. Challenges to address in this age group are ensuring adherence to therapy, optimizing self-care, addressing psychological issues and obtaining a support system.[1]

Individuals are considered to have *clinically significant allergy* or *allergic disease*, when they develop symptoms upon exposure to substances containing that allergen and have an allergen-specific IgE. Mere sensitization to an allergen should not be equated with clinical allergy. When a sensitised person is exposed to the same allergen again, there occurs binding between specific allergen and IgE antibodies lying on the surface of mast cells and basophils. This is followed by cross linking of IgE molecules. This clustering generates a signal for activation of mast cells and basophils. A number of mediators are released (histamine, prostaglandins, leukotrienes, platelet activating factors, cytokines, etc.), that directly or indirectly lead to the clinical manifestation of allergic disorders.

Mast cells are widely distributed but are most concentrated in the skin, lungs and gastrointestinal (GI) mucosa; histamine facilitates inflammation and is the primary mediator of clinical atopy. The sequence of events in an allergic-reaction are as follows. First, an aero allergen enters into the tonsils. Antigen presenting cells interact with T helper Type 2 cells and B cells in lymph nodes, leading to allergen-specific IgE production. The IgE then enters into the bloodstream and spreads into different tissues to bind to high affinity Fc receptors in those local tissue mast cells and basophils. Second, exposure of the same allergen then elaborates a florid allergic reaction (Figure 27.1).

Atopy is defined as the production of specific IgE in response to exposure to common environmental allergens. Atopic individuals are associated with various forms of allergic disease. *Atopic March* is an entity that explains the probable chronology in which these allergic manifestations are noted in an atopic individual. Usually, atopic dermatitis starts in infancy and progresses to allergic rhinitis or allergic asthma by childhood and young adulthood. This phenomenon is called "atopic march" or "allergic march".

A large proportion, up to 80%, of children with atopic dermatitis subsequently develop allergic rhinitis or asthma in a future course[3–7]. It has been noted that when children reach adolescence asthmatic manifestations and airway hyper responsiveness improve, which

DOI: 10.1201/9781003125785-27

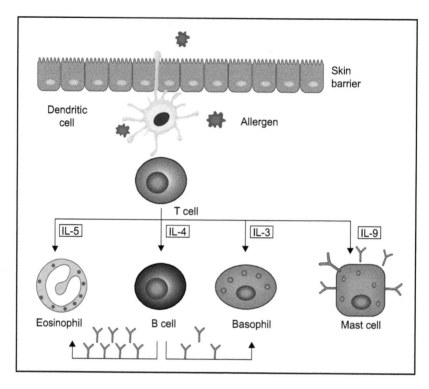

Figure 27.1   Allergen-induced sensitization and inflammation.[2]

is not very well explained. This phenomenon has been attributed to hormonal changes at puberty. Risk factors for allergic diseases have been established as genetic predisposition, early age, male gender and persistent sensitization due to smoking or pollution.

ROLE OF CORTICOSTEROIDS

Corticosteroids are therapeutic agents predominantly used to treat inflammation, allergy and inappropriate immune dysfunction. Their anti-inflammatory effect is extremely useful in managing allergic disorders.

MECHANISM OF ACTION

The steroid molecule diffuses across the cell membrane and binds to intracellular glucocorticoid receptors to cause conformational changes at the receptor level. This complex then moves inside the nucleus to interact with Glucocorticoid Response Element (GRE). These GREs have specific genes to suppress or trigger the transcription followed by protein synthesis, as depicted in Figure 27.2. These genes then inhibit several transcription factors that control synthesis of pro-inflammatory mediators. Additionally, corticosteroids lead to suppression of Phospholipase A2, cyclooxygenase 2 and

pro-inflammatory cytokines like tumour necrosis factor and interleukins. Thus, steroids suppress the inflammatory response at all levels, starting from promotor sites, genes, gene products, stimulatory factors and finally end products causing the allergic response at target sites. Specifically, for allergic responses, they lead to impaired functioning of eosinophils by causing early apoptosis of eosinophils, sequestration to extravascular tissue and inhibition of their degranulation. They also suppress degranulation of mast cells and basophils, leading to a reduced quantum of cytokines.

Corticosteroids can be used in different forms, depending upon the site and extent of inflammation. They are available as systemic formulation (intravenous and oral) or local formulation (topical and inhalation). There are different types of corticosteroids like cortisone, prednisolone, hydrocortisone, dexamethasone, etc. Onset of action of systemic steroids is 3–8 hours (intravenous or oral). They vary as per potency, mineralocorticoid activity and hypothalamic-pituitary-adrenal axis suppression. They can be classified as short-, medium- and long-acting agents based on the duration of hypothalamic-pituitary-adrenal axis suppression, as shown in Table 27.1.

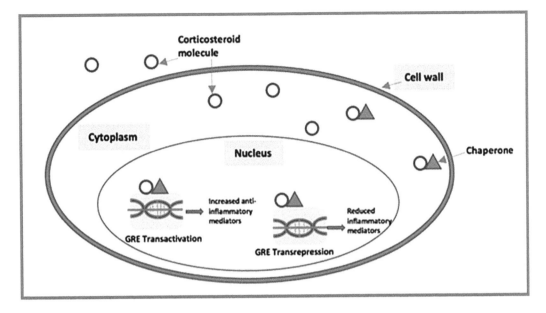

Figure 27.2 Anti-inflammatory action of corticosteroids.[8]

Therapeutic action may last longer than the duration of suppression of HPA axis, due to the intracellular mechanism of action. Thus, the effects persist even when circulatory levels fall.

ALLERGIC DISORDERS
Allergic Rhinitis

Allergic rhinitis (AR) is a symptomatic disorder of the nose, induced after exposure to allergens via IgE-mediated hypersensitivity reactions, which are characterized by the four cardinal symptoms of watery rhinorrhoea, nasal obstruction, nasal itching and sneezing[10]. Sinusitis is a frequent complication, which may manifest as a frontal headache. On exposure to allergens, allergic reactions develop in two different patterns, according to time sequence. Early reaction is noted within 30 minutes, with sneezing and rhinorrhoea due to mast cell degranulation. Late reaction occurs approximately 6 hours after exposure to allergens with nasal obstruction due to eosinophil chemotaxis. Table 27.2 shows classification of severity of allergic rhinitis, which depends upon the pattern of disease and severity of illness. In patients with a persistent severe form of AR, asthma should be ruled out. Approximately, 10–40% of patients with AR have concomitant asthma.[11]

The most effective first-line treatment is nasal steroids with or without oral anti-histaminics and oral decongestants. Intranasal corticosteroids inhibit both early and late reactions and reduce IgE production and eosinophilia by inhibiting the secretion of cytokines, including IL-4, 1L-5 and IL-13. When intranasal corticosteroids are administered, eosinophils and basophils decrease in 1 week[12]. The therapeutic effect of intranasal corticosteroids is encountered 7 hours after

Table 27.1: Systemic Corticosteroid Properties[9]

Medication	Anti-Inflammatory Potency (Relative)	Equivalent Potency (mg)	Duration of Effect (Hours)*	Mineralo-Corticoid Potency (Relative)
Short-acting				
Hydrocortisone	1	20	8–12	1
Intermediate-acting				
Prednisone	4	5	18–36	0.8
Prednisolone	4	5	18–36	0.8
Methylprednisolone	5	4	18–36	0.5
Long-acting				
Dexamethasone	25	0.75	>36	0

*Duration of effect on hypothalamic-pituitary-adrenal axis.

Table 27.2: ARIA Classification of Severity of Allergic Rhinitis

Intermittent
Symptoms
• < 4 days per week
• Or < 4 consecutive weeks

Persistent
Symptoms
• > 4 days per week
• And > 4 consecutive weeks

Mild
All of the following
• Normal sleep
• No impairment of daily activities, sport, leisure
• No impairment of work and school
• Symptoms present but not troublesome

Moderate -Severe
One or more items
• Sleep disturbance
• Impairment of daily activities, sports, leisure
• Impairment of school or work
• Troublesome symptoms

administration and reaches the maximal level after 2 weeks. Various molecules are available currently, as shown in Table 27.3. Efficacy is nearly comparable, but systemic side effects vary. Systemic absorption rates of flunisolide, triamcinolone acetonide and beclomethasone dipropionate are 20–50%. On the contrary, minimal systemic absorption is seen with mometasone furoate and fluticasone propionate (≤0.1% and ≤2%, respectively). Intranasal corticosteroids are eliminated by first-pass hepatic metabolism. Intranasal steroids are safe for children above 6 years of age and are known to additionally benefit asthmatics by reducing bronchial hyper responsiveness.

ALLERGIC ASTHMA

Asthma comprises episodes of wheezy breathlessness due to airway narrowing which are partially, or totally, reversible. Airway hyper-responsiveness is an almost invariable accompanying feature. The majority of asthmatics are atopic and responsive to inhaled steroids. A smaller proportion has intrinsic, non-atopic disease, which is often later onset and has a worrisome course. Inhaled

corticosteroids, when administered correctly, are highly effective and virtually free from side effects. However, a minority of chronic asthmatics are 'corticosteroid-dependent' and require oral medication to control their symptoms.

INHALED CORTICOSTEROIDS (ICS) IN ASTHMA

ICS reduces morbidity and mortality in asthma[13]. After inhalation, only 10–15% of ICS reaches the lung for therapeutic benefits[14]. A larger proportion goes to the gastrointestinal system. Ancillary devices like spacers or holding chambers typically increase the proportion of drug deposition in the airway rather than oropharynx (Figure 27.3).

Epithelial cells may be major cellular targets for ICS, which are the mainstay of modern asthma management. ICS suppress many activated inflammatory genes in airway epithelial cells (Figure 27.2). Epithelial integrity is restored by regular ICS. The suppression of mucosal inflammation is relatively rapid with a significant reduction in eosinophils detectable within 6 hours and associated with reduced airway hyperresponsiveness.

Significant therapeutic benefits are demonstrated within 1–2 weeks of initiation of ICS[15]. An ideal ICS should have sharp receptor selectivity, potency and targeting of the lung with reduced oral bioavailability and high systemic clearance. ICS enjoys a state of high potency, but struggles with poor dose response relationship. They surely have a better therapeutic index than systemic formulations. Challenges with ICS include myths surrounding the therapy and lack of adherence. As per Global Initiative for Asthma (GINA) 2020 guidelines, ICS in combination with beta-2 agonists should be started even in mild

Table 27.3: Intranasal Corticosteroids for Adolescents and Adults (>12 years)

Drug	Dose per Spray (mcg)	Initial Dose (Sprays per Nostril)
Beclomethasone	42	1 spray twice a day to 4 times a day
Budesonide	32	1 spray once a day
Fluticasone	50	2 sprays once a day
Mometasone	50	2 sprays once a day
Triamcinolone	55	2 sprays once a day

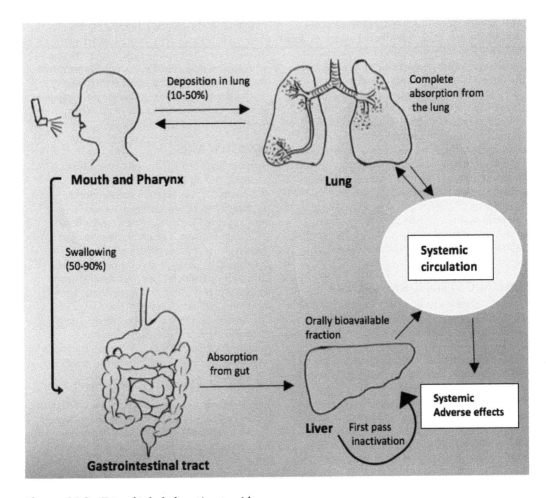

Figure 27.3 Fate of inhaled corticosteroids.

to moderate asthma. Dose increment should be done in stepwise manner, as per the clinical status. Systemic steroids are required in severe asthma when patient is not controlled despite high dose of ICS or while acute exacerbation.

Table 27.4 shows different ICS preparations available with their dosages used in asthma, as per GINA 2020.

Small-particle aerosols, such as hydrofluoroalkane-134a (HFA) beclomethasone

Table 27.4: Total Daily Dose (mcg) of Inhaled Corticosteroids (GINA 2020)[16] for >12 Years of Age

Inhaled Corticosteroids	Low Dose	Medium Dose	High Dose
Beclomethasone dipropionate (pMDI, standard particle, HFA)	200–500	>500–1000	>1000
Beclomethasone dipropionate (pMDI, extrafine particle HFA)	100–200	>200–400	>400
Budesonide (DPI)	200–400	>400–800	>800
Ciclesonide (pMDI, extrafine particle, HFA)	80–160	>160–320	>320
Fluticasone furoate (DPI)	100	100	200
Fluticasone propionate (DPI)	100–250	>250–500	>500
Fluticasone propionate (pMDI, standard particle, HFA)	100–250	>250–500	>500
Mometasone furoate (DPI)	200	200	400
Mometasone furoate (pMDI, standard particle, HFA)	200–400	200–400	>400

Abbreviations: DPI—dry powder inhaler, pMDI—pressurized meter dose inhaler, HFA—hydrofluroalkane propellent.

and ciclesonide—which have particle sizes around 1 mm—have recently become available for use. These are promising molecules that ensure activation of molecules after reaching the lung with high pulmonary deposition and low systemic exposure. Ciclesonide shows superiority with high affinity for the glucocorticoid receptor, high lipophilicity and fatty acid conjugation and high protein binding and systemic clearance.[16] Likewise, HFA beclomethasone has shown improvement in acinar airway function when compared to large molecule aerosol preparations[17]. Side effects of ICS include sore throat, oral candidiasis, pharyngitis and reflex cough locally; systemically, it can cause adrenal crisis, cataract, glaucoma, reduced bone mineral density, etc.

SYSTEMIC STEROIDS IN ASTHMA

Systemic steroids have a definite role in asthma. They can be used as well as a controller medication, in an emergency situation with acute worsening of symptoms. As per the Asthma Action plan, Oral Corticosteroids (OCS) should be used when patients clinically progress beyond moderate grade i.e steps 4–5. In all such situations, tapering is not needed if OCS are prescribed for <2 weeks. Importantly, the oral and intravenous route are equally effective[18]. The oral route is less costly, non- invasive and more comfortable for use with usual onset of action being 4 hours. However, if the patient is unable to accept medications orally in situations of extreme breathlessness, vomiting or non-invasive or invasive mechanical ventilatory support, the intravenous route should be preferred.

In a scenario of acute worsening, a short course of OCS is used (e.g. 40–50 mg/day usually for 5–7 days[19]) for patients who:

- Fail to respond to an increase in reliever and controller medication for 2–3 days

- Deteriorate rapidly or who have a PEF or FEV_1 <60% of their personal best or predicted value

- Have a history of sudden severe exacerbations

OCS as controller medication is considered in a smaller sicker subset of asthma; i.e Severe Asthma patients[20]. In approximately 30% of severe Asthma patients, OCS are required in addition to ongoing high/medium dose ICS to achieve better control[21]. Usually, low dose should be used; i.e ≤7.5 mg/day prednisone equivalent[22]. A word of caution is mandatory for all such patients regarding the possible side effects. Thus, one has to be extremely careful to add OCS in limited scenarios, such as adults with inadequate symptom control and/or frequent exacerbations despite appropriate inhaler technique and adherence to therapy with Step 4 treatment, and after the exclusion of other contributory factors and other add-on treatments including biologics.

ANAPHYLAXIS

Anaphylaxis is a severe systemic allergic reaction due to the massive release of histamine. It consists of a constellation of symptoms of which the most serious are laryngeal oedema or asthma (or both) and hypotension. The common causes of anaphylaxis are IgE-mediated sensitivity to foods (e.g. peanuts, tree nuts, fish, shellfish and dairy products), bee and wasp stings, drugs (e.g. penicillin and anaesthetic agents) and latex rubber. Treatment for Anaphylaxis is immediate adrenaline, bronchodilators—if bronchoconstriction is seen—and anti-histaminics. Intravenous corticosteroids can be given primarily to curb late phase reaction.

ADVERSE EFFECTS OF STEROIDS

These agents have an effect on every organ of body. Dose and duration of steroid therapy decides probable side effects. Long-term usage leads to suppression of hypothalamic pituitary adrenal axis, which is usually seen with long-term systemic therapy. Short-term usage may lead to hyperglycaemia, oedema, gastrointestinal bleeding, blood pressure fluctuation, psychiatric issues, increased risk of infection and electrolyte imbalance.

CONCLUSION

Corticosteroids are extremely important drugs in management of allergies, for all the forms of allergic disorders across all the age groups. Allergic disorders have an overwhelmed immune response at various sites in the body like skin, nose, airway and gastrointestinal tract leading to manifestation at respective sites. Corticosteroids are available in various forms and can be delivered through possibly all routes. They are potent anti-inflammatory and immunosuppressive agents. One must understand that they are double-edged swords and have equally significant side effects involving almost all the systems. Thus, decisions regarding the rationale for initiation, route of administration, dosage and duration should be strictly supervised by experts only. On principle, for chronic allergic states, local formulations should be preferred over systemic formulations to avoid side effects.

The minimum possible dose should be used as most of the side effects are dose related. In the scenario of allergies, corticosteroids are effective and safe to be used with caution under guidance.

REFERENCES

1. Roberts G, Vazquez-Ortiz M, Knibb R, et al. EAACI Guideline on the effective transition of adolescents and young adults with allergy and asthma. Allergy 2020;75:2734–2752.

2. Broide DH. The pathophysiology of allergic rhinoconjunctivitis. Allergy Asthma Proc 2007; 28:398–403.

3. Zheng T, Yu J, Oh MH, Zhu Z. The atopic march: progression from atopic dermatitis to allergic rhinitis and asthma. Allergy Asthma Immunol Res 2011;3:67.

4. Spergel JM. From atopic dermatitis to asthma: the atopic march. Ann Allergy Asthma Immunol 2010; 105:99.

5. Ker J, Hartert TV. The atopic march: what's the evidence? Ann Allergy Asthma Immunol 2009;103:282.

6. von Kobyletzki LB, Bornehag CG, Hasselgren M, et al. Eczema in early childhood is strongly associated with the development of asthma and rhinitis in a prospective cohort. BMC Dermatol 2012;12:11

7. Leung DY, Nicklas RA, Li JT, et al. Disease management of atopic dermatitis: an updated practice parameter. Joint Task Force on Practice Parameters. Ann Allergy Asthma Immunol 2004;93:S1.

8. Derendorf H, Nave R, Drollmann A, Cerasoli F, Wurst W. Rele vance of pharmacokinetics and pharmacodynamics of inhaled corti- costeroids to asthma. Eur Respir J 2006;28(5):1042–1050.

9. Swartz SL, Dluhy RG. Corticosteroids: clinical pharmacology and therapeutic use. Drugs 1978; 16(3):238–255.

10. Bousquet J, Van Cauwenberge P, Khaltaev N. Allergic rhinitis and its impact on asthma. J Allergy Clin Immunol 2001;108:S147–334.

11. Min YG, Choi BY, Kwon SK, Lee SS, Jung YH, Kim JW, Oh SJ. Multi-center study on the prevalence of perennial allergic rhinitis and allergy-associated disorders. J Korean Med Sci 2001;16:697–701.

12. Lee BJ, Kim YJ, Kim JH, Shin HS, Chung YS. A comparative study of intranasal budesonide and oral terfenadine in perennial allergic rhinitics: effect on the symptom score and nasal secretion eosinophils. J Asthma Allergy Clin Immunol 2001;21:216–22. Korean.

13. Raissy HH, Kelly HW, Harkins M, Szefler SJ. Inhaled corticosteroids in lung diseases. Am J Respir Crit Care Med 2013;187(8):798–803.

14. Derendorf H. Pharmacokinetic and pharmacodynamic properties of inhaled corticosteroids in relation to efficacy and safety. Respir Med 1997; 91: Suppl. A, 22–28.

15. Phillips K, Oborne J, Lewis S, Harrison TW, Tattersfield AE. Time course of action of two inhaled corticosteroids, fluticasone propionate and budesonide. Thorax 2004;59(1):26–30.

16. Global Initiative for Asthma (GINA) A Global strategy of Asthma management and Prevention 2020.

17. Verbanck S, Schuermans D, Paiva M, Vincken W. The functional benefit of anti-inflammatory aerosols in the lung periphery. J Allergy Clin Immunol 2006;118: 340–346.

18. Ratto D, Alfaro C, Sipsey J, Glovsky MM, Sharma OP. Are intravenous corticosteroids required in status asthmaticus? JAMA 1988;260:527–529.

19. Reddel HK, Barnes DJ. Pharmacological strategies for self-management of asthma exacerbations. Eur Respir J 2006;28:182–199.

20. Kian Fan Chung et al. International ERS/ATS guidelines on definition, evaluation and treatment of severe asthma. Eur Respir J 2014;43: 343–373.

21. Ten Brinke A, Zwinderman AH, Sterk PJ, et al. Factors associated with persistent airflow limitation in severe asthma. Am J Respir Crit Care Med 2001;164: 744–748.

22. Chung KF, Wenzel SE, Brozek JL, Bush A, Castro M, Sterk PJ, Adcock IM, et al. International ERS/ATS Guidelines on Definition, Evaluation and Treatment of Severe Asthma. Eur Respir J 2014;43:343–373.

28 Inhaler Therapy for Asthma in Adolescents and Young Adults

Shajahan P Sulaiman

CONTENTS

INTRODUCTION

Asthma is one of the oldest diseases known to mankind and still a substantial health problem among all age groups across the world. More than 300 million people suffer from asthma, and it is predicted that a further 100 million will be added to this number by the year 2025.[1] The disease burden of asthma in India is largely unknown. Many studies have shown a prevalence of 3% among the adult population; i.e. more than 40 million asthmatics at present. But, considering the poor data retrieval system in our country, these figures may be a gross underestimate of the real problem.

Asthma nearly account for 500,000 hospitalizations and 250,000 deaths worldwide annually.[2] India contributes a major share to the total asthma related deaths accounting for 22.3% of all global asthma deaths as per the report by the World Health Organization in 2004.

The introduction of medications in the inhaled form as the primary treatment for asthma has led to remarkable achievements in asthma control.[3] Despite this fact, uncontrolled asthma is very common and represents a heavy burden to patients and society, especially in developing countries.[4]

Irrespective of age, the aim of asthma therapy is to achieve good symptom control and to minimize the risk of future exacerbations, fixed airflow limitations and side effects of treatment.[5] Treatment strategies recommended by the Global Initiative for Asthma (GINA) are tailored according to age, with separate recommendations for adults, adolescents and children aged 6–11 years versus those ≤5 years.[5] However, despite the availability of effective treatments such as inhaled corticosteroids (ICS), long-acting β2-agonists and long-acting muscarinic antagonists, many children and adolescents with asthma remain uncontrolled.[6] Poorly controlled asthma is often associated with significant morbidity, mortality and socioeconomic burden.[7]

The percentage of asthmatics opting for inhalers as the preferred choice of treatment seems to be low across the globe.[8] The key factors attributed to poor asthma control with respect to inhalers include poor supply of inhaled medications at affordable cost, lack of training given to patients on the correct usage of inhaled devices and the barriers created by the cultural beliefs, attitudes and misconceptions of patients on the use of inhalers.

INHALED THERAPY IN ASTHMA
The History

The concept of inhaled therapy is not new, and the delivery of therapeutic vapours and aerosols through inhalation has been used for

DOI: 10.1201/9781003125785-28

thousands of years in various cultures. The word 'inhaler' was first used by John Mudge in his book *A Radical and Expeditious Cure for a Recent Catarrhous Cough*,[9] where he disclosed the invention of an inhaler adapted from a pewter tankard and the use of opium vapour to treat cough.

Long before, the inhalation of the vapour of black henbane is recorded in the Ancient Egyptian Ebers papyrus (1,554 BC); Egyptian physicians threw the weed onto hot bricks to vapourize the alkaloid contents of the plant, which could subsequently be inhaled by the patient having breathlessness.

In China metal inhalers and incense burners were used for opium inhalation. The practice of inhaling the fumes of stramonium and hemp was common, and Hippocrates advocated the inhalation of vapours of herbs and resins boiled with vinegar and oil for respiratory ailments. Maimonides (1135–1204 AD), the physician to the Arab King, wrote the first book on asthma *A Treatise on Asthma* in 1190 and recommended numerous treatments which included the inhalation of vapours generated from herbs thrown onto a fire.[10]

Inhalation therapy was practiced in the ancient civilizations of India as well. The inhalation of therapeutic aerosols for the treatment of asthma is described in the writings of Charaka and Sushruta, which provide detailed instructions for preparing herbals, including datura that could be smoked in a pipe or a cigarette to relieve asthma symptoms.[11]

The first MDI was introduced in 1956 and since then much advancement has been made, especially in the development of inhaler devices. Now, we have hundreds of such devices with much sophistication and precision to suit individual preferences and needs.

Types of Inhalers[12,13]

There are a number of devices that deliver medications directly to the airways. Pressurised metered-dose inhalers (pMDIs), dry powder inhalers (DPIs), breath actuated inhalers (BAIs) and nebulizers are the commonly available inhaled devices.

pMDI

The pressurized metered dose inhaler (pMDI) consists of a pressurized canister of medicine in a plastic case with a mouthpiece. A holding chamber consists of a plastic tube with a mouthpiece, a valve to control aerosol delivery and a soft sealed end to hold the MDI. The holding chamber assists delivery of medication to the lungs.

DPI

Dry powder inhalers consist of a plastic device used to inhale powdered medication. The dry powder inhalers are breath activated; i.e. the device automatically releases the medication while the patient inhales. There are different types of DPIs, which include capsule inhalers, the multiple unit dose inhalers and the reservoir devices.

BAI

A breath actuated inhaler (BAI) is a modified version of a metered dose inhaler that delivers medications to the airways during inhalation. It consists of a pressurized canister of medication in a plastic case with a mouthpiece. When the patient inhales, the device automatically releases a mist of medication. It can be very useful to people who have problems with the timing and coordination required to use a pMDI device.

NEBULIZERS

A nebulizer delivery system consists of a nebulizer and a source of compressed air. These are electric or battery powered machines that turn medications in the liquid form into a fine mist. The airflow to the nebulizer changes the medication solution to a mist that is inhaled. Different types of nebulizers are available for clinical use; e.g. jet nebulizers which use compressed gas to make an aerosol, ultrasonic nebulizers which make aerosol through high frequency vibrations and mesh nebulizers in which the liquid passes through a very fine mesh to form the aerosol.

SPACERS

A spacer is an add-on device used often with a pressurized metered dose inhaler (pMDI). It is a type of holding chamber that attaches to the inhaler and slows the delivery of medication. Spacers are intended to make inhalers easier to use and to deliver medication more efficiently.

Each of these devices can be used to inhale various medications and has its own merits and demerits (Table 28.1).[13]

INITIATING INHALED THERAPY IN ASTHMA

Many international scientific groups advise that mild asthmatics are to be treated with short-acting beta-2 agonists (SABA) alone on an as needed basis. However, airway inflammation, which is the hallmark of asthma, is present in most patients even among those with intermittent, infrequent or trivial symptoms.

The idea of treating mild forms of asthma with reliever medications alone dates back

Table 28.1: Advantages and Disadvantages of Different Inhaler Devices

Device	Advantages	Disadvantages
pMDI	Compact Portable Cheaper than DPIs Minimal preparation Quick to use	Contains propellants Not breath-actuated Many patients cannot use it correctly (e.g. coordination difficulties, "cold Freon" effect) Usually low lung deposition/high oropharyngeal deposition
pMDI with spacer	Quick to use Easy to coordinate Tidal breathing is often enough Less oropharyngeal deposition Usually higher lung deposition than a pMDI	Contains propellants Not very portable or convenient Not breath actuated Plastic spacers may acquire static charge
Breath-actuated pMDI	Compact Portable Minimal preparation Quick to use Breath actuated (no coordination needed)	Contains propellants 'Cold Freon' effect Low lung deposition/high oropharyngeal deposition
DPI	Compact Portable Quick to use Breath actuated (no coordination needed) Usually higher lung deposition than a pMDI Do not contain propellants	Work poorly if inhalation is not forceful enough Many patients cannot use them correctly (e.g. capsule handling problems for elderly) Most types are moisture sensitive
Nebulizers	Minimal coordination is sufficient Can be used in very young or old, debilitated patients or those in acute distress Works with low inspiratory flows or volumes Breath hold is not required Drug concentration can be adjusted if desired	Expensive and cumbersome Chances of infection from unsterile chambers or tubings into the respiratory tract. Drug wastage is more Aerosolization to the surroundings—concerns of spread of infection to health care workers and others. Less portable

50 years when the condition was thought to be a disease with mere bronchoconstriction. SABA provides immediate relief of symptoms but obviously it will not address the very basic pathology of airway inflammation. Treating with SABA alone is associated with increased risk of exacerbations and deterioration of lung function. Its regular and unabated use is likely to enhance the allergic response and inflammation of the airways and over a period of time decreases the bronchodilator response needed. Over use of these agents is also associated with increased risk of asthma related deaths.[5]

ICS containing treatment protocol is preferred once the diagnosis of asthma is established, irrespective of the stage/severity of the disease. There are multiple reasons for opting for this modality which include the following. Any patients with asthma irrespective of their symptoms can develop severe exacerbations at any point of time and low dose ICS significantly decreases symptoms, exercise-induced bronchoconstriction, asthma exacerbations, hospitalizations and asthma related deaths. It also helps to improve lung function. It is essential to establish the diagnosis of asthma before a treatment plan is initiated. Documentation of the level of control, presence of modifiable risk factors and assessment of lung function are also equally important. Patients should be trained to use the inhaler properly and at each visit it should be rechecked.

Apart from corticosteroids, short-acting beta-2 agonists such as salbutamol and terbutaline, long-acting beta-2 agonists like salmeterol and formoterol, and antimuscarinic agents like ipratropium and tiotropium are used as inhaled medications in the management of asthma under varying circumstances. The low, medium, and high doses of inhaled corticosteroids are given in Table 28.2. It is not a table of equivalence but is based on available studies and product literature.

INHALER THERAPY—ISSUES THAT MATTER

Inhalers are the mainstay of therapy for any stage of asthma. Medications in the inhaled forms are the best therapeutic options

Table 28.2: Low, Medium and High Daily Doses of Inhaled Corticosteroids

Adults and Adolescents Inhaled Corticosteroid	Total Daily ICS Dose (mcg)		
	Low	Medium	High
BDP (pMDI*, HFA as propellent)	200–500	>500–1000	>1000
BDP (pMDI, extrafine particle, HFA as propellent)	100–200	>200–400	> 400
Budesonide (DPI)	200–400	>400–800	>1000
Ciclesonide (pMDI, extrafine particle, HFA as propellent)	80–160	> 160–320	>1000
Fluticasone furoate (DPI)	100		200
Fluticasone propionate (DPI)	100–250	>250–500	>500
Fluticasone propionate (pMDI*, HFA as propellent)	100–250	> 250–500	>500
Mometasone furoate (DPI)	200		400
Mometasone furoate (pMDI*, HFA as propellent)	200–400		400

*Standard (non-fine) particle.
Abbreviations: ICS: inhaled cortico steroids; BDP: beclomethasone diproprionate; HFA: hydrofluoroalkane propellent (non-CFC).

currently available for asthma. Despite this, the percentage of patients opting for inhalers as the preferred modality of treatment seems to be low. The patient's ability to use the device correctly and the adherence to the treatment regimen are likely to be influenced by their beliefs, attitudes and concerns about the use of inhalers as the preferred mode of treatment.

Non-adherence is a major issue especially among adolescents, who have age-specific barriers for following a regular therapeutic schedule. This can have a detrimental effect on asthma control and subsequent outcomes.[14–16]

Non-adherence is not always deliberate. It may be accidental too. Deliberate or intentional non-adherence refers to patients missing or altering doses to suit their own needs, and includes an unwillingness to take medication owing to beliefs or cultural preferences. Accidental or unintentional non-adherence, however, includes unknowingly using the inhalation device incorrectly or forgetting to take medication as prescribed, or non-adherence due to practical issues like non affordability and non availability. There can be pseudo adherence too which causes poor asthma control. Beyond the labelled number of actuations, the propellant can release an aerosol plume that contains little or no drug and patients may believe that they are taking medications as per schedule. The dose of delivered drug per actuation may be highly inconsistent and unpredictable after the labelled number of actuations. This phenomenon is called tail off.[17]

DETERMINANTS OF NON-ADHERENCE

Asthma regimens often require intake of appropriate medications at regular intervals of time. Inadequate instructions, or a complex regimen which is time-consuming (eg, multiple inhalers or dosing 3–4 times a day) are important issues that affect adherence. The hectic schedules of patients and family members with insufficient communication and coordination between them can all affect adherence.[15,16] Lack of education and negative perceptions about treatment also frequently influence adherence.

The patient's beliefs, cultural preferences, attitude towards disease and their health seeking behaviour are significant issues in understanding and responding to various heath conditions, including asthma. Misconceptions about the use of inhalers may constitute a major obstacle in the proper management of asthma, which result in adverse treatment outcomes and poor asthma control. Concerns for patients with asthma include worries about the addictive nature of inhaled medications, the misconception that they are stronger than medications in the tablet or parenteral form, fear of side effects and the belief that once started, they cannot be stopped for life. Moreover, patients may also be less inclined to take medication to prevent or reduce risks, than to take medication for immediate symptoms.[15]

Many patients are not aware of the fact that various drugs are available in the inhaled form and they do not know the difference between a reliever and a controller. This ignorance of controller medications is of great concern with regard to asthma control. Studies show that 64% of asthmatics in India believed that regular controller medications are not really needed for asthma, and about 50% of the asthmatics had fears on the use of inhaled steroids.[18] This observation emphasizes the fact that all asthmatics need to be educated on the importance of using optimal doses of inhaled steroids for the adequate control of asthma.

Many studies have shown that females were more reluctant to use inhalers for social reasons. The majority preferred to keep inhaler use a secret to avoid social stigma and preferred oral medications over inhalers, if possible.[19]

Most patients do not know how to take an inhaler medication properly. The major factor leading to these errors is the lack of formal training by trained personnel on the proper usage of inhaled devices. A few believe that the particles in the DPI can block the already narrowed respiratory passages and aggravate the asthma and cause lung damage.[20] Studies have shown that asthma education programmes focussing on self-management and behavioural modification improves inhaler device usage, adherence to proper treatment and thereby asthma control.[21]

These issues are compounded by physician related issues, such as a poor rapport with patients.[16] Most doctors/nurses/trainers themselves do not know how to demonstrate and educate patients in the proper use of their inhaler devices.[22] Asthma has also been found to affect the mental health of affected individuals, and studies have shown that depression and anxiety disorders are associated with an adverse impact on adherence.[23] In terms of symptom perception, many accept mild asthma exacerbations as normal, or attribute them to other causes,[24] and these events are associated with emergency visits and hospitalizations.

As children with asthma become adolescents, the barriers impeding good adherence begin to change. While younger children rely largely on parents for the administration of asthma medication, at age 16, children typically begin to claim more independence and responsibility, which may in turn affect adherence.[25] They begin to form individual opinions and beliefs about their health, and develop self-regulatory behaviour that can significantly contribute to adherence. However, since adolescents often reject parental monitoring and support at this stage, conflict and confusion over responsibility for ensuring proper administration of medications may occur, with adherence commonly suffering.[25] In contrast, some adolescents still rely on their parents and struggle to take responsibility for their asthma management,[26] and so parental motivation may still remain important for adherence.

Intentional non-adherence is associated with other factors, such as not being bothered, finding it time-consuming or conflicting with other activities, as well as a perception of the lack of effect of asthma medications.[27] Stigma around using inhalers can affect adherence at the level of initiation, implementation or persistence.[15] For adolescents with asthma, embarrassment in front of friends is a predominant reason for non-adherence, including a desire to hide their condition and treatment from their peers.[14] Addictive behaviours such as smoking and drinking alcohol can also have a significant negative impact on adherence.

PROBLEMS OF NON-ADHERENCE

The major issues of non-adherence to medications include decrease in asthma control, poor symptom control, higher rates of exacerbations and reduced quality of life.[16,22] Uncontrolled asthma, resulting from poor adherence and other factors is a major cause of mortality and disability, particularly in adolescents.[16] If non-adherence remains undetected, the dose of medication may be increased or extra treatment may be prescribed unnecessarily in order to try to achieve disease control, thus further increasing the cost and complexity of the regimen.[28] Other consequences may include sleep disruption and a limited ability to do sports or recreational activities.[29] Poorly controlled asthma is also one of the leading causes of school absenteeism.

HOW TO ADDRESS NON-ADHERENCE?
Refining the Inhaler Technique

Poor inhaler instruction and technique represent a primary cause of medication non-adherence in asthma, resulting in ineffective/insufficient drug delivery to the airways and decreased medication efficacy. Improving understanding of the need for inhaled therapy and advice on optimal technique for using the inhaler device should increase patient adherence.[22] The ease of use and acceptance of the inhaler device is of paramount importance in adherence among adolescents. If a patient does not like the inhaler device or is unable to use it correctly, it is useless. A preferred device that is taken by the patient and is effective represents a better device. Almost all inhaler devices like pMDI, DPI, breath actuated inhalers (BAI) can effectively be used by adolescents and adults with asthma. Patient preference should be taken into account when choosing the inhaler device if there are no compelling reasons to adopt the physician's choice. Assessments of inhaler technique should be carried out regularly, and retraining and/or alternative treatment options considered where appropriate.[22,30]

Some studies suggest that specific inhaler types may be associated with better adherence, although further investigation is needed to confirm this.[31] Many factors, including age, dexterity, inspiratory capacity, cognitive ability, health literacy and ethnicity, affect the ability and motivation of patients to use their inhaler devices, and it is most important that the inhaler device which is most appropriate to each individual patient be chosen in order to achieve good adherence. Adherence can be affected by the choice of medications as well.

Enhancing Patient–Physician Communication

The collaboration of patients and physicians to ensure understanding of asthma and its treatment will likely enhance adherence.[32] Clear and open patient–physician communication that builds empathy and incorporates motivational interviewing techniques and shared decision making/treatment goals is vital, particularly for adolescents.[32] This approach can address patient-specific concerns, evaluate their beliefs, engage patients in the management of their disease and ensure family members are able to support the patient. It is also important to ensure that regular follow-up appointments are arranged with the treating physician, with reminders and other organizational factors to help improve adherence.[32]

Other Approaches to Improve Adherence

Several methods of adherence monitoring are available, which include subjective monitoring tools such as physician assessment of adherence, or self-report questionnaires like the recently developed adolescent asthma self-efficacy questionnaire. Objective monitoring strategies include analysis of prescriptions, weighing inhaler canisters, dose counters, directly observed therapy and nursing home visits.[33] Other approaches that may help to influence adherence among adolescents include peer support, medication reminders via smartphone applications and user-friendly online support systems with messaging facilities.[34] These measures may help to identify patients with poor asthma control despite good adherence who may be considered for escalation of inhaled medications or newer therapies, such as biologics.[35]

Poor adherence and inhaler technique are not the sole reasons for poor response to asthma therapy. A list of major causes and possible solutions for poor response are given in Table 28.3. Management needs to focus on and address the reasons for poor adherence,

Table 28.3: Major Causes and Possible Solutions to Poor Response to Inhaled Medications

Causes/Condition	Possible Solution
Wrong diagnosis	Exclude other causes
Avoidable factors	Control environmental factors
Inappropriate devices	Choose appropriate device, training and education
Non-adherence	Education, monitoring strategies
Wrong dose/medicine	Reassess dose/medication
Use of concomitant medicines	Try safer medicines
Presence of exacerbating conditions	Address issues like reflux, sinusitis, rhinitis
Deterioration of disease	Adopt possible preventive strategies

rather than simply escalating the prescribed treatment.[35]

CONCLUSION

The advent of medications in the inhaled form revolutionized the management of asthma. The use of inhaled corticosteroids alone, or in combination with long-acting beta-2 agonists, is the treatment of choice in most cases of asthma. They are safe, cost effective and the best agents available at present for the control of asthma. These medications can also considerably reduce hospitalizations due to asthma, if taken as per direction. However, the effectiveness of inhaled medication largely depends on the ability of the patient to use the inhaler device properly and adhere to the treatment schedule advised. This is highly influenced by their opinions and beliefs about the use of inhalers as the preferred and most suitable mode of treatment. Medication adherence in asthma faces many challenges. Identifying the reasons for poor disease control and adherence is essential to reduce morbidity, mortality and to improve patient quality of life. Patient education and communication between patients and health care personnel are key elements for effective and comprehensive patient assessment and for tailoring treatment to individual needs.

REFERENCES

1. Braman SS. The global burden of asthma. Chest 2006; 130(1 suppl):4S-12S.

2. World Health Organization. Global surveillance, prevention and control of chronic respiratory diseases: a comprehensive approach. 2007. https://www.who.int/gard/publications/GARD_Manual/en/

3   British Thoracic Society, Scottish Intercollegiate
    Guidelines Network. British guideline on
    the management of asthma. Thorax 2008; 63
    Suppl. 4:iv1–iv121.

4. Peters SP, Ferguson G, Deniz Y, et al. Uncontrolled
    asthma: a review of the prevalence, disease burden
    and options for treatment. Respir Med 2006;
    100:1139–1151.

5. Global Initiative for Asthma. Global Strategy for
    Asthma Management and Prevention (2020 Update).
    2020. Available from www.ginaasthma.org

6. Hamelmann E, Szefler SJ, Lau S. Severe asthma in
    children and adolescents. Allergy 2019;74: 2280–2282..
    https://doi.org/10.1111/all.13862

7. Kwong KYC, Morphew T, Scott L. Asthma control
    and future asthmarelated morbidity in innercity
    asthmatic children. Ann Allergy Asthma Immunol
    2008; 101(2):144–152.

8. Riccioni G, Bucciarelli T, Mancini B, et al. Compliance
    therapy with anti-inflammatory antiasthmatic drugs:
    inhaled corticosteroids and leukotriene receptor
    antagonists. Clin Ter 2007; 158(4):363–370.

9. Mudge J. *A Radical and Expeditious Cure for a Recent
    Catarrhous Cough*. London Publishers: Allen;1778.

10. Muntner S. *Treatise on Asthma by Maimonides*.
    Philadelphia: Lippincott, 1963.

11. Sanders M: Inhalation therapy: An historical review.
    Prim Care Respir J 2007;16:71–81.

12. Ayah Shakshuki, Remigius U. Agu. Improving the
    efficiency of respiratory drug delivery: A review of
    current treatment trends and future strategies for
    asthma and chronic obstructive pulmonary disease.
    Pulm Ther 2017; 3:267–281.

13. Omar S Usmani. Choosing the right inhaler for your
    asthma or COPD patient. Therapeutics and Clinical
    Risk Management 2019; 15:461–472.

14. De Simoni A, Horne R, Fleming L, et al. What
    do adolescents with asthma really think about
    adherence to inhalers? Insights from a qualitative
    analysis of a UK online forum. BMJ Open 2017;7:
    e015245. https://doi.org/10.1136/bmjopen-2016-015245

15. Naimi DR, Freedman TG, Ginsburg KR, et al.
    Adolescents and asthma: why bother with our meds?
    J Allergy Clin Immunol 2009; 123:1335–1341. https://
    doi.org/10.1016/j.jaci.2009.02.022

16. Desai M, Oppenheimer JJ. Medication adherence
    in the asthmatic child and adolescent. Curr
    Allergy Asthma Rep 2011; 11:454–464. doi:10.1007/
    s11882-011-0227-2

17. Conner JB, Buck PO. Improving asthma management:
    The case for mandatory inclusion of dose counters on
    all rescue bronchodilators. J Asthma 2013; 50:658–663.
    doi: 10.3109/02770903.2013.789056.

18. Salvi SS, Apte KK, Dhar R, et al. Asthma insights
    and management in India: lessons learnt from the
    Asia Pacific—asthma insights and management
    (AP-AIM) study. Journal of the Association of
    Physician of India 2015; 63:36–41.

19. Gupta VK, Bahia JS, Maheshwari A, et al. To study
    the attitudes, beliefs and perceptions regarding
    the Use of inhalers among patients of obstructive
    pulmonary diseases and in the general population in
    Punjab. J Clin Diagn Res 2011;5(3):434–439.

20. Sulaiman SP, Panicker V. Attitudes of patients with
    asthma on inhaler use. A cross sectional study
    from south Kerala. J. Evid. Based Med. Healthc
    2017;4(19):1505–1509. https://doi.org/10.18410/
    jebmh/2017/1.

21. Takemura M, Kobayashi M, Kimura K, et al. Repeated
    instruction on inhalation technique improves
    adherence to the therapeutic regimen in asthma.
    J Asthma 2010;47(2):202–208.

22. Braido F, Chrystyn H, Baiardini I, et al. "Trying, but
    failing" – the role of inhaler technique and mode
    of delivery in respiratory medication adherence.
    J Allergy Clin Immunol 2016;4:823–832. https://doi.
    org/10.1016/j.jaip.2016.03.002

23. McCauley E, Katon W, Russo J, et al. Impact of
    anxiety and depression on functional impairment
    in adolescents with asthma. Gen Hosp Psychiatry
    2007;29:214–222. https://doi.org/10.1016/j.
    genhosppsych.2007.02.003

24. Yawn BP. The role of the primary care physician
    in helping adolescent and adult patients improve
    asthma control. Mayo Clin Proc 2011;86:894–902.
    https://doi.org/10.4065/mcp.2011.0035

25. Costello RW, Foster JM, Grigg J, et al. The seven
    stages of man: the role of developmental stage
    on medication adherence in respiratory diseases.
    J Allergy Clin Immunol 2016;4:813–820. https://doi.
    org/10.1016/j.jaip.2016.04.002

26. Blaakman SW, Cohen A, Fagnano M, et al. Asthma
    medication adherence among urban teens: a
    qualitative analysis of barriers, facilitators and
    experiences with school-based care. J Asthma
    2014;51:522–529. https://doi.org/10.3109/02770903.
    2014.885041

27. Edgecombe K, Latter S, Peters S, et al. Health
    experiences of adolescents with uncontrolled severe
    asthma. Arch Dis Child 2010;95:985–991. https://doi.
    org/10.1136/adc.2009.171579

28. Burgess S, Sly P, Devadason S. Adherence with
    preventive medication in childhood asthma.
    Pulm Med 2011;2011:973849. https://doi.
    org/10.1155/2011/973849

29. Ahmad A, Sorensen K. Enabling and hindering
    factors influencing adherence to asthma treatment
    among adolescents: a systematic literature review.
    J Asthma 2016;53:862–878. https://doi.org/10.3109/
    02770903.2016.1155217

30. Kaplan A, Price D. Matching inhaler devices with patients: the role of the primary care physician. Can Respir J 2018;2018:9473051. https://doi.org/10.1155/2018/9473051

31. Laube BL, Janssens HM, de Jongh FH, et al. What the pulmonary specialist should know about the new inhalation therapies. Eur Respir J 2011;37:1308–1331. https://doi.org/10.1183/09031936.00166410

32. Plaza V, Fernández-Rodríguez C, Melero C, et al. Validation of the 'Test of the Adherence to Inhalers' (TAI) for asthma and COPD patients. J Aerosol Med Pulm Drug Deliv 2016;29:142–152. doi:10.1089/jamp.2015.1212

33. Pearce CJ, Fleming L. Adherence to medication in children and adolescents with asthma: methods for monitoring and intervention. Expert Rev Clin Immunol 2018;14:1–9. https://doi.org/10.1080/1744666X.2018.1532290

34. Koster ES, Philbert D, de Vries TW, et al. "I just forget to take it": asthma self-management needs and preferences in adolescents. J Asthma 2015;52:831–837. https://doi.org/10.3109/02770903.2015.1020388

35. Panzera AD, Schneider TK, Martinasek MP, et al. Adolescent asthma self-management: patient and parent-caregiver perspectives on using social media to improve care. J School Health 2013;83:921–930. https://doi.org/10.1111/josh.12111

29 Management of Chronic Severe Asthma

Saleel Punnilath Abdulsamad and Mohammed Munavvar

CONTENTS

INTRODUCTION

Severe asthma may account for only about 5–10% of asthmatics[1], but its impact on healthcare costs and patient burden is tremendous. In the United Kingdom, asthma related expenditures were estimated to be around £1,111,837,000 in the year 2011–2012 alone, and undoubtedly a major proportion of this can be attributed to Severe Asthma[2]. The seemingly uncontrollable and fast growing nature of this subset of asthmatics is indeed worrying and calls for a systematic, scientific and, more importantly, cost-effective way of managing these patients.

DEFINITION

As with every other entity in medicine, the first step towards addressing an issue at hand is to try and define the very nature and characteristics of the same as clearly as possible, which in simple language means to have a good definition. A proper definition leads to better understanding of the disease and paves the way forward for meaningful research in that area.

As severe asthma is a complex and heterogeneous condition[3,4], and with personalised and precision medicine opening up new horizons and changing the way modern patient care is delivered all around the world, the need to classify and characterise various 'phenotypes' (observable physiological traits) and 'endotypes' (underlying mechanisms) of severe asthma

cannot be over emphasised. Ever since the introduction of the concept of severe/refractory asthma in ERS/ATS guidelines released in 1999, various taskforces and organisations over the years have continued addressing this complex issue, which also meant the coining of different terminologies such as 'Brittle asthma, Refractory asthma, Corticosteroid-resistant asthma, Difficult to treat/control asthma,' etc. Some of these definitions are no longer used in clinical practice, and currently the most widely accepted definition is derived from ERS/ATS taskforce report on severe asthma in 2014[5].

Their working definition of severe asthma, which undoubtedly remains the cornerstone for current concepts of severe asthma, stated:

"When a diagnosis of asthma is confirmed and comorbidities have been addressed, severe asthma is defined as "asthma which requires treatment with high-dose inhaled corticosteroids (ICS) plus a second controller (and/or systemic corticosteroids) to prevent it from becoming 'uncontrolled' or which remains 'uncontrolled' despite this therapy".

It also defines 'uncontrolled asthma', as illustrated in Table 29.1.

For the clinician, differentiation between 'uncontrolled' and 'severe asthma' is very important, as therapeutic approaches in these populations are not the same. A recent study from the Netherlands[6] showed prevalence of difficult-to-control asthma from the national pharmacy database to be 17.4%; however when adherence issues to high-dose ICS and proper

DOI: 10.1201/9781003125785-29

Table 29.1: Definition of Severe Asthma for Patients Aged ≥6 Years

Asthma that requires treatment with guideline-suggested medications for GINA steps 4–5 asthma (high-dose ICSs# and LABA or leukotriene modifier/theophylline) for the previous year or SCSs for ≥50% of the previous year to prevent it from becoming "uncontrolled" or which remains "uncontrolled" despite this therapy.

Uncontrolled asthma is diagnosed when at least one of the following is present:

Poor symptom control: ACQ consistently ≥1.5, ACT <20 (or "not well controlled" by NAEPP/GINA guidelines)

1. Frequent severe exacerbations: 2 or more bursts of SCSs (≥3 days each) in the previous year
2. Serious exacerbations: at least 1 hospitalisation, ICU stay or mechanical ventilation in the previous year
3. Airflow limitation: after appropriate bronchodilator withhold FEV_1 <80% predicted (in the face of reduced FEV_1/FVC defined as less than the lower limit of normal)

Or

4. Controlled asthma that worsens on tapering of these high doses of ICSs or SCSs (or additional biologics)

(ACT: Asthma Control Test; NAEPP: National Asthma Education and Prevention Program; SCSs: systemic corticosteroids; #: the definition of high-dose ICSs is age specific.)

inhalation techniques were addressed, the figure representing 'true' severe asthma went down to 3.6%.

INITIAL ASSESSMENT AND EVALUATION

The first point of patient contact, which can either be in an outpatient clinic setting or as an inpatient in hospital remains very crucial in the management of severe asthma. Detailed assessment is the key, and it starts with questioning the very diagnosis of asthma itself: *Is this bronchial asthma, or is this one of the asthma mimics? Or is this one of the many comorbidities associated with asthma?* This is often challenging and not very straightforward. The 'Severe Asthma Checklist' for systematic assessment of severe asthma developed by the 'Centre of Excellence in Severe Asthma' serves as an excellent tool for this purpose (Table 29.2).

DIAGNOSIS, SEVERITY ASSESSMENT AND TREATMENT OPTIMIZATION

Asthma is one of the most over diagnosed conditions, with up to 30–35%[8] of patients falling into this category. This is often attributed to the fact that treatment is initiated in the community without even performing basic spirometry to confirm the diagnosis. Evaluation of such patients (most of them already on long-term ICS/LABA and even on maintenance OCS) can be particularly challenging, as the sensitivity of diagnostic testing is low, especially if they already have persistent airflow limitation. Patients who may actually have underlying corticosteroid resistance would unfortunately already have had high-dose ICS/OCS treatment and present with various complications, adding onto the difficulty in reaching a diagnosis.

The most characteristic feature with regards to symptoms and airflow limitation in asthma

is its *variability*. When there is no variability in airflow limitation, a repeat bronchodilator reversibility testing after withholding bronchodilators (SABA for 4 hours and LABA for 12 hours) or during symptoms may be considered. Alternative diagnoses need to be considered if this is normal. A bronchial provocation test may be needed if FEV_1 is >70% predicted, which if negative will need stepping down of controller treatment and a reassessment in 2–4 weeks. If at that point the symptoms re-emerge, accompanied by a fall in FEV_1, a diagnosis of asthma can be confirmed, and the controller treatment may be stepped up to the lowest previous effective dose.

Poor symptom control in asthma is when there are[9]:

- 3 or more days a week with symptoms; or

- 2 or more days a week with required use of a rescue SABA inhaler for symptomatic relief; or

- 1 or more nights a week with awakening due to asthma

Two of the most commonly used 'tools' for this purpose are the ACQ (Asthma Control Questionnaire) and the ACT (Asthma Control Test), and can be easily used in a clinic setting. The ACQ score is calculated as the average of 5, 6 or 7 items over a 1-week period: all versions of the ACQ include 5 symptom questions; ACQ-6 includes reliever use; and in ACQ-7, a score for pre-bronchodilator FEV_1 is averaged with symptom and reliever items[10]. Lower the score the better will be symptom control. ACQ score of 1.5 or more is indicative of poor symptom control.

ACT involves five different domains covering symptoms over a 4-week period, scored on a 5-point scale[11]. The higher the score, the better

Table 29.2: Severe Asthma Assessment Checklist[7]

Serial No.	Clinical Question	Assessment
1.	Has the diagnosis of asthma been confirmed	Compatible history and objective evidence of variability in symptoms and lung function over time, either spontaneously, by treatment or by bronchial provocation testing
2.	Is it severe?	Demonstration of: • Poor control • Airflow obstruction • Frequent exacerbations • Life-threatening episodes
3.	Is treatment optimal?	Treatment with: • High-dose ICS and LABA or other controller OR • Moderate dose ICS with more than one controller
4.	Are self-management skills optimal?	Optimized: • Inhaler device technique • Adherence • Self-monitoring • Asthma knowledge • Written action plan
5.	Are trigger factors identified and managed?	Examples: • Allergen • NSAIDs • Cigarette smoke • Respiratory viral infections • Emotional stress • Mould or dampness • Patient-reported triggers
6.	Is comorbidity identified and managed?	Examples: • Sino-nasal disease • Dysfunctional breathing • Paradoxical vocal fold movement/VCD • Obstructive sleep apnoea • Anxiety and/or depression • Gastroesophageal reflux disease • Obesity
7.	What is the pattern of airway inflammation?	Eosinophilic: sputum assessment, FeNO, blood eosinophils Noneosinophilic: sputum assessment
8.	What is the optimal individualized management plan?	Developed with evidence based interventions that targets clinical issues identified during a systematic and multidimentional assessment, in partnership with patients and clinicians, considering patient preferences

the symptom control - and an ACT of < 20 is reflective of poor symptom control (Table 29.3).

As mentioned previously in this chapter, severe asthma is diagnosed when patients are already on GINA steps 4/5 treatment (medium or high dose ICS with a second controller; maintenance OCS) (Figure: BOX 3-5A from GINA 2020[12]), once comorbidities and adherence issues have been identified and addressed. ICS are the recommended preventer drug for both adults and children, and the first choice as an add-on therapy to ICS in adults is an inhaled LABA, which should be considered before increasing the dose of ICS. A minimum of >/= 3 months is recommended by GINA for a trial of high dose ICS as sufficient time to assess whether there is any improvement in symptoms and/or lung function. If asthma control remains suboptimal after the addition of an inhaled LABA, then the next step will be to increase the dose of ICS, and to consider adding a LTRA. ICS-formoterol is the preferred reliever therapy for patients prescribed maintenance and reliever therapy. For other ICS-LABAs, reliever is a SABA. Step 4 mentions add-on tiotropium to high-dose ICS, or medium dose ICS-LABA. For patients on step 5, referral for phenotypic assessment and identifying the inflammatory pathway is advised, an area which has shown tremendous

Table 29.3: Asthma Control Test for Patients >12 Years

Questions	Score				
1—During the *last 4 weeks*, how much of the time has your asthma kept you from getting much done at work, school or home?	All of the time	Most of the time	Some of the time	A little of the time	None of the time
2—During the *last 4 weeks*, how often have you had shortness of breath?	More than once a day	Once a day	3–6 times a week	1–2 times a week	Not at all
3—During the *last 4 weeks*, how often have your asthma symptoms (wheezing, coughing, shortness of breath, chest tightness or pain) woken you up at night or earlier than usual in the morning?	4 or more nights a week	2–3 nights a week	Once a week	Once or Twice	Not at all
4—During the *last 4 weeks*, how often have you used your rescue inhaler or nebuliser medication (such as Salbutamol)?	3 or more times per day	Once or twice per day	2–3 times per week	Once a week or less	Not at all
5—How would you rate your asthma control during the *last 4 weeks*?	Not Controlled at all	Poorly Controlled	Somewhat Controlled	Well Controlled	Completely Controlled

potential in the management of chronic severe asthma especially with the advent of anti-IgE, IL5/5R, IL4R agents.

ADDRESSING NON-ADHERENCE, TRIGGER FACTORS AND COMORBITITIES

WHO defines 'adherence' as *the extent to which a person's behaviour, taking medication, following a diet, and/or executing/lifestyle changes, corresponds with agreed recommendations from a healthcare provider*[13]. For a better understanding of non-adherence, it is worthwhile classifying them as 'intentional' and 'non-intentional'. Intentional non-adherence is when a patient chooses not to be on a particular treatment, which could be commonly due to medication side effects, social or psychological factors, or cost of the medication itself. Non-intentional non-adherence are the more easily correctable ones, as they are most often due to lack of understanding of proper inhaler technique, or something more simple as forgetting to take medications. It is essential to show empathy to the patient in order to better understand the type of non-adherence (which could even be a combination of both intentional and non-intentional)[14] and the reasons behind it and work towards a more personalised and acceptable management plan. Poor healthcare outcome have been consistently associated with poor adherence in many studies[14–17]. The need to employ more objective and surrogate measures like electronic inhaler monitoring, blood prednisolone level, monitoring of dispensing records, etc., and also the potential use of FeNO suppression in the severe asthma

population can be found in the latest GINA guidelines[12]. Documented evidence of adequate FeNO suppression in such patients with improved adherence to ICS can be extremely useful in identifying those with prior poor adherence to ICS, who will potentially benefit from optimised inhaled treatment. This will also on the other hand help identify the subset of patients who will most likely benefit from biological treatment if they fail to adequately suppress the type 2 markers (FeNO, blood eosinophils) whilst on optimised ICS treatment[18,19]. Patient education, a written action plan and self-monitoring are all proven ways of improving adherence, but their impact on clinical outcomes, including measures of asthma control is not very clear[20].

Avoidance of environmental allergens and irritants known to trigger symptoms is an important factor for prevention of future exacerbations[1]. Allergens, NSAIDs, cigarette smoke, emotional stress, mould or dampness and respiratory viral infections are some of the commonly known trigger factors. In committed families with evidence of house dust mite allergy and who wish to try mite avoidance, interventions such as complete barrier bed covering systems, removal of carpets, removal of soft toys from bed, high temperature washing of bed linen, ascaricides to soft furnishings, dehumidification, etc., are recommended[21].

For clinicians dealing with severe asthma, dealing with the comorbidities is perhaps as important as dealing with the disease itself. Not only do they represent potential targets for therapy, but they are now also increasingly

Table 29.4: Major Comorbidities Associated with Severe Asthma

Comorbidities	Management
Rhinitis, Chronic Rhinosinusitis and Nasal Polyposis	Sinus rinses, topical steroid, surgery
Vocal cord dysfunction/ Inducible laryngeal obstruction	Language therapy, counselling, Psychotherapy
Obesity and OSA	Weight loss, bariatric surgery, nasal CPAP, Adeno-tonsillectomy (Children)
GERD	Proton pump inhibitor
Bronchiectasis and ABPA	Chest physiotherapy, postural drainage Corticosteroids, antifungal agents
ACO (Asthma COPD Overlap)	ICS/LABA, Targeted therapy

recognised as treatable traits[22-24] (Table 29.4). The evaluation and investigative approach to severe asthma thus should not be stopped as soon as a diagnosis of severe asthma is made, and every effort should be made to identify any comorbidities associated with it, which is crucial for its effective management.

Studies have attributed prevalence rates of >/= 30% for some of the comorbidities among severe asthma cohorts, which includes obesity, dysfunctional breathing, upper airway disorders, vocal cord dysfunction, OSA and GERD. Often there are multiple comorbidities in a single patient, with one study by Radhakrishna et al. showing the presence of a mean of 3 per patient[25]. Similarly, the prevalence of anxiety and depression in many severe asthma cohorts has been found to be 30%[26]. A detailed discussion on all the comorbidities is beyond the scope of this chapter, but a brief description of some of the important ones from a management perspective is as follows.

RHINITIS, CHRONIC RHINOSINUSITIS AND NASAL POLYPOSIS

Allergic rhinitis is far more prevalent (55%) than non-allergic rhinitis (15%) in both non-severe and severe asthma[27]. In coexisting rhinitis and asthma, the possibility of a common or shared pathophysiology has been proposed, even in non-allergic rhinitis[28-31]. Intranasal corticosteroid therapy has been found to improve asthma symptoms, but its effect in those already on ICS is not very clear[32-36]. Allergen immunotherapy is effective

in improving symptoms of mild to moderate asthma but in severe uncontrolled asthma it is an absolute contraindication[37,38]. The prevalence of both chronic rhinosinusitis (45%) and nasal polyposis have been found to be greater in severe asthma than non-severe asthma[39,40]. Nasal polyposis may be accompanied by Aspirin-exacerbated respiratory disease (AERD) and can affect 15% of severe asthma patients[41]. Even though there are no large studies in severe asthma, both medical (mainly with intranasal coticosteroids) and surgical therapy are associated with improved asthma control[42-44].

VCD/ILO

Vocal cord dysfunction is a frequently under diagnosed and under treated condition in severe asthmatics, with a prevalence as high as 30–50%[45,46]. It is also known by a different term PVFM (paradoxical vocal fold movement), but a recent task force has suggested a new name -ILO (inducible laryngeal obstruction)[47]. VCD is the paradoxical adduction of otherwise structurally normal vocal cords, often brought about by triggers such as scents, odours or phonation, and can mimic asthma symptoms. Screening can be done by the use of questionnaires like Pittsburgh VCD index, VCDQ, etc.[48,49], but diagnosis often requires direct visualisation of the larynx either via nasal endoscopy or dynamic CT scan of the neck, or with the evidence of variable extrathoracic airflow obstruction on inspiratory flow volume curves. Very careful evaluation is often required to distinguish this condition from the otherwise physiologically occurring expiratory vocal fold adduction in patients with airflow obstruction[50]. There are still no randomised control trials showing supportive evidence to pharmacological therapy in VCD, and speech retraining remains the mainstay of treatment.

OBESITY AND OSA

Obesity (BMI > 30 kg.m^{-2}) is more prevalent in severe asthma than non-severe asthma (39% versus 18%)[51]. There is evidence for a worsening quality of life and airflow obstruction with central adiposity, thereby underlining the significance of pattern of fat distribution as well[52,53]. Obesity can also be associated with other comorbidities like type 2 diabetes, metabolic syndrome, cardiovascular diseases, OSA, corticosteroid insensitivity, etc. Weight loss by the means of dietary changes and regular exercise is of paramount importance and losing as much as 5–10% of body weight has been associated with improvement in asthma symptoms. It is worth mentioning that being underweight (BMI<18.5 kg.m[-2]) also has been linked to increased risk of exacerbations[54].

The prevalence of OSA in severe asthma is extremely high, with data from polysomnography showing it to be as much as 80%[55]. Unsurprisingly, CPAP treatment has been shown to improve symptoms and quality of life and patients should be carefully assessed and started on treatment at the earliest.

GERD

Increased rate of exacerbations have been recognised in severe asthmatics with reflux symptoms, with a prevalence rate of around 40%[40,51]. However, apart from a couple of older studies showing improved asthma control following surgical reflux treatment[56,57], there are no convincing data in either the non-severe or severe asthma cohorts that medical or surgical treatments improve outcomes.

EXCESSIVE CENTRAL AIRWAY COLLAPSE

Two separate entities namely TBM (tracheobronchomalacia) and EDAC (excessive dynamic airway collapse) constitute 'excessive central airway collapse'. TBM is increased collapsibility of the tracheal and bronchial walls due to cartilaginous weakness whereas EDAC causes excessive forward movement of the posterior membrane of airways without any underlying cartilaginous abnormality. Certain risk factors like female sex, increasing age, obesity and thyroid disorders have been identified with excessive central airway collapse[58,59]. Presentation is usually very similar with cough, wheeze and recurrent infections due to sputum retention and as a result diagnosis is often delayed. Functional bronchoscopy or a dynamic CT is often required to confirm the disease[60]. Management revolves around treating infections, physiotherapy, CPAP, but stenting or tracheoplasty may be required in more severe cases.

BRONCHIECTASIS AND ABPA

Bronchiectasis is much more prevalent in severe asthma than mild asthma, with prevalence rates ranging from 24–40% and 30% respectively[61]. Airflow limitation is found to be more severe in patients with frequent exacerbations as well. Radiological evidence of airway dilatation alone without bronchiectasis symptoms can be seen in severe asthma, which often confirms the diagnosis. For established bronchiectasis, management should be as usual with emphasis on airway clearance and treating infections with appropriate antibiotics.

Prevalence of ABPA in asthma has been reported to be 13% in one study[62]. Serum IgE level measurement is a very useful test in the setting of characteristic clinical and radiological features. However, the presence of other allergic conditions like allergic rhinitis and atopic asthma can make diagnosis difficult if based solely on a raised IgE level[63,64], as they can also be frequently associated with IgE levels more than 1000 IU mL[-1]. Itraconazole has been found to be effective in treatment now with RCT evidence[65], but the mainstay of management remains to be corticosteroids.

ACO (ASTHMA COPD OVERLAP)

Prevalence of COPD in severe asthma is thought to be around 20%, and ACO (Asthma COPD overlap) is now being increasingly recognised as a separate entity with many overlapping features. The previous concept of describing it as a syndrome (ACOS) changed with the release of GINA 2017 guidelines, which proposed the term ACO. A detailed description of this interesting entity is beyond the scope of this chapter. ACO shares many similar features with severe asthma, and the concept of ACO as a distinct phenotype of severe asthma has also been proposed[66]. Compared to COPD, ACO subjects have been shown to have frequent and more severe exacerbations, but less smoking packs history[67-69]. Th2 inflammatory response was enhanced in ACO subjects with high levels of IL-4 and immunoglobulin E (IgE). Airway hyper reactivity, and also CT findings of increased bronchial wall thickness have been described in ACO compared to COPD[68,70]. ICS based treatment combined with LABA as for severe asthma is the general recommendation for management in ACO, however the response to ICS/LABA in such patients with severe airway limitation is often very dismal. Wenzel SE et al. showed that Dupilumab, a human anti-IL-4 receptor α monoclonal antibody, resulted in elevated FEV$_1$, improved symptom control and reduced annual rates of exacerbation in patients with severe asthma. After performing a post-hoc analysis of possible ACO subjects in their study, the authors later concluded that Dupilumab may function in ACO patients as well[71,72]. The striking similarity of ACO with severe asthma also makes it suitable for bronchial thermoplasty (mentioned later on in this chapter) in carefully selected cohorts.

INFLAMMATORY PHENOTYPES AND PRECISION MEDICINE APPROACH

Broadly asthma phenotypes are divided in two for treatment purposes—as 'T2-high' and 'T2-low'. This is based on sputum

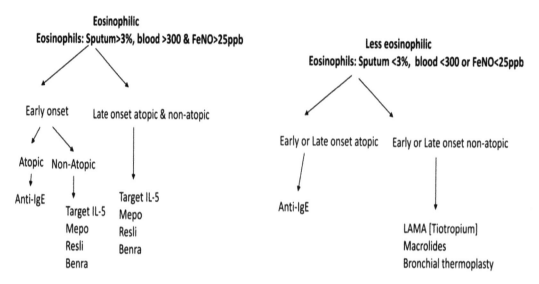

Figure 29.1 Severe asthma algorithm approach: A simple approach.

eosinophil count, blood eosinophilia and FeNO levels. According to the inflammatory phenotype, four categories have been recognised namely **eosinophilic** (high eosinophil count), **neutrophilic** (high neutrophil count), **mixed** (both eosinophil and neutrophil count raised) and **paucigranulocytic** (normal eosinophil and neutrophil counts with airflow limitation and symptoms). Currently, multiple biological agents are available with most of them showing good satisfactory outcomes in patients with persistent T2 inflammation despite treatment with high-dose ICS and/ or OCS. Biologics targeting IgE, IL-4, IL-5, IL-13 are the mainstay of treatment (discussed in detail in chapter). For anti-IgE-based therapy (Omalizumab), IgE levels >/30 IU mL⁻¹ is generally taken as an inclusion criteria. For drugs targeting IL-5, IL-4 an IL-13, absolute eosinophil counts >/300 cells/micro litre in patients who are not on OCS, has shown good response to treatment[73–76].

As mentioned earlier in this chapter, the precision medicine approach has opened up new horizons in terms of treatment and allows tailoring of available management options based on individual patients rather than a 'one size fits all' approach. A simple algorithm has been proposed by Andriana I et al.[77], which is summarised below (Figure 29.1).

BRONCHIAL THERMOPLASTY

Bronchial thermoplasty is the only US FDA approved non pharmacological intervention in the treatment of severe asthma. It involves bronchoscopic administration of thermal energy to bronchial walls via a disposable electrode catheter, and is usually done under sedation or general anaesthesia. Three sessions with an interval of at least 3 weeks between each session is required to complete the procedure, which delivers radio frequency energy to the bronchial walls in a circumferential manner by moving from the distal to the proximal bronchi. The rationale behind this interventional modality is to reduce the airway smooth muscle mass (ASM), which is a well-recognized feature of airway remodelling and thought to contribute to bronchial hyperreactivity[78]. Increased ASM mass is also linked to an increased accumulation of fibroblast in bronchial biopsies, fall in FEV₁, and potentially to glucocorticoid insensitivity as well, as a result of expression of certain chemokines (CCL5, CCL11, CX3CL2) responsible for recruiting eosinophils and mast cells[79–81]. As per the NICE guidance on bronchial thermoplasty in severe asthma[82], it is still unclear which patient group will benefit most from this procedure. Hence careful patient selection is of utmost importance, and the procedure should only be carried out by experienced and competent interventional pulmonologists, in centres with access to intensive care treatment.

CONCLUSION

■ Severe asthma, though accounting for only 5–10% of cases of asthma, causes a significant burden on the healthcare system

■ Identifying and addressing the various comorbidities in a timely manner remains the cornerstone of management of severe asthma

- A well-co-ordinated multi-disciplinary team comprising a pulmonologist, specialist asthma nurse, chest physiotherapist, speech and language therapist is key to effective management

- Differentiation and categorisation into various inflammatory phenotypes (eosinophilic vs non-eosinophilic) has now made it possible to have a more personalised and targeted approach to such patients, which along with the advent of biological agents have tremendously improved the prospects in the management of severe asthma

REFERENCES

1. European Academy of Allergy and Clinical Immunology (EAACI). Global Atlas of Asthma 2013.

2. M Mukherjee, A Stoddart, R P Gupta, B I Nwaru, A Farr, M Heaven, et al. The epidemiology, healthcare and societal burden and costs of asthma in the UK and its member nations: analyses of standalone and linked national databases. BMC Med 2016;14: 113. https://10.1186/s12916-016-0657-8

3. Israel E, Reddel HK. Severe and difficult-to-treat asthma in adults. N Engl J Med 2017;377: 965–976.

4. Papi A, Brightling C, Pedersen SE, et al. Asthma. Lancet 2018;391: 783–800.

5. Chung KF, Wenzel SE, Brozek JL, et al. International ERS/ATS guidelines on definition, evaluation and treatment of severe asthma. Eur Respir J 2014;43: 343–373.

6. Hekking PP, Wener RR, Amelink M, et al. The prevalence of severe refractory asthma. J Allergy Clin Immunol 2015;135: 896–902.

7. Severe Asthma Assessment Checklist. https://www.severeasthma.org.au/tools-resources/toolkits/

8. Aaron SD, Boulet LP, Reddel HK, et al. Underdiagnosis and overdiagnosis of asthma. Am J Respir Crit Care Med 2018;198: 1012–1020.

9. National Institute for Health and Care Excellence (NICE). Asthma: diagnosis, monitoring and chronic asthma management. NICE guideline [NG80]. November 2017.

10. https://bmjopen.bmj.com/content/bmjopen/7/1/e013935/DC1/embed/inline-supplementary-material-1.pdf?download=true

11. https://www.thoracic.org/members/assemblies/assemblies/srn/questionaires/act.php

12. Global Initiative for Asthma (GINA). Difficult-to-treat and Severe Asthma in Adolescent and Adult Patients. Diagnosis and Management 2018. https://ginasthma.org/wp-content/uploads/2018/11/GINA-SA-FINAL-wms.pdf

13. World Health Organization. Adherence to long-term therapies: Evidence for action. Geneva, World Health Organization, 2003.

14. Heaney LG, Horne R. Non-adherence in difficult asthma: time to take it seriously. Thorax 2012;67: 268–270.

15. Gamble J, Stevenson M, McClean E, et al. The prevalence of nonadherence in difficult asthma. Am J Respir Crit Care Med 2009;180: 817–822.

16. Murphy AC, Proeschal A, Brightling CE, et al. The relationship between clinical outcomes and medication adherence in difficult-to-control asthma. Thorax 2012;67: 751–753.

17. Royal College of Physicians. National Review of Asthma Deaths. www.rcplondon.ac.uk/projects/national-review-asthma-deaths

18. Heaney LG, Busby J, Bradding P, et al. Remotely monitored therapy and nitric oxide suppression identifies non-adherence in severe asthma. Am J Respir Crit Care Med 2019;199: 454–464.

19. Bender BG. Sorting out nonadherence and airway inflammation in treatment escalation for severe asthma. Am J Respir Crit Care Med 2019;199: 400–402.

20. Normansell R, Kew KM. Interventions to improve adherence to inhaled steroids for asthma. Cochrane Database Syst Rev 2017;4: CD012226.

21. British guideline on the management of asthma. Thorax. 2003 Feb; 58 Suppl 1(Suppl 1):i1–94. https://10.1136/thorax.58.suppl_1.1i.24.

22. Agusti A, Bel E, Thomas M, et al. Treatable traits: toward precision medicine of chronic airway diseases. Eur Respir J 2016; 47: 410–419.

23. Fingleton J, Hardy J, Beasley R. Treatable traits of chronic airways disease. Curr Opin Pulm Med 2018; 24: 24–31.

24. Tay TR, Hew M. Comorbid "treatable traits" in difficult asthma: current evidence and clinical evaluation. Allergy 2018; 73: 1369–1382.

25. Radhakrishna N, Tay TR, Hore-Lacy F, et al. Profile of difficult to treat asthma patients referred for systematic assessment. Respir Med 2016; 117: 166–173.

26. Heaney LG, Conway E, Kelly C, et al. Predictors of therapy resistant asthma: outcome of a systematic evaluation protocol. Thorax 2003; 58: 561–566.

27. Shaw DE, Sousa AR, Fowler SJ, et al. Clinical and inflammatory characteristics of the European U-BIOPRED adult severe asthma cohort. Eur Respir J 2015; 46: 1308–1321.

28. Braunstahl GJ, Kleinjan A, Overbeek SE, et al. Segmental bronchial provocation induces nasal inflammation in allergic rhinitis patients. Am J Respir Crit Care Med 2000; 161: 2051–2057.

29. Braunstahl GJ, Overbeek SE, Kleinjan A, et al. Nasal allergen provocation induces adhesion molecule expression and tissue eosinophilia in upper and lower airways. J Allergy Clin Immunol 2001; 107: 469–476.

30. Kanani AS, Broder I, Greene JM, et al. Correlation between nasal symptoms and asthma severity in patients with atopic and nonatopic asthma. Ann Allergy Asthma Immunol 2005; 94: 341–347.

31. Leynaert B, Bousquet J, Neukirch C, et al. Perennial rhinitis: an independent risk factor for asthma in nonatopic subjects: results from the European Community Respiratory Health Survey. J Allergy Clin Immunol 1999; 104:301–304.

32. Scichilone N, Arrigo R, Paterno A, et al. The effect of intranasal corticosteroids on asthma control and quality of life in allergic rhinitis with mild asthma. J Asthma 2011; 48: 41–47.

33. Baiardini I, Villa E, Rogkakou A, et al. Effects of mometasone furoate on the quality of life: a randomized placebo-controlled trial in persistent allergic rhinitis and intermittent asthma using the Rhinasthma questionnaire. Clin Exp Allergy 2011; 41: 417–423.

34. Dahl R, Nielsen LP, Kips J, et al. Intranasal and inhaled fluticasone propionate for pollen-induced rhinitis and asthma. Allergy 2005; 60: 875–881.

35. Lohia S, Schlosser RJ, Soler ZM. Impact of intranasal corticosteroids on asthma outcomes in allergic rhinitis: a meta-analysis. Allergy 2013; 68: 569–579.

36. Nair A, Vaidyanathan S, Clearie K, et al. Steroid sparing effects of intranasal corticosteroids in asthma and allergic rhinitis. Allergy 2010; 65: 359–367.

37. Pitsios C, Demoly P, Bilo MB, et al. Clinical contraindications to allergen immunotherapy: an EAACI position paper. Allergy 2015; 70: 897–909.

38. Abramson MJ, Puy RM, Weiner JM. Injection allergen immunotherapy for asthma. Cochrane Database Syst Rev 2010; 8: CD001186.

39. Micheletto C, Visconti M, Trevisan F, et al. The prevalence of nasal polyps and the corresponding urinary LTE4 levels in severe compared to mild and moderate asthma. Eur Ann Allergy Clin Immunol 2010; 42: 120–124.

40. Moore WC, Bleecker ER, Curran-Everett D, et al. Characterization of the severe asthma phenotype by the National Heart, Lung, and Blood Institute's Severe Asthma Research Program. J Allergy Clin Immunol 2007; 119:405–413.

41. Rajan JP, Wineinger NE, Stevenson DD, et al. Prevalence of aspirin-exacerbated respiratory disease among asthmatic patients: a meta-analysis of the literature. J Allergy Clin Immunol 2015; 135: 676–681.

42. Ragab S, Scadding GK, Lund VJ, et al. Treatment of chronic rhinosinusitis and its effects on asthma. Eur Respir J 2006; 28: 68–74.

43. Batra PS, Kern RC, Tripathi A, et al. Outcome analysis of endoscopic sinus surgery in patients with nasal polyps and asthma. Laryngoscope 2003; 113: 1703–1706.

44. Al Badaai Y, Valdes CJ, Samaha M. Outcomes and cost benefits of functional endoscopic sinus surgery in severely asthmatic patients with chronic rhinosinusitis. J Laryngol Otol 2014; 128: 512–517.

45. Tay TR, Radhakrishna N, Hore-Lacy F, et al. Comorbidities in difficult asthma are independent risk factors for frequent exacerbations, poor control and diminished quality of life. Respirology 2016; 21: 1384–1390.

46. Low K, Lau KK, Holmes P, et al. Abnormal vocal cord function in difficult-to-treat asthma. Am J Respir Crit Care Med 2011; 184: 50–56.

47. Halvorsen T, Walsted ES, Bucca C, et al. Inducible laryngeal obstruction: an official joint European Respiratory Society and European Laryngological Society statement. Eur Respir J 2017; 50: 1602221.

48. Fowler SJ, Thurston A, Chesworth B, et al. The VCDQ – a questionnaire for symptom monitoring in vocal cord dysfunction. Clin Exp Allergy 2015; 45: 1406–1411.

49. Traister RS, Fajt ML, Landsittel D, et al. A novel scoring system to distinguish vocal cord dysfunction from asthma. J Allergy Clin Immunol Pract 2014; 2: 65–69.

50. Denlinger LC, Phillips BR, Ramratnam S, et al. Inflammatory and comorbid features of patients with severe asthma and frequent exacerbations. Am J Respir Crit Care Med 2017; 195: 302–313.

51. Shaw DE, Sousa AR, Fowler SJ, et al. Clinical and inflammatory characteristics of the European U-BIOPRED adult severe asthma cohort. Eur Respir J 2015; 46: 1308–1321.

52. Goudarzi H, Konno S, Kimura H, et al. Impact of abdominal visceral adiposity on adult asthma symptoms. J Allergy Clin Immunol Pract 2019; 7: 1222–1229.

53. To M, Hitani A, Kono Y, et al. Obesity-associated severe asthma in an adult Japanese population. Respir Investig 2018; 56: 440–447.

54. McDonald VM, Hiles SA, Godbout K, et al. Treatable traits can be identified in a severe asthma registry and predict future exacerbations. Respirology 2019; 24: 37–47.

55. Julien JY, Martin JG, Ernst P, et al. Prevalence of obstructive sleep apnea–hypopnea in severe versus moderate asthma. J Allergy Clin Immunol 2009; 124: 371–376.

56. Larrain A, Carrasco E, Galleguillos F, et al. Medical and surgical treatment of nonallergic asthma associated with gastroesophageal reflux. Chest 1991; 99: 1330–1335.

57. Sontag SJ, O'Connell S, Khandelwal S, et al. Asthmatics with gastroesophageal reflux: long term results of a

randomized trial of medical and surgical antireflux therapies. Am J Gastroenterol 2003; 98: 987–999.

58. Del Negro RW, Tognella S, Guerriero M, et al. Prevalence of tracheobronchomalacia and excessive dynamic airway collapse in bronchial asthma of different severity. Multidiscip Respir Med 2013; 8: 32.

59. Boiselle PM, Litmanovich DE, Michaud G, et al. Dynamic expiratory tracheal collapse in morbidly obese COPD patients. COPD 2013; 10: 604–610.

60. Murgu S, Colt HG. Tracheobronchomalacia and excessive dynamic airway collapse. Clin Chest Med 2013; 34:527–555.

61. Porsbjerg C, Menzies-Gow A. Comorbidities in severe asthma: clinical impact and management. Respirology 2017; 22: 651–661.

62. Agarwal R, Aggarwal AN, Gupta D, et al. Aspergillus hypersensitivity and allergic bronchopulmonary aspergillosis in patients with bronchial asthma: systematic review and meta-analysis. Int J Tuberc Lung Dis 2009; 13: 936–944.

63. Tay TR, Bosco J, Aumann H, et al. Elevated total serum immunoglobulin E (>1000 IU/mL): implications? Intern Med J 2016; 46: 846–849.

64. Tay TR, Bosco J, Gillman A, et al. Co-existing atopic conditions influence the likelihood of allergic bronchopulmonary aspergillosis in asthma. Ann Allergy Asthma Immunol 2016; 117: 29–32.

65. Stevens DA, Schwartz HJ, Lee JY, et al. A randomized trial of itraconazole in allergic bronchopulmonary aspergillosis. N Engl J Med 2000; 342: 756–762.

66. Yang Xia, Yuan Cao, Lexin Xia, Wen Li, and Huahao Shen. Severe asthma and asthma-COPD overlap: a double agent or identical twins?

67. Caillaud D, Chanez P, Escamilla R, et al. Asthma-COPD overlap syndrome (ACOS) vs 'pure' COPD: a distinct phenotype? Allergy 2017;72:137-45. 10.1111/all.13004

68. Hardin M, Cho M, McDonald ML, et al. The clinical and genetic features of COPD-asthma overlap syndrome. Eur Respir J 2014;44:341-50. 10.1183/09031936.00216013

69. Kumbhare S, Pleasants R, Ohar JA, et al. Characteristics and Prevalence of Asthma/Chronic Obstructive Pulmonary Disease Overlap in the United States. Ann Am Thorac Soc 2016;13:803–810. 10.1513/AnnalsATS.201508-554OC

70. Bumbacea D, Campbell D, Nguyen L, et al. Parameters associated with persistent airflow obstruction in chronic severe asthma. Eur Respir J 2004;24:122–128. 10.1183/09031936.04.00077803.

71. Wenzel S, Castro M, Corren J, et al. Dupilumab efficacy and safety in adults with uncontrolled persistent asthma despite use of medium-to-high-dose inhaled corticosteroids plus a long-acting beta2 agonist: a randomised double-blind placebo-controlled pivotal phase 2b dose-ranging trial. Lancet 2016;388:31–44. 10.1016/S0140-6736(16)30307-5

72. Wenzel SE, Jayawardena S, Graham NM, et al. Severe asthma and asthma-chronic obstructive pulmonary disease syndrome - Authors' reply. Lancet 2016;388:2742. 10.1016/S0140-6736(16)31720-2

73. Ortega HG, Yancey SW, Mayer B, et al. Severe eosinophilic asthma treated with mepolizumab stratified by baseline eosinophil thresholds: a secondary analysis of the DREAM and MENSA studies. Lancet Respir Med 2016; 4: 549–556.

74. Bleecker ER, Fitzgerald JM, Chanez P, et al. Efficacy and safety of benralizumab for patients with severe asthma uncontrolled with high-dosage inhaled corticosteroids and long-acting β2-agonists (SIROCCO): a randomised, multicentre, placebo-controlled phase 3 trial. Lancet 2016;388: 2115–2127.

75. FitzGerald JM, Bleecker ER, Nair P, et al. Benralizumab, an anti-interleukin-5 receptor α monoclonal antibody, as add-on treatment for patients with severe, uncontrolled, eosinophilic asthma (CALIMA): a randomised, double-blind, placebo-controlled phase 3 trial. Lancet 2016; 388:2128–2141.

76. Castro M, Corren J, Pavord ID, et al. Dupilumab efficacy and safety in moderate-to-severe uncontrolled asthma. N Engl J Med 2018; 378:2486–2496.

77. Papaioannou AI, Diamant Z, Bakakos P, Loukides S. Towards precision medicine in severe asthma: Treatment algorithms based on treatable traits. Respir Med 2018 Sep;142:15–22. doi: 10.1016/j.rmed.2018.07.006. Epub 2018 Jul 17.

78. Benayoun L, Druilhe A, Dombret MC, et al. Airway structural alterations selectively associated with severe asthma. Am J Respir Crit Care Med 2003;167:1360–1368.

79. El-Shazly A, Berger P, Girodet PO, et al. Fraktalkine produced by airway smooth muscle cells contributes to mast cell recruitment in asthma. J Immunol 2006;176:1860–1868.

80. Ghaffar O, Hamid Q, Renzi PM, et al. Constitutive and cytokine-stimulated expression of eotaxin by human airway smooth muscle cells. Am J Respir Crit Care Med 1999; 159: 1933–1942.

81. Berkman N, Krishnan VL, Gilbey T, et al. Expression of RANTES mRNA and protein in airways of patients with mild asthma. Am J Respir Crit Care Med 1996;154:1804–1811.

82. Bronchial thermoplasty for severe asthma Interventional procedures guidance Published: 19 December 2018 www.nice.org.uk/guidance/ipg635

30 Biologics for Asthma in Adolescents and Young Adults

Arjun Padmanabhan and Soofia Mohammed

CONTENTS

INTRODUCTION

Asthma is a heterogeneous disease with multiple phenotypes caused by a variety of endotypes. Most of the patients with asthma achieve good disease control with standard controller therapy. Approximately 5% have severe asthma that remains inadequately controlled despite adherence to standard treatment[1]. As compared to patients with well-controlled disease, patients with severe asthma have disproportionally high morbidity and healthcare utilization. Currently, these patients are routinely considered as candidates for biologic therapies.

It is important to distinguish two specific endotypes, **T2 high and T2 low,** when considering biologic therapy. These endotypes are defined based on their level of expression of cytokines such as IL-4, IL-5, and IL-13 that may be secreted by the classic T-helper cell type 2 (Th2) cells, or the innate lymphoid cells–type 2 (ILC-2). T2 inflammation occurs in around 50% of patients with severe asthma[2].

Biologic therapies target inflammatory modulators that have been identified to play a key role in the pathogenesis of asthma predominantly in the T2-high subset of patients (Figure 30.1). Approval of some of these biologicals in adolescents and young adults offer a new, very promising and more personalized therapy option.

BIOLOGICS USED IN THE TREATMENT OF ASTHMA (TABLE 30.1)

Table 30.1: Summary of the Biologics Currently Approved for the Treatment of Moderate to Severe Persistent Asthma

Drug	Mechanism of Action
Omalizumab	Anti-IgE: Prevents IgE from binding to its receptors n mast cells and basophils
Mepolizumab	Anti-IL-5: Binds to IL-5 ligand. Prevents IL-5 from biding to its ligand
Roslizumab	Anti-IL-5: Binds to IL-5 ligand. Prevents IL-5 from binding to its ligand
Benralizumab	Anti-IL-5: Binds to IL-5 receptor. Causes apoptosis of eosinophils and basophils
Dupilumab	Anti-IL-4R: Binds to IL-4 receptor. Blocks signaling of IL-4 and IL-13

DOI: 10.1201/9781003125785-30

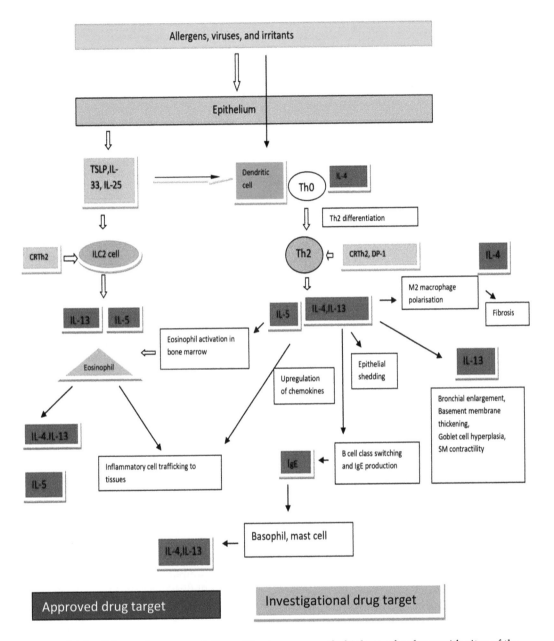

Figure 30.1 Schematic representation of the immune pathobiology of asthma with sites of the targeted treatment marked.

ANTI-IgE: OMALIZUMAB

Omalizumab is a humanized anti-IgE monoclonal antibody (mAb). It was the first biologic approved for the treatment of severe persistent allergic asthma in adults and adolescents.

Mechanism of Action

IgE is essential in the inflammatory pathway of allergic asthma that is found in approximately 70% of patients with asthma[3,4]. Omalizumab

prevents IgE from binding to its high affinity receptor (FcεR1) found on mast cells and basophils, which reduces the release of pro-inflammatory mediators and blunts the allergic response[5,6]. It also downregulates the expression of the IgE receptor on mast cells, further reducing inflammation.

Efficacy (Table 30.2)

Omalizumab has been used successfully for the treatment of allergic asthma for more than

Table 30.2: Efficacy of the Biologics That Are U.S. Food and Drug Administration Approved for the Treatment of Moderate to Severe Persistent Asthma with T2–High Phenotype

Therapy	Asthma Exacerbation	Lung Function	Corticosteroid Weaning	Special Considerations
Omalizumab	Reduces by 25%	Minimal or equivocal improvement	Decreases use of ICS, but no data that it helps with OCS weaning	Biologic approved for allergic asthma
Mepolizumab	Reduces by 50%	Inconsistent effect	Decreases total use of OCS and has been shown to facilitate complete weaning from chronic OCS	Standard sc. dosing has not been shown to decrease sputum eosinophilia; approved at higher dosing for EGPA
Reslizumab	Reduces by about 50–60%	Improved	Has not been specifically evaluated for this indication	Only weight-based dosing iv. biologic approved for asthma
Benralizumab	Reduces by 25–60%	Improved	Decreases total use of OCS and has been shown to facilitate complete weaning from chronic OCS	Only sc. biologic that offers every 8-wk dosing
Dupilumab	Reduces by 50–70%	Improved	Decreases total use of OCS and has been shown to facilitate complete weaning from chronic OCS	Only biologic that can be self-administered sc. showed benefit with FeNO >25 ppb regardless of eosinophil count

15 years. Clinical trials of asthmatic children and adolescents treated with omalizumab as an add-on therapy demonstrated a significantly reduced number of exacerbations[78] and a reduced rate of hospitalization. Furthermore, a reduction of respiratory symptoms and improvement in asthma control have been shown. The PROSE study demonstrated a decreased susceptibility to infection with rhinovirus in asthmatic children treated with omalizumab, resulting in a reduction of viral asthma exacerbations[9,10]. In another study, omalizumab decreased the expression of FcεR1 on basophils in patients with nonatopic asthma, suggesting a possible role of omalizumab in a nonallergic phenotype[11]. There have been no clear data that support a reduction in OCS in patients treated with omalizumab.

Indications, Administration, and Safety

Omalizumab is currently approved for ages ≥6 years, given subcutaneously every 2–4 weeks, with dose and frequency based on body weight and pretreatment IgE level. Self-administration may be an option[2].

Eligibility criteria: These vary between payers but usually include:

- Sensitization to inhaled allergen(s) on skin prick testing or specific IgE.

- Total serum IgE and body weight within local dosing range.

- More than a specified number of exacerbations within the last year.

Monitoring of IgE levels during treatment is not recommended. A trial of 3–6 months should be given to assess for clinical response, and treatment should be continued indefinitely if a patient has a favourable response as supported by the XPORT (Xolair Persistency of Response after Long-Term Therapy) trial[12].

Omalizumab is generally well tolerated with a risk of anaphylaxis of 0.1–0.2%. The most commonly reported adverse reactions were headaches and injection site reactions, including injection site pain, swelling, erythema, and pruritus during clinical trials in adult and adolescent patients ≥12 years. Patients should be observed for 2 hours after the first 3 injections and then 30 minutes with subsequent injections. Also, they should be monitored for helminthic infections.

Potential predictors of good asthma response[2]: Baseline IgE levels don't predict likelihood of response. A greater reduction in exacerbation is reported in randomized controlled trials, if blood eosinophils ≥260/μl,

FeNO ≥20 ppb, it is a case of childhood onset asthma, and there is a clinical history suggesting allergen driven symptoms.

ANTI-IL-5

Anti-IL-5 drugs reduce eosinophilic airway inflammation because IL-5 is the primary cytokine involved in the recruitment, activation, and survival of eosinophils[13]. Mepolizumab and reslizumab bind and inhibit IL-5, thus preventing IL-5 from binding to its receptor on eosinophils. Benralizumab binds the α-subunit of the IL-5 receptor on eosinophils and basophils, thereby preventing IL-5 binding and the subsequent recruitment and activation of eosinophils. Also afucosylation of the benralizumab enhances its ability to engage with FcγRIIIa on natural killer cells and results in antibody-directed cell-mediated cytotoxicity and eosinophil apoptosis followed by phagocytosis by macrophages[14].

Eligibility criteria: These vary between the products and patients but usually include:

1. More than a specified number of severe exacerbations in the last year and

2. Blood eosinophils above specified level (eg ≥300/μl). In some cases there is a different cut off point for patients who take OCS.

MEPOLIZUMAB

Efficacy (Table 30.2)

Mepolizumab has been studied in patients with uncontrolled eosinophilic asthma who have increased sputum (>3%) or AEC (≥150 or ≥300 cells/ml). The MENSA trial demonstrated that mepolizumab can significantly reduce the risk for asthma exacerbations and improve asthma control in adolescents (>12 years) and adults with severe eosinophilic asthma[15]. In the SIRIUS trial, treatment with mepolizumab led to a reduction in OCS dosage by 50% in patients with eosinophilic asthma on chronic OCS[16].

Indications, Administration, and Safety

Mepolizumab is currently approved for patients ≥6 years of age with severe asthma with an eosinophilic phenotype. It is administered subcutaneously every 4 weeks at 100 mg per dose in patients ≥12 years. For ages ≥6 years, the dose is 40 mg by SC injection every 4 weeks[2].

A clinical response should be seen within 4 months, and treatment with mepolizumab should be continued indefinitely if a clinical response is achieved.

The most frequently reported adverse reactions were headache, injection site reactions, back pain, and fatigue. In patients treated with mepolizumab, herpes zoster virus infections have been detected[17]. This led to the recommendation to vaccinate against varicella before the initiation of mepolizumab treatment.

Mepolizumab is also approved for the treatment of eosinophilic granulomatosis with polyangiitis (Churg–Strauss syndrome) at a higher dose of 300 mg every 4 weeks.

RESLIZUMAB

Efficacy (Table 30.2)

In studies including adolescents ≥12 years and adults with uncontrolled asthma and an eosinophil count of ≥400 μg, a reduction of the exacerbation rate, improvement in lung function, and quality of life were reported[17-19].

Indications, Administration, and Safety

Reslizumab is approved as add-on treatment for patients aged 18 years or older with severe eosinophilic asthma (AEC>400 cells/ml). Reslizumab is the only biologic delivered intravenously using weight-based dosing at 3 mg/kg dose every 4 weeks.

Reslizumab is well tolerated, with adverse events similar to the placebo group. The most common adverse effects are worsening asthma symptoms, upper respiratory tract infections, and nasopharyngitis[18]. However, 3 cases of anaphylaxis occurred during RCTs, and thus reslizumab carries an FDA black box warning.

BENRALIZUMAB

Efficacy (Table 30.2)

Benralizumab has been shown to reduce asthma exacerbation rates and improve lung function in patients with uncontrolled eosinophilic asthma. In the ZONDA trial, benralizumab was shown to significantly reduce OCS use by 75% inpatients on long-term OCS with AEC≥150 cells/ml, while reducing annualized asthma exacerbations by 70%[20]. Benralizumab appears to be equally effective independent of atopy[21].

Indications, Administration, and Safety

Benralizumab is approved for patients ≥12 years with uncontrolled eosinophilic asthma (AEC ≥300 cells/ml)[22,23]. It is administered at a dose of 30 mg subcutaneously every 4 weeks for the first 3 doses as an induction phase (to reduce tissue eosinophilia), followed by every 8 weeks thereafter for maintenance. A trial of 4 months should be given to assess for response. Benralizumab is generally well tolerated but has led to hypersensitivity reactions, including anaphylaxis, angioedema, and urticaria.

Potential predictors of good asthma response[2]:

1. Higher blood eosinophils (strongly predictive)

2. Higher number of severe exacerbations in previous year (strongly predictive)

3. Adult onset asthma

4. Nasal polyposis

5. Maintenance OCS at baseline

ANTI–IL-4/IL-13

Dupilumab
Mechanism of Action

IL-4 and IL-13 are the key cytokines that promote production of IgE and recruitment of inflammatory cells. These cytokines also stimulate goblet cell hyperplasia and modulate airway hyper responsiveness and airway remodelling. Dupilumab is a mAb that targets the IL-4α receptor and blocks signaling of both IL-4 and IL-13.

Efficacy

It has been shown to reduce asthma exacerbations, rapidly improve lung function, and decrease OCS use, while decreasing levels of T2 inflammation in moderate to severe asthma. In the Liberty Asthma QUEST Study[24,] patients who received dupilumab had a greater reduction in symptom scores and improvement in mean FEV$_1$. The Liberty Asthma VENTURE study demonstrated the effectiveness of dupilumab in reducing OCS use in 210 patients with CS-dependent severeasthma. Dupilumab has improved outcomes in patients with symptomatic chronic rhinosinusitis and nasal polyposis and should be considered in patients asthma with this comorbidity[25].

Indications, Administration, and Safety

Dupilumab is currently approved for patients ≥12 years, 200 mg or 300 mg SC injection every 2 weeks for severe eosinophilic/T2 asthma; 300 mg SC injection every 2 weeks for OCS dependant severe asthma or if there is concomitant moderate/severe atopic dermatitis. Self-administration may be an option.

Eligibility criteria: These vary between payers but usually include:

1. More than a specified number of severe exacerbations in the last year, and

2. Type 2 biomarkers above a specified level (e.g: blood eosinophils ≥300/µl or FeNO ≥25 ppb); OR

3. Requirement for maintenence OCS.

As the actions of IL-4 and IL-13 are more pleiotropic, the beneficial effects of anti–IL-4/13 treatment would be expected in a broader population of patients and not necessarily only in those with significant airway eosinophilia[26]. Dupilumab has a favourable safety profile, with common side effects, including injection site reaction and transient blood eosinophilia.

Potential predictors of good asthma response:

1. Higher blood eosinophils (strongly predictive)

2. Higher FeNO

It is suggested to have an initial trial of at least 4 months to know the response to treatment.

Since eosinophils are involved in the immune response to some helminthic infections, caution is advised in patients with a high risk of parasitic infections. It is recommended to sufficiently treat a helminthic infection before initiating a therapy with biologicals. If helminthiasis occurs during antibody therapy and does not sufficiently respond to antihelminthic therapy, discontinuation of antibody treatment is recommended[16].

REVIEW RESPONSE TO AN INITIAL TRIAL OF ADD-ON TYPE 2 TARGETED THERAPY

At present, there are no well-defined criteria for a good response, but frequency of exacerbations, symptom control, lung function, side effects, treatment intensity including OCS dose, and patient satisfaction need to be considered. If the clinical response is unclear, consider extending the trial for 6–12 months. If there is no response, biologic therapy should be stopped and switching to another biologic in light of availability and patient eligibility should be considered.

FUTURE BIOLOGICS

Researchers are studying various upstream targets of T2 inflammation, including IL-25, IL-33, and TSLP. Anti-IL-33 is currently, on phase 1 trial [AMG 282 (RG 6149)] and phase 2 trial (ANB020) in patients affected by asthma[27].

ANTI-THYMIC STROMAL LYMPHOPOIETIN (TSLP)

Tezepelumab, a mAb against TSLP, has shown to reduc asthma exacerbations unrelated to baseline AEC, and decreased markers of T2 inflammation, IgE and FeNO[28]. Studies evaluating use of tezepelumab in adolescents are ongoing[29].

Other molecules undergoing clinical trials are Prostaglandin D2 antagonist (asapiprant), CRTh2 antagonists (Timapiprant, fevipiprant), Anti GATA3 DNAzyme, and IL-13R antagonist[30].

Alternative modes of delivery of biologic therapies besides subcutaneous or intravenous are being evaluated. To increase drug concentration in the terminal bronchioles while decreasing systemic toxicity, researchers are studying nebulized biologic therapy.

CONCLUSION

Biologics ensure a precise way of treating the particular phenotypes and also help reduce the unwanted adverse effects of the non-phenotypic add-on drugs, which we currently use to treat difficult to control and severe asthma. In those patients who truly have severe asthma and whose airway obstruction and asthma severity are predominantly mediated by eosinophils, anti–IL-5 mAbs are the therapy of choice. In patients whose airway obstruction and severity may be driven by factors such as mucus production, eosinophils, and smooth muscle contraction and remodelling, an anti–IL-4R mAb may be the drug of choice. Finally, patients with asthma that is clearly driven by a clinical history of allergies (rather than just an elevated IgE level) are candidates for anti-IgE therapy; however, anti–IL-5 mAbs may also be effective in some of these patients. In patients who require maintenance OCS, there is insufficient evidence to recommend anti-IgE therapy[30]. There is a need to study and develop new biologics that will improve outcomes in patients with non-eosinophilic or T2-low disease.

REFERENCES

1. Moore WC, Bleecker ER, Curran-Everett D, Erzurum SC, Ameredes BT, Bacharier L, et al.; National Heart, Lung, Blood Institute's SevereAsthma Research Program. Characterization of the severe asthma phenotype by the National Heart, Lung, and Blood Institute's Severe Asthma Research Program. J Allergy Clin Immunol 2007; 119:405–413.

2. Global Initiative for Asthma. Global Strategy for Asthma Management and Prevention, 2020.

3. Humbert M, Busse W, Hanania NA, Lowe PJ, Canvin J, Erpenbeck VJ, et al. Omalizumab in asthma: an update on recent developments. J Allergy Clin Immunol Pract 2014; 2:525–536.e1.

4. Novak N, Bieber T. Allergic and nonallergic forms of atopic diseases. J Allergy Clin Immunol 2003; 112:252–262.

5. Manka LA, Wechsler ME. Selecting the right biologic for your patients with severe asthma. Ann Allergy Asthma Immunol 2018; 121:406–413.

6. McCracken JL, Tripple JW, Calhoun WJ. Biologic therapy in the management of asthma. Curr Opin Allergy Clin Immunol 2016; 16:375–382.

7. Berger W, Gupta N, McAlary M, Fowler-Taylor A. Evaluation of long-term safety of the anti-IgE antibody, omalizumab, in children with allergic asthma. Ann Allergy Asthma Immunol 2003; 91:182–188. https://doi.org/10.1016/S1081-1206(10)62175-8

8. Busse WW, Morgan WJ, Gergen PJ, Mitchell HE, Gern JE et al. Randomized trial of omalizumab (anti-IgE) for asthma in inner city children. N Engl J Med 2011; 364:1005–1015. https://doi.org/10.1056/NEJMoa1009705

9. Esquivel A, Busse WW, Calatroni A, Togias AG, Grindle KG et al. Effects of omalizumab on rhinovirus infections, illnesses, and exacerbations of asthma. Am J Respir Crit Care Med 2017; 196:985–992. https://doi.org/10.1164/rccm.201701-0120OC

10. Teach SJ, Gill MA, Togias A, Sorkness CA et al. Preseasonal treatment with either omalizumab or an inhaled corticosteroid boost to prevent fall asthma exacerbations. J Allergy Clin Immunol 2015; 136:1476–1485. https://doi.org/10.1016/j.jaci.2015.09.008

11. Garcia G, Magnan A, Chiron R, Contin-Bordes C, Berger P, Taillé C, et al. A proof-of-concept, randomized, controlled trial of omalizumab in patients with severe, difficult-to-control, nonatopic asthma. Chest 2013; 144:411–419.

12. Ledford D, Busse W, Trzaskoma B, Omachi TA, Rosén K, Chipps BE, et al. A randomized multicenter study evaluating Xolair persistence of response after long-term therapy. J Allergy Clin Immunol 2017; 140:162–169.e2.

13. Walsh GM. An update on biologic-based therapy in asthma. Immunotherapy 2013; 5:1255–1264.

14. Pelaia C, Calabrese C, Vatrella A, Busceti MT et al. Benralizumab: from the basic mechanism of action to thepotential use in the biological therapy of severe eosinophilicasthma. BioMed Res Int 2018; 2018:4839230

15. Ortega HG, Yancey SW, Mayer B, Gunsoy NB et al. Severe eosinophilic asthma treated with mepolizumab stratified by baseline eosinophilthresholds: a secondary analysis of the DREAM and MENSA studies. Lancet Respir Med 2016; 4:549–556. https://doi.org/10.1016/S2213-2600(16)30031-5

16. Deeks ED. Mepolizumab: A review in eosinophilic asthma. BioDrugs 2016; 30:361–370. https://doi.org/10.1007/s40259-016-0182-5

17. Corren J, Weinstein S, Janka L, Zangrilli J, Garin M. Phase 3 study of reslizumab in patients with poorly controlled asthma: effects across a broad range of eosinophil counts. Chest 2016; 150:799–810. https://doi.org/10.1016/j.chest.2016.03.018

18. Castro M, Zangrilli J, Wechsler ME, Bateman ED, Brusselle GG et al. Reslizumab for inadequately controlled asthma with elevated bloodeosinophil counts: Results from two multicentre, parallel, double-blind, randomised, placebo controlled, phase 3 trials. Lancet Respir Med 2015; 3:355–366. https://doi.org/10.1016/S2213-2600(15)00042-9

19. Bjermer L, Lemiere C, Maspero J, Weiss S, Zangrilli J, Germinaro M. Reslizumab for inadequately controlled asthma with elevated blood eosinophil levels: A randomized phase 3 study. Chest 2016; 150:789–798. https://doi.org/10.1016/j.chest.2016.03.032

20. Nair P, Wenzel S, Rabe KF, Bourdin A, Lugogo NL, Kuna P, et al. ZONDA Trial Investigators. Oral glucocorticoid-sparing effect of benralizumab in severe asthma. N Engl J Med 2017; 376:2448–2458.

21. Chipps BE, Newbold P, Hirsch I, Trudo F, Goldman M. Benralizumabefficacy by atopy status and serum immunoglobulin E for patientswith severe, uncontrolled asthma. Ann Allergy Asthma Immunol 2018; 120:504–511.e4.

22. Farne HA, Wilson A, Powell C, Bax L, Milan SJ. Anti-IL5 therapies forasthma. Cochrane Database Syst Rev 2017; 9:CD010834.

23. FitzGerald JM, Bleecker ER, Nair P, Korn S, Ohta K, Lommatzsch M, et al. CALIMA Study Investigators. Benralizumab, an antiinterleukin-5 receptor a monoclonal antibody, as add-on treatment for patients with severe, uncontrolled, eosinophilic asthma (CALIMA): A randomised, double-blind, placebo-controlled phase 3 trial. Lancet 2016; 388:2128–2141.

24. Castro M, Corren J, Pavord ID, et al. Dupilumab efficacy and safety in moderate-to-severe uncontrolled asthma. N Engl J Med. 2018; 378.

25. Bachert C, Mannent L, Naclerio RM, Mullol J, Ferguson BJ, Gevaert P, et al. Effect of subcutaneous dupilumab on nasal polyp burden in patients with chronic sinusitis and nasal polyposis: a randomized clinical trial. JAMA 2016; 315:469–479.

26. Robinson D, Humbert M, Buhl R, Cruz AA, Inoue H, Korom S, et al. Revisiting Type 2-high and Type 2-low airway inflammation in asthma: current knowledge and therapeutic implications. ClinExpAllergy 2017; 47:161–175.

27. Lawrence MG, Steinke JW, Borish L. Cytokine-targeting biologics for allergic diseases. Ann Allergy Asthma Immunol 2018; 120:376–81. https://doi.org/10.1016/j.anai.2018.01.009

28. Corren J, Parnes JR, Wang L, Mo M, Roseti SL, Griffiths JM, et al. Tezepelumab in adults with uncontrolled asthma. N Engl J Med 2017; 377:936–946.

29. Menzies-Gow A, Colice G, Griffiths, JM, Almqvist G, Ponnarambil S, Kaur P, et al. NAVIGATOR: a phase 3 multicentre, randomized, double-blind, placebo-controlled, parallel-group trial to evaluate the efficacy and safety of tezepelumab in adults and adolescents with severe, uncontrolled asthma. Respir Res 2020; 21:1.

30. McGregor MC, Krings JG, Nair P, Castro M. Role of biologics in asthma. Am J Respir Crit Care Med 2019;199(4):433–45. https://doi.org/10.1164/rccm.201810-1944

31 Allergen Immunotherapy

Jyothi Edakalavan and Ravindran Chetambath

CONTENTS

INTRODUCTION

Allergic diseases are common clinical manifestations affecting all age groups. This group of diseases includes atopic dermatitis, urticaria, asthma, allergic rhinitis, allergic rhino-conjunctivitis, food allergy and venom allergy. The symptoms usually start in early childhood and continue throughout life. Allergen avoidance and pharmacotherapy with antihistamines and corticosteroids remain the mainstay of treatment. But there are limitations for this approach, as symptoms often recur once treatment is stopped.

Allergen immunotherapy (AIT) is an immunomodulatory method for the treatment of IgE mediated allergic diseases, to decrease sensitivity to allergens and thus control the symptoms. Allergen immunotherapy was first described for the treatment of hay fever in 1911 by Leonhard Noon and John Freeman[1]. This treatment is known by various names such as allergen-specific immunotherapy (SIT), desensitization, hypo-sensitization or allergy vaccination. It is a disease modifying intervention. The treatment consists of administering a sequentially increasing dose of the offending antigen to shift the immunological response from TH2 to TH1[2].

This form of treatment is currently used to treat allergic rhinitis, rhino-conjunctivitis, asthma, food allergy and venom hypersensitivity. The commonly preferred route of administering an antigen for immunotherapy is subcutaneous and sublingual. The success of AIT depends on proper selection of patients, quality of antigen used, adequate dose and duration and, above all, compliance of the patient. The initiation of AIT must always be done after discussing with the patient/family the benefits, harm, disadvantages, cost and route of delivery.

INDICATIONS FOR AIT

AIT is currently used in conditions such as:

- Allergic rhinitis, conjunctivitis and asthma due to aeroallergens sensitivity

- Food allergy

- Venom hypersensitivity due to bee sting and wasp bite

- Atopic dermatitis sensitive to aeroallergens

DIAGNOSTIC TESTS FOR ALLERGENS

Identification of specific allergens is the most important step in allergen immunotherapy of

DOI: 10.1201/9781003125785-31

patients with IgE mediated allergic diseases. A history and physical examination are the primary modalities for diagnosing allergic diseases, as well as identifying possible allergens for the symptoms. Both in vitro and in vivo tests have been recommended for the identification of specific allergens.

In vivo tests available for identifying the offending allergen are the **skin prick test**, **intradermal test** and **mucosal challenge test**. Mucosal challenge tests are nasal or bronchial challenge tests and food challenge tests. These are seldom done in routine clinical practice.

In vitro tests are used to quantify level of serum IgE and allergen-specific IgE. The available tests are radio immune-sorbent test (RAST) and enzyme linked immune-sorbent assay (ELISA).

SKIN TESTS

Skin tests are convenient, simple, reproducible, easy and rapid to perform and have high sensitivity. Two methods are used.

- **Skin Prick Test (SPT)**: It is the gold standard diagnostic method to detect the allergen and is reproducible and minimally invasive. It has high specificity and lower systemic effects compared to the intradermal test[3].

- **Intradermal Test**: It is more sensitive than SPT, but less specific and has more systemic effects and a higher false positive rate. The intradermal test may be used when the SPT is negative and there is strong history of exposure and symptoms.

The preparation of a high-quality allergen extract is essential for skin tests. In addition to allergen extracts, there should be a positive control (histamine) and negative control (buffered saline). Positive controls are used to ensure that the patient is suitable for an allergy test and is not taking any medication that may suppress the skin tests. Similarly, the diluent used to prepare the allergen extract is used as a negative control. Negative control is used to avoid false positive skin tests due to dermographism or traumatic reactivity induced by the skin test device.

Patients having any chronic skin disease like dermographism, eczema and severe dermatitis are not suitable for skin testing. The antigens are administered on the volar aspect of arm or over the back of the patient. The distance between the 2 tests should be 5 cm for intradermal test and 3 cm for SPT. Tests should be done 5 cm away from the wrist and 3 cm away from the antecubital fossae[4]. The wheal diameter is measured 15–20 minutes later and is expressed in millimetres. A skin reaction ≥3 mm than that produced by the negative control is considered as positive.[5]

When testing in a patient with severe systemic allergic reactions, skin test should first be done with diluted allergens. It should ideally be done 4–6 weeks following an allergic reaction.[4]

Certain drugs can suppress skin reactivity, leading to false negative skin tests. These include antihistamines, glucocorticoids and omalizumab and antidepressants like imipramine, amitriptyline and doxepin[6]. Topical steroids at the test site and systemic steroids should be stopped for at least 1 week[7]. Topical antihistamine, nasal and inhaled steroid, leukotriene receptor antagonists, beta-2 agonists or theophylline do not have any suppressant effect. Treatment with long-term steroids at a dose of less than 10 mg daily does not interfere with skin allergy testing.

MUCOSAL CHALLENGE TEST

Both bronchial and nasal provocation test are of limited clinical value. These tests are mainly used for research purposes.

IN VITRO TESTS

The commonly done in vitro tests for diagnosing allergic diseases are estimation of total IgE and allergen-specific IgE. The measurement of allergen-specific IgE gives information about patients' sensitivity to various aeroallergens. In vitro tests are considered as a back up to skin tests and should only be done when skin tests cannot be done.

ALLERGEN PREPARATIONS

Aqueous extract of the allergenic material obtained from natural sources is routinely used as an allergen extract for immunotherapy. The composition and biologic properties depend on the quality of source material, extraction and preparation. The manufacturing process includes crushing raw material, extracting allergenic protein by adding solvents that release them from the raw material into the liquid solvent. This is followed by purification of the allergen extract. In addition to the aqueous preparations, new hypoallergenic depot preparations are available. Here, the allergen is physically adsorbed to a carrier like aluminium hydroxide, tyrosine or calcium phosphate[8]. The advantage of hypoallergenic preparation is that it causes less systemic reactions and less frequent dosing.

The common aeroallergens incorporated in AIT are pollens, fungi, house dust mite, animal dander and insects. Th selection, total number and proportion of allergens that are included in a therapeutic mixture are critical aspects of success of allergen immunotherapy. In choosing the allergens for immunotherapy, familiarity with local and regional aerobiology and indoor and outdoor allergens is needed. Special attention should be given to potential allergens in the patient's own environment. If a greater number of allergens are incorporated in a single therapeutic mixture, it can lead to reduced concentrations of individual allergens and hence reduce the efficacy. Another problem with combining multiple allergens is that it creates a chance for potential interactive effects, thus changing their allergenic and immunogenic properties. Some fungi and whole-body insect extracts contain proteolytic enzymes, and this can reduce the efficacy of grass pollens allergens. So, it is advisable that fungal and insect allergen extracts be separated from pollen allergen[9].

TYPES OF ALLERGEN IMMUNOTHERAPY

Allergen immunotherapy typically involves administration of gradually increasing dose of relevant allergens until a dose is reached that is effective in inducing immunological tolerance to the allergen. The usual routes for providing allergen immunotherapy are:

- Subcutaneous
- Sublingual
- Oral
- Bronchial
- Nasal
- Epicutaneous

Before starting immunotherapy, patients should understand its benefits and risks. Counselling should also include the expected onset of efficacy, duration of treatment and risk of systemic reactions, including anaphylaxis and importance of adhering to the immunotherapy schedule. The protocol for immunotherapy can be conventional, or consist of accelerated protocols like rush, ultra-rush and cluster immunotherapy. In conventional immunotherapy the build-up phase will last up to 5–8 months. When rapid desensitization is needed, rush, ultra-rush or cluster immunotherapy is practised. The use of accelerated protocols also provides the advantage of reduced hospital visit and increased compliance. The disadvantage of accelerated protocols includes a higher risk of systemic reactions.

SUBCUTANEOUS IMMUNOTHERAPY

This is the most preferred route for administering allergen immunotherapy. Aqueous extracts of allergenic material are used for providing subcutaneous immunotherapy. Typically, AIT consists of two phases:

- **Build-up phase:** This is also known as the up-dosing phase and lasts for 5–8 months: AIT is started with 1:5000 w/v diluted antigen and injections are given twice weekly initially, and the dose is increased by 0.1 ml every visit. The concentration of the antigen is increased gradually from 1:5000 to 1: 500 till it reach a concentration of 1:50. The frequency of injections is gradually decreased to once a week and then once in 2 weeks. If there is high local reaction after the first injection, then the schedule is restarted with 1: 50000 dilutions. Injection should be postponed in the presence of respiratory infection, intercurrent illness or asthma exacerbation. The first injection should always be given from the hospital having the facility to manage anaphylaxis.

- **Maintenance phase:** In this phase the highest concentration of 1:50 is used Maintenance injection is given at a frequency of once a month. Dosage reduction should be done in case of previous systemic or large local reaction, and if there is an extended break after the last injection. Usually, the maintenance phase is continued up to 3–5 years.

ACCELERATED SCHEDULES

Apart from conventional immunotherapy, there are accelerated schedules to build up tolerance rapidly in certain situations. These involve administration of several injections at increasing doses on a single visit. The advantage of these types of schedules is that patients develop symptomatic improvement earlier. But may also be associated with increased risk of systemic reactions. So, premedication with oral steroid and antihistamines is advisable.

- **Cluster immunotherapy:** In cluster immunotherapy 2 or 3 injections at increasing doses are given sequentially in a single day at 30 minute- to 2 hour-intervals. These are given in non-consecutive days[10]. Usually, the maintenance dose is reached in 2 months.

■ **Rush immunotherapy**: This schedule involves administering incremental doses of the allergen at intervals varying between 15–60 minutes over 1–3 days until the target maintenance dose is achieved[11].

Pre-seasonal immunotherapy preparations that are administered on an annual basis are also available for seasonal allergic rhino-conjunctivitis and asthma.

CONTRAINDICATIONS FOR AIT
I. Absolute Contraindications

- Co-existent uncontrolled asthma (FEV_1 < 70% with regular treatment)
- Malignancy
- Children below the age of 2 years
- Pregnancy- AIT must not be started during pregnancy, but if already on maintenance injection, it may be continued
- AIDS (CD4 <200 cells)

II. Relative Contraindications

- Beta-blocker use
- Cardiovascular diseases
- HIV (CD4 > 200 cells)
- Children between 2–5 years
- Psychiatric illness
- Chronic infections
- Autoimmune diseases.
- Immunodeficiencies or use of immunosuppressives

SAFETY OF ALLERGEN IMMUNOTHERAPY

A limitation of subcutaneous immunotherapy is the risk of serious adverse events including systemic allergic reactions, occasional anaphylaxis and death. Risk factors for systemic reactions are a history of asthma, extreme high sensitivity and a history of previous systemic reactions.

SUBLINGUAL IMMUNOTHERAPY (SLIT)

Even though subcutaneous immunotherapy is the accepted form of AIT, its greatest disadvantage is that the patient must visit a health care facility for regular injections for a period of 3–5 years. Sublingual immunotherapy is an alternative way of AIT without injections. This route of immunotherapy is gaining increasing popularity. The allergens are absorbed through the rich vascular lymphoid network of oral mucosa. The allergen extract for sublingual immunotherapy contains a higher concentration of antigen extract. It is available in the form of drops, mono dose vials and tablets. It can be self-administered by patients or caregivers and carries a lower risk of anaphylaxis compared to subcutaneous immunotherapy[12].

SLIT doses are available in the form of rapidly dissolving tablets that is held under the tongue until it is completely dissolved. It is also available in the form of aqueous or glycerinated liquid allergen extracts. The drops are held under the tongue for a specified period and then swallowed. As an alternative, oral drops can be held in the mouth for a specified period and then spit out.

FOOD ALLERGY

For the past several years food allergy has been on the rise, seriously affecting the quality of life of those involved. It affects up to 8% children and 5% of adults in westernised societies[13]. The most common food allergens are milk, egg, peanuts, soy and other seeds, shellfish and fish. It is found that milk, egg, soy and wheat related allergic reactions can be outgrown, but peanut, other nuts, fish and shellfish related allergy is usually persistent.

The main treatment for food allergy is strict avoidance of the offending food and the use of rescue medications in the event of an allergic reaction. It has been found that early introduction of food allergens in high risk infants can prevent the development of food allergy[14,15]. But recently, AIT has been studied extensively for patients with evidence of an IgE-mediated food allergy and in whom avoidance measures are ineffective or undesirable. Immunotherapy for food allergy was first introduced by AT Schofield for hens' egg allergy in 1908[16]. The ultimate goal of food allergen immunotherapy is to achieve post discontinuation effectiveness so that the patient can eat the trigger food without any symptoms and improve the quality of life.

Prior to initiating AIT, confirming the diagnosis of IgE-mediated food allergy is mandatory. This requires a recent, clear clinical history of an acute reaction(s) after consumption of the triggering food. The presence of IgE to the triggering food should be established with a skin prick test and/or serum-specific IgE. When the diagnosis is unclear, an oral food challenge is considered.

Food allergen immunotherapy has been tried with various delivery methods, including subcutaneous, oral, sublingual and epicutaneous. But due to concern of increased side effects and safety of treatment, the subcutaneous route has mostly been abandoned. The most frequent route of administration of AIT for food allergy is the oral route[17]. The allergen is either immediately swallowed (oral immunotherapy) or held under the tongue for a specified period (sublingual immunotherapy). The other route of AIT for food allergy is epicutaneous, where a patch is applied to the forearm[18]. It is a new method of allergen administration that has a high rate of adherence and safety.

Most of the trials for food allergy immunotherapy have focused on hens' egg, cow's milk and peanut, the most common allergens. Food allergen immunotherapy aims at increasing the threshold of reactivity to the food allergen by administering a gradually increasing dose (oral, sublingual) or fixed dose (epicutaneous) of the allergen on a daily basis. To maintain desensitization to the food allergen, a daily maintenance dose of immunotherapy is needed.

IMMUNOTHERAPY SCHEDULE

Like aeroallergens, an immunotherapy schedule consists of an initial up-dosing phase and a maintenance phase. The oral dose of the allergen is gradually increased as per protocol, until a maintenance dose is reached. In the epicutaneous route, the medicinal patch contains a fixed dose of the allergen, but the dose of allergen exposure is increased by extending the duration of patch application. During the maintenance phase the patch is applied for up to 24 hours.

The daily dose of food allergen protein by various routes of AIT varies widely. The daily dose for oral allergen immunotherapy in various studies is between 300 and 4000 mg. For sublingual immunotherapy it varies between 2–7 mg and by epicutaneous route it is 100–500 µg[19]. Successfully desensitized individuals will likely be protected from accidental ingestion of the allergens and resultant life-threatening reactions. It may also be possible to tolerate the food allergen after years of desensitization.

Local side effects are common with food allergen immunotherapy. Oropharyngeal itching, perioral rash and abdominal pain are the most common symptoms reported with oral immunotherapy[20]. The local side effects of sublingual immunotherapy are limited to oral and pharyngeal symptoms. Mild local reaction at the patch site has been reported in epicutaneous immunotherapy[21]. Systemic side effects—including anaphylaxis—are less common with oral immunotherapy, rare with sublingual immunotherapy and have not been reported with epicutaneous immunotherapy.

Food allergen immunotherapy protocols also vary widely in different studies. Certain factors increase the risk of allergic reactions to food immunotherapy. These include uncontrolled asthma, allergic rhinitis, eczema and urticaria. Poor compliance to medication and concomitant viral infections are also unfavourable factors. If the patient is having recurrent symptoms while on immunotherapy during the build up phase, then the dose escalation maybe stopped, or the doses may be reduced. If there are severe systemic reactions, an individualized dosing schedule with longer and slower up-dosing phase combined with antihistamines or omalizumab may be tried.

Although food allergen immunotherapy does not provide a cure for food allergy, protection against anaphylaxis from accidental exposure to food allergen has been reported.

VENOM IMMUNOTHERAPY

Hymenoptera venom allergy is a potentially life-threatening allergic reaction following a honeybee, wasp or ant sting. It has been described in up to 7.5% adults and 3.4% of children[22]. The reaction can be restricted to skin or can be severe with a risk of life-threatening anaphylaxis.

Venom immunotherapy is the only treatment available to prevent the development of further serious systemic reactions. There should be a documented sensitization to the venom of the culprit insect with either skin prick tests or raised specific serum IgE. Incidental finding of sensitization to insect venom using a multiplex system without a history of insect venom hypersensitivity is not an indication for venom immunotherapy. Patients with recurrent troublesome large local reactions may also benefit from venom immunotherapy.

VENOM PREPARATIONS

Purified aqueous preparation, non-purified aqueous preparation and aluminium hydroxide adsorbed depot preparations are available for subcutaneous venom immunotherapy. Aqueous preparations can be used for the rush, ultra-rush or conventional build up phase as well as for the maintenance phase. The depot preparations are used only for the conventional build up phase and maintenance phase of immunotherapy. Treatment can also be shifted from aqueous to depot preparation once the rapid build up phase is over. Depot preparations are associated with few local side effects compared to aqueous preparations[23].

Selection of correct venom is important for the success of VIT. Sensitization to venom of more than 1 Hymenoptera species is common in insect venom allergic patients. It maybe due to true sensitization to multiple allergens or cross-reactivity due to shared allergenic determinants[24]. It is not always possible to differentiate between asymptomatic sensitization and true allergy with the help of currently available tests. If the initial sting reaction was severe, and tests show equal reaction to both honeybee and wasp, then VIT with both venoms should be considered.

IMMUNOTHERAPY PROTOCOLS

The route of venom immunotherapy is subcutaneous. Similar to other AIT, there is a build up phase followed by a maintenance phase. In the conventional protocol the maintenance phase is reached after several weeks to months and is done on an out-patient basis. Rush and ultra-rush protocols are available to reach the maintenance phase faster, usually within hours to days and this is done in hospitals[25]. Conventional immunotherapy is well tolerated compared to rush and ultra-rush protocols.

The starting dose of venom immunotherapy ranges from 0.001 to 0.1 μg. A starting dose of 1 μg is also tolerated. Usually accepted maintenance dose is 100 μg. But if a patient develops systemic allergic reactions to insect sting while on 100 μg maintenance dose, then the dose should be increased to 200 μg. An increased maintenance dose is also recommended for high risk individuals, like beekeepers who are at risk of multiple stings[26].

The interval for maintenance dose for VIT is 4–6 weeks for aqueous preparations and 6–8 weeks for depot preparations. Usual consensus is to give injections every 4 weeks in the first year of treatment, every 6 weeks in the second year of treatment and thereafter every 8 weeks in a 5-year treatment schedule. If lifelong treatment is needed interval between doses maybe extended to once in 3 months in the maintenance phase. It has been found that a 3-month interval does not reduce the efficacy or increase the side effects and will be more convenient and economical for the patient[27].

The usually recommended duration of treatment is 5 years. But lifelong treatment maybe needed for patients with severe initial systemic reactions, systemic adverse reactions during VIT and those with honeybee allergic reactions with future high risk of honeybee stings.

Many studies have shown that pre-treatment with H_1 antihistamines improves the tolerability of VIT. The effectiveness of VIT does not decrease with antihistamines. Antihistamines can be given 1–2 hours before VIT, or twice daily. Pre-treatment with omalizumab is recommended if there are severe adverse reactions during the intensive up dosing phase.

EFFECTIVENESS OF VIT

Treatment with ant venom is effective in 97–98% of patients. The efficacy of honeybee VIT is around 77–84% and for wasp VIT, it is 91–96%[22]. The exact reason for reduced efficacy for honeybee VIT is not known. It has been proposed that the venom injected by a honeybee sting is large, resulting in more systemic reactions. The effectiveness of aqueous and aluminium hydroxide adsorbed preparation is found to be similar.

Performing sting challenges is the most reliable method for monitoring the effectiveness of VIT. VIT is usually effective after reaching the first maintenance dose[28]. At this stage the sting challenge test should be done to identify those patients who are not protected with 100 μg of maintenance dose. In such patients, a higher maintenance dose may be needed[29]. If the sting challenge cannot be done, information on field stings can be useful. But here it is not always possible to identify the insect.

Relapse is more common for honeybee VIT, after stopping the maintenance phase. A relapse rate of 17% has been reported 1 year after stopping VIT. A severe systemic reaction prior to VIT has a higher risk for relapse compared to mild reactions[30]. Patients who had a systemic adverse event while on VIT have a higher chance of relapse compared to those with no reaction.

ADVERSE EVENTS

Systemic adverse events have been reported with VIT. The most important risk factor is treatment with honeybee venom. A 3.1–6-fold risk for systemic adverse events has been reported for honeybee VIT[22]. Rapid dose escalation during the build up period is also an established risk factor. Severe initial sting reaction, positive skin tests, ACE inhibitor or beta-blocker treatments do not carry an increased risk for systemic reactions.

Mild allergic reactions during VIT can be managed with standard antiallergic treatment. But if there are systemic adverse events, then a dose reduction is advised. Going 1 or 2 steps back in the treatment protocol can be done. Premedication with antihistamine has been found to reduce systemic adverse events.

Pre-treatment with omalizumab may be beneficial in patients when systemic adverse events prevent reaching the maintenance dose[31].

GENETIC VACCINES

Recently, research is being conducted to develop peptide or DNA vaccines by encoding allergens. This is shown to induce T helper1 as well as T regulatory responses, which modulate allergic T helper 2–based reactions. Currently, evaluated DNA-based vaccines are being designed for therapeutic interventions. However, the safety and efficacy of genetic vaccines encoding allergens will have to be demonstrated in healthy as well as sensitized adults beforehand.

CONCLUSION

Allergen avoidance is considered as the best intervention to prevent the development of allergic symptoms. However, it is practically not possible in all circumstances. Drug therapy with antihistamines and corticosteroids give only temporary relief. When these treatment approaches fail to achieve satisfactory disease control, one should consider allergen immunotherapy. Immunotherapy is effective in controlling symptoms and reducing the requirement for medications. The therapeutic benefits of immunotherapy manifest late, but once established, the beneficial effect persists long after discontinuation of treatment. Immunotherapy can also prevent the development of new sensitivities and asthma. Newer forms of immunotherapy, such as peptide immunotherapy and DNA vaccination, are considered to be even safer and more effective.

REFERENCES

1. Ring J Gutermuth J. 100 years of hyposensitization: history of allergen-specific immunotherapy (ASIT). Allergy 2011; 66(6):713–724.

2. Ihara F, Sakurai D, Yonekura S, et al. Identification of specifically reduced Th2 cell subsets in allergic rhinitis patients after sublingual immunotherapy. Allergy 2018;73(9):1823–1832.

3. Nevis IF, Binkley K, Kabali C. Diagnostic accuracy of skin-prick testing for allergic rhinitis: a systematic review and meta-analysis. Allergy Asthma Clin Immunol 2016;12:20. doi:10.1186/s13223-016-0126-0

4. Bernstein L Li JT, Bernstein DI, et al. Allergy diagnostic testing: An updated practice parameter. Ann Allergy Asthma Immunol 2008;100(3.3):S1–148.

5. Roberts G, Pfaar O, Akdis CA, Ansotegui IJ. EAACI Guidelines on Allergen Immunotherapy: Allergic rhinoconjunctivitis Allergy 2018;73(4):765–798.

6. Ebbesen AR, Riis LA, Gradman J. Effect of Topical Steroids on Skin Prick Test: A Randomized Controlled Trial. Dermatol Ther (Heidelb) 2018;8(2):285–290.

7. Heinzerling L, Mari A, Bergmann K, et al. The skin prick test-European standards. Clin Transl Allergy 2013;3(1):3. doi: 10.1186/2045-7022-3-3

8. Gunawardana NC, Durham SR. Reviews New approaches to allergen immunotherapy. Ann allergy Asthma Immunol 121 (2018) 293–305.

9. Daigle BJ, Rekkerth DJ. Practical recommendations for mixing allergy immunotherapy extracts. Allergy Rhinol (Providence) 2015;6(1):e1–e7.

10. Tabar AI, Echechipia S, Garcia BE, Olaguibel JM, Lizaso MT, Gomez B, et al. Double-blind comparative study of cluster and conventional immunotherapy schedules with ermatophagoides pteronyssinus J Allergy Clin Immunol 2005;116(1):109–18.

11. Nagata M, Yamamoto H, Tabe K, et al. Effect of rush immunotherapy in house dust mite-sensitive adults with bronchial asthma: changes in in-vivo and in-vitro responses to HDM. Intern Med 1993;32:702–709.

12. Ciprandi G, Marseglia GL. Safety of sublingual immunotherapy. J Biol Regul Homeost Agents 2011;25(1):1–6.

13. Sicherer, SH, Sampson HA. Food allergy: Epidemiology, pathogenesis, diagnosis, and treatment. J Allergy Clin Immunol 2014;133(2):291–307.

14. Du Toit G, Katz Y, Sasieni P, Mesher D, Maleki SJ, Fisher HR, Fox AT, Turcanu V, Amir T, Zadik-Mnuhin G, Cohen A, Livne I, Lack G. Early consumption of peanuts in infancy is associated with a low prevalence of peanut allergy. J Allergy Clin Immunol 2008;122(5):984–991.

15. Koplin JJ, Osborne NJ, Wake M, Martin PE, Gurrin LC, Robinson MN, Tey D, Slaa M, Thiele L, Miles L, Anderson D, Tan T, Dang TD, Hill DJ, Lowe AJ, Matheson MC, Ponsonby AL, Tang ML, Dharmage SC, Allen KJ. Can early introduction of egg prevent egg allergy in infants? A population-based study. J Allergy Clin Immunol 2010;126(4):807–813.

16. Deol S, Bird JA. Current opinion and review on peanut oral immunotherapy. Hum Vaccin Immunother 2014;10(10): 3017–3021.

17. Pajno, GB Fernandez-Rivas M, Arasi S, et al. EAACI Guidelines on allergen immunotherapy: IgE-mediated food allergy. Allergy 2018;73(4):799–815.

18. Dupont C, Kalach N, Soulaines P, Legoue-Morillon S, Piloquet H, Benhamou PH. Cow's milk epicutaneous immunotherapy in children: a pilot trial of safety, acceptability, and impact on allergic reactivity. J Allergy Clin Immunol 2010;125:1165–1167.

19. Varshney P, Jones SM, Scurlock AM. A randomized controlled study of peanut oral immunotherapy:

clinical desensitization and modulation of the allergic response. J Allergy Clin Immunol 2011;1 (27):654–660.

20. Martorell, A, De la Hoz, B, Ibáñez MD, et al. Oral desensitization as a useful treatment in 2-year-old children with cow's milk allergy. Clin Exp Allergy: Special Centenary Edition on Immunotherapy 2011;14(9):1297–1304.

21. Jones SM, Sicherer SH, Burks AW, et al. Consortium of Food Allergy Research. Epicutaneous immunotherapy for the treatment of peanut allergy in children and young adults. J Allergy Clin Immunol 2017;139(4):1242–1252.

22. G. J. Sturm, GJ, Varga E-M, Roberts G, et al. EAACI guidelines on allergen immunotherapy: Hymenoptera venom allergy. Allergy 2018;73(4):744–764.

23. Mosbech H, Müller U. Side effects of insect venom immunotherapy: results from an EAACI multicenter study. Allergy 2000;55: 1005–1010.

24. Johanna Stoevesandt, J, Hofmann B, Hain J, et al. Single venom-based immunotherapy effectively protects patients with double positive tests to honey bee and Vespula venom. Allergy, Asthma Clin Immunol 2013;9:33.

25. Ruëff F, Wenderoth A, Przybilla B. Patients still reacting to a sting challenge while receiving conventional Hymenoptera venom immunotherapy are protected by increased venom doses. J Allergy Clin Immunol 2001;108:1027–1032.

26. Goldberg A, Confino-Cohen R. Maintenance venom immunotherapy administered at 3-month intervals is both safe and efficacious. J Allergy Clin Immunol 2001;107:902–906.

27. Bożek A, Kołodziejczyk K. Safety of specific immunotherapy using an ultra-rush induction regimen in bee and wasp allergy. Hum Vaccin Immunother 2018;14(2):288–291.

28. Goldberg A, Confino-Cohen R. Bee venom immunotherapy—how early is it effective? Allergy 2010;65:391–395.

29. Ruëff F, Wenderoth A, Przybilla B. Patients still reacting to a sting challenge while receiving conventional Hymenoptera venom immunotherapy are protected by increased venom doses. J Allergy Clin Immunol 2001;108(6):1027–1032.

30. Golden DB.Discontinuing venom immunotherapy, Curr Opin Allergy Clin Immunol 2001;1(4):353–356.

31. Ricciardi L. Omalizumab: A useful tool for inducing tolerance to bee venom immunotherapy. Int J Immunopathol Pharmacol 2016;29(4):726–728.

32 Management Guidelines for Asthma in Young Adults

Nishtha Singh and Virendra Singh

CONTENTS

INTRODUCTION

Asthma is a disease that can start at an early age and affects all age groups, from small children to the elderly. At every age group, asthma carries with it general features and the features that are unique to that age group, such as presentation, phenotype, triggers and treatment response.[1–3] Management at every step is very crucial especially when we look at the magnitude of morbidity of asthma.

Proper assessment is the first step in asthma treatment. The assessment of asthma depends on the patient's symptomatic control, risk of future exacerbations, challenges that are faced by the patient in following the correct inhaler techniques and any associated comorbidities, such as rhinosinusitis, gastroesophageal reflux disease, obesity, depression and obstructive sleep apnoea. The management should also aim to minimize medication side effects on the patient.

SEVERITY CATEGORIZATION OF ASTHMA

The severity of asthma can be described in many ways, but those most accepted are described by GINA and NIH.

A. Global Initiative of Asthma (GINA)

An important goal of asthma management is to achieve complete asthma control. Asthma control depends on the severity of symptoms. Reduction of future risk is the second goal of asthma management.

A.1 Symptom control

GINA assesses asthma control of a patient by answering 4 questions.[2] These questions evaluate the ability of a patient in performing overall activities at normal or near normal level (Table 32.1).

A2. Future risk of the patient

The asthmatic patient is at risk for disease exacerbations, decline in lung function and adverse effects associated with medications. Poor symptom control and more than one exacerbation episode in the last year are associated with an increased risk of asthma exacerbations in the future.[4] Forced expiratory volume in 1sec (FEV_1) is an important parameter to assess the risk of future exacerbations. The normal rate of decline in FEV_1 is 15–20 ml/year in non-smoking, healthy adults. This rate of decline is increased in some asthmatic subjects and slowly leads to non-reversible airflow limitation. Risk factors for rapid decline include cigarette smoke exposure, mucus hyper-secretion and under treatment or if the patient is not taking inhaled corticosteroids (ICS).

- The risk of medication side effects occurs with high doses of medicines such as ICS. Long-term ICS use may be associated with glaucoma, easy bruising, cataracts and osteoporosis. Locally, ICS causes oral thrush and hoarseness of voice.

DOI: 10.1201/9781003125785-32

Table 32.1: Criteria to Assess Asthma Control (GINA)

During the past month, did the patient have	Yes	No	Asthma Control Interpretation
i. any night time awakening			
ii. daytime asthma symptoms more than twice per week			**None yes**: Well controlled
iii. a need for the use of reliever medicines more than twice per week			**Any yes (1–2)**: Partly controlled **Many yes (3–4)**: Uncontrolled
iv. any Activity Limitation			

- Preventing repetitive exacerbations, loss of lung function and administering proper pharmacotherapy can be set as goals for reducing risk.

- Lung functions should be measured at the start of treatment and 6 months later to assess control; then once every 1–2 years.

Asthma exacerbation is associated with factors described in the following table (Table 32.2).

The presence of these risk factors increases the chances of a patient having an exacerbation, even if the asthma symptoms are well controlled. This occurs especially in cases where the patient gets symptomatic relief by taking SABA alone repeatedly or when controlled by other placebo drugs. In these cases, because the airway inflammation is not controlled properly, the patients are prone to frequent exacerbations.[15]

Screening tools like the GINA symptom control tool, 30-second Asthma Test and Primary Care Asthma Control Screening Tool (PACS) are used to assess asthma control.[16] The Asthma Control Questionnaire (ACQ)[17]

and Asthma Control Test (ACT)[18] are other useful tests.

B. Severity categorization based on treatment

Apart from symptom evaluation and pulmonary function tests, asthma severity can also be assessed by the treatment given to control the symptoms. Based on the treatment, asthma severity can be categorized as follows:[19]

1. *Mild Asthma*: Patients who are following GINA Step 1 or 2 asthma treatment

2. *Moderate Asthma*: Patients who are following GINA Step 3 asthma treatment

3. *Severe Asthma*: Patients who are following GINA Step 4 asthma treatment or who remain uncontrolled. It is also called as refractory asthma[19]

Patients often think that their asthma is severe when they develop frequent and severe symptoms. Mostly symptoms of these patients are controlled within a few weeks of starting ICS.

C. National Institutes of Health (NIH) categorization

NIH guidelines also use these 4 parameters and spirometric indices to categorize asthma into four categories; mild intermittent, mild persistent, moderate persistent and severe persistent.[1]

i. Mild persistent asthma is characterized by the following:

Table 32.2: Factors Associated with Asthma Exacerbation

S. No.		Risk Factors
i.	Treatment related	Increased SABA* use[5] Insufficient ICS dosage Low adherence to treatment[6] Incorrect Inhaler technique[7]
ii.	Comorbidities	Rhinosinusitis[8,9] Gastroesophageal reflux disease[8] Obesity[8,10] Depression Obstructive sleep apnoea Pregnancy[11]
iii.	Environment	Air Pollution[12] Asthmatic triggers Smoking[13]
iv.	Lung functions	FEV_1<60% predicted[13] High bronchodilator reversibility[8]
v.	Other tests	Elevated blood eosinophils[8] and FeNO[14]

*SABA—Short-acting beta agonists.

- Symptoms more than twice weekly (although less than daily)

- Approximately 3–4 nocturnal awakenings per month due to asthma (but fewer than every week)

- Use of SABAs to relieve symptoms more than 2 days out of the week (but not daily)

- Minor interference with normal activities

- FEV_1 measurements within normal range (≥80% of predicted)

ii. Moderate persistent asthma characteristics include:

- Daily symptoms of asthma

- Nocturnal awakenings as often as once per week

- Daily need for SABAs for symptom relief

- Some limitation in normal activity

- FEV_1 between ≥60 and <80% of predicted and FEV_1/FVC below normal

iii. In severe persistent asthma, patients need prompt initiation with asthma therapy. Severe persistent asthma is manifested as follows:

- Presence of asthma symptoms throughout the day

- Nocturnal awakenings daily

- Reliever medicine needed for symptoms several times a day

- Activity limitation due to asthma

PATIENT EDUCATION

The patient should become an active partner in the asthma management. Both doctor related and patient related goals must be directed to achieve complete symptom control and to help the patient lead a normal life. This can be achieved by taking proper steps to reduce asthma related deaths, activity limitation and exacerbations.

When planning management of a patient with asthma, keeping the patient's family in the decision-making process favours a good outcome. It has been shown that a partnership between the patient and the healthcare system in treatment decisions produces good results.[20] It has also been seen that improved outcomes and decreased morbidity occurs when patients take part in their own treatment.[21]

Another important parameter is good communication with the patient. Educating asthma patients about their illness, allergic trigger factors and medications used can increase the patient's satisfaction, reduce the morbidity of the patient and the burden on the healthcare system.[22]

A communication gap with the patient can be bridged with the help of few strategies. These include:

i. Simplified explanation of asthma and its triggers

ii. Understanding the expectations and goals of the patient

iii. Motivating behaviour and action plan

iv. Rectifying any queries or doubts

Investigations

At the time of the first visit, the diagnosis of asthma should be confirmed. Severity of symptoms and frequency of exacerbation should be evaluated. Spirometry is a key investigation in establishing diagnosis and assessing the severity of airway obstruction.

SPIROMETRY

Spirometry is a useful test in making the diagnosis, assessing the severity and knowing the risk of exacerbation in a patient with asthma. A low FEV_1 signifies a higher chance of exacerbation.[23] It is also useful in calculating the age related lung function decline[24] and in measuring bronchodilator reversibility. Bronchodilator reversibility is denoted by a change in FEV_1 of greater than 12% and 200 ml after inhalation of 2 puffs of salbutamol metered dose inhaler. If a patient is having bronchodilator reversibility, even when taking controller medications or having taken SABA (short-acting beta agonists) within 4 hours, then a diagnosis of uncontrolled asthma can be made.

PEAK EXPIRATORY FLOW (PEF)

Peak expiratory flow rate measurement is useful in making a diagnosis of asthma, identifying trigger factors, assessing the severity of asthma and evaluating response to treatment. PEF reaches its personal best after approximately 2 weeks of starting ICS. PEF charting is usually indicated for those suffering from severe asthma or those who are unable to calculate the airflow limitation.[25]

INVESTIGATING UNCONTROLLED ASTHMA

When symptoms of asthma are not controlled, it is usually called uncontrolled asthma. Uncontrolled asthma occurs for a variety of reasons such as:

1. Compliance is inadequate[26]

2. The technique of taking the inhaler is incorrect.[7] Check the inhaler technique of the patient. Demonstrate the correct method and ask him to perform it in front of you. Inhaler technique should be checked at every visit

3. Presence of comorbidities like obesity, chronic rhinosinusitis, gastroesophageal reflux and obstructive sleep apnea[8]: A thorough search should be made of the presence of potential risk factors such as contact with the suspected triggers or allergens, smoking or intake of medicines

aggravating asthma such as beta-blockers or NSAIDs and the presence of comorbidities such as obesity, gastroesophageal reflux, chronic rhinosinusitis, depression, etc.

4. Continuous exposure to allergens or triggers

5. The diagnosis of asthma is not correct: If the patient is not responding, the dose of ICS can be halved and a spirometry recheck can be performed after 2–3 weeks to confirm the diagnosis

6. After excluding all causes of uncontrolled asthma, the treatment can be stepped up or some alternate regime of the present step can be tried

7. Specific strategies

    i. Induced sputum eosinophils— This is a good marker to guide the asthma therapy. Monitoring sputum eosinophils has been shown to result in better control of symptoms and reduces exacerbations in patients as compared to guideline based treatment alone.[27] Although the number of centres having this facility is limited, it can be used in the treatment of moderate to severe asthmatic patients.[19]

    ii. Fractional concentration of exhaled nitric oxide (FeNO)—The symptom control of patients varies with the use of FeNO to guide treatment. In young adults, it has shown significant effect as compared to guideline-based treatment.[28] But in non-smoking adults, no such improvement has been seen.[29] Further studies are required to prove its role in guiding management of asthma.

Initiating Pharmacologic Treatment

The medicines advised at each step consists of two approaches:

1. **Population approach**: This includes medicines that have shown good results for the majority of the population. This approach has been deciphered looking at the mean data from studies.[30]

2. **Individual approach**: This approach includes medicines that are advised for individual patients, looking at their particular characteristics, cost factors and other preferences of the patient. This approach is mainly used for patients whose asthma remains uncontrolled despite all routine asthma medications.[31]

The medicines used in asthma treatment are divided into:

1. **Controller medications**: These are generally used to reduce airway inflammation, thereby decreasing chances of future exacerbations. For mild asthma, this treatment is given in the form of low dose ICS-formoterol inhaler.

2. **Reliever medications**: These are also called rescue medications. These are used to give immediate relief to the patients. The aim of well-controlled asthma is the complete stoppage in usage of reliever medications.

3. **Add-on therapies**: These are treatment options for patients with severe asthma not controlled by the usage of high dose controller drugs.

TREATMENT INITIATION

It is advisable to start patients on controller therapies such as ICS at the earliest date. It has been seen that the patients who start ICS early have less lung function decline than those who started ICS later.[32] It has also been seen that patients not on ICS, show greater lung function decline after exacerbation.[33] This has also been seen in patients having occupational asthma.[34] A step-wise approach is advised for the management of asthma. The treatment should be dictated according to symptoms of the patient.

1. **STEP 1**: When asthmatic symptoms occur less than 2 times per month, and the patient does not have any risk factor for exacerbation. Low-dose ICS-formoterol is used as needed treatment. It is also a recommended strategy for stepping down therapy from Step 2 patients.
    Alternate therapies: ICS with SABA

2. **STEP 2**: When asthmatic symptoms occur more than 2 times/month, low-dose daily ICS is taken regularly. SABA or Low-dose ICS-formoterol may be used on as needed basis.
    Alternate therapies: LTRA (Leukotriene receptor antagonist), ICS with SABA

3. **STEP 3**: When asthmatic symptoms persist on most days of the month or on waking up. It is more important when risk factors of exacerbation are present. Low-dose ICS with Formoterol are used as maintenance and reliever. Alternatively, ICS with LABA can be used as maintenance with SABA reliever or medium-dose ICS with SABA reliever.

4. **STEP 4**: Patient has symptoms on most days or is waking with asthma once a week or more. Medium-dose ICS-LABA or High-dose ICS-LABA with add-on tiotropium or LTRA.

5. **STEP 5**: Severe uncontrolled asthma or if the patient has an acute exacerbation. High-dose ICS-LABA (with as needed short course of oral steroids and add-on therapy). Add-on treatment is advised at this step. It includes the following treatment modalities.

   a. *High-dose ICS-LABA combination:* It is advised only for 3–6 months, given the high amount of side effects with steroids.[35]

   b. *Tiotropium:* It is a long-acting anti-muscarinic antagonist. It modestly improves the exacerbation time and spirometric readings. It is to be used for patients older than 6 years of age.

   c. *Azithromycin:* Azithromycin is taken 3 times a week. It is given for a minimum duration of 6 months. However, long-term side effects include ototoxicity and arrythmias. Therefore, patients with hearing problems and those with prolonged QTc interval should be prescribed this therapy cautiously. Sputum for acid fast bacilli examination is advisable before initiation of this therapy. In tuberculosis, single use of this drug can lead to the development of resistance.

   d. *Anti-immunoglobulin E:* Also called Omalizumab. It is prescribed for patients older than 6 years of age with severe asthma. It is a humanized monoclonal antibody. Various studies have shown and proven its role in reducing the exacerbation rate and asthma symptoms.[36]

   e. *Anti-interleukin-5:* Include subcutaneous Mepolizumab and intravenous Reslizumab. Benralizumab used subcutaneously is an anti-interleukin 5 receptor therapy. IL4 and IL5 are chemoattractants for eosinophils.

   f. *Anti-interleukin-4R or Dupilumab* is used subcutaneously in patients older than 12 years age. It prevents binding of IL-4 to IL-4Rα.

   g. *Induced sputum eosinophils:* The asthma treatment guided with sputum eosinophils has shown better results in cases of severe asthma. The target sputum eosinophils are >3%.

   h. *Low-dose oral corticosteroids:* A dose of less than 7.5 mg is used. However, patient counselling with lifestyle changes should be implemented before starting this treatment. These are associated with a good number of side effects.

   i. *Immunotherapy:* It is a technique where an increasing dose of the allergen is given. It is of 2 types: Subcutaneous and Sublingual. Subcutaneous immunotherapy is administered subcutaneously with the concentration of allergen progressively increased.[37] Sublingual immunotherapy is a mode where the allergen is administered sublingually.[38]

   j. *Vaccination:* An influenza vaccination is given to reduce the risk of asthma exacerbation.[39]

   k. *Bronchial thermoplasty:* This is a Step 5 treatment in patients with severe uncontrolled asthma. Three sittings of radiofrequency pulse are given to the patient involving the bronchial tree.[40] It has been shown to have increased the exacerbation rate in the first 3 months but later is followed by a decrease in the exacerbations.[40]

   l. *Vitamin D:* It has been seen that vitamin D deficiency leads to greater exacerbation rates and lung function impairment.[41] Studies have shown that vitamin D supplementation reduced the frequency of exacerbations in patients having vitamin D levels less than 25nmol/L.[42]

DOSAGES OF INHALED CORTICOSTEROIDS

The ICS can be divided into low-, medium- and high-dose corticosteroids on the basis of strengths of the dosages (Table 32.3). The majority of asthmatics require only low dose steroids. Some patients who do not get complete control with low doses of steroids are advised to try medium and high dose steroids. However, high-dose steroids taken for a long time are associated with significant side effects. These include diabetes mellitus, hypertension, cataracts, decreased bone density, adrenal suppression, etc. Therefore, the benefits of using high doses of ICS should always be balanced against their side effects.

Table 32.3: Dosages of Various Formulations of Inhaled Corticosteroids

ICS	Low Dose	Medium Dose	High Dose
Beclomethasone dipropionate	200–500	>500–1000	>1000
Budesonide	200–400	>400–800	>800
Ciclesonide	80–160	>160–320	>320
Fluticasone furoate	100		200
Fluticasone propionate (DPI)	100–250	>250–500	>500
Mometasone furoate	200		400
Mometasone furoate	200–400		>400

FOLLOW-UP OF ASTHMA PATIENTS

After commencement of asthma treatment, further stepping up or down depends on the individual patient. Once asthma control is achieved, the treatment can reviewed and stepped down. FeNO may be useful in predicting the response of ICS in patients of mild asthma.[2] When used in non-smoking adults, it becomes a good predictor of ICS response, especially when its value is more than 50 parts per million.[43] The maximum benefit of treatment in asthma is seen in around 3 months. Therefore, ideal follow up of the patient is done 1–3 months after starting the treatment.[44] If asthma is well controlled for 3 months, the treatment is stepped down. After the first visit, patient may visit again after a gap of 3–12 months. The correct inhaler technique should be taught to the patient at each visit. If the patient gets an exacerbation, a follow-up visit should be done within 1 week.

STEPPING UP TREATMENT

If a patient continues to have symptoms despite being on controller medications for 2–3 months, stepping up of treatment is needed. However, before stepping up, the following issues should be addressed:

1. Treatment adherence
2. Inhaler technique
3. Accuracy of diagnosis
4. Presence of comorbidities
5. Exposure to allergens or triggers at home or work
6. Concomitant medicines such as non-steroidal anti-inflammatory drugs, beta-blockers, etc.

METHOD OF STEPPING UP

1. **Sustained step up:** This is done for a patient who is not controlled on a low dose ICS-LABA combination. The inhaler technique and adherence to treatment should be checked before the treatment is stepped up. The result of stepping up the treatment should be reviewed after 2–3 months.

2. **Short-term step up:** This can be done by the patient himself or herself, according to their asthma plan. This stepping up is usually done when the patient suffers from a viral infection or is exposed to some allergen and may benefit from a short-term increase in dose of ICS-LABA for 1–2 weeks.

3. **Reliever drug adjustments:** These can be made on a daily basis by the patient, while keeping the maintenance medicines constant.

STEPPING DOWN TREATMENT

Stepping down in asthma treatment is generally done when the asthma has been well controlled for the past 3 months and the spirometry also shows a plateau. The advantage of stepping down is that the patient is stabilized on the the minimum required medicines. Moreover, it reduces the cost of treatment and results in fewer side effects.

Before stepping down, risk of exacerbation should be analyzed. If baseline FEV_1 is low[45] or patient is having history of exacerbation in the last 12 months[46] then the risk of getting another exacerbation increases on stepping down the treatment.

HOW TO STEP DOWN TREATMENT

While stepping down the treatment, there are two options—to reduce ICS and to reduce LABA. A reduction in the dose of LABA has been associated with greater chances of exacerbation. The timing of stepping down of the treatment should also be carefully chosen. The time of seasonal exacerbation, pregnancy, travelling or viral infection should be avoided.

General principles of treatment step down of a patient are:

- If patient is on a high-moderate dose of ICS: Stepping down the dose of ICS to 25–50% of the original dose over a 3-month gap has shown good results.[47]

- If low-dose ICS is being used: Stepping down the dose to once daily.

- If patient is on oral corticosteroids: Switch to a high dose of ICS.

- LTRAs can be added: They help in allowing the step down of ICS dose.

MANAGING OTHER RISK FACTORS

If a patient has a history of exacerbation, he or she is at risk of getting another exacerbation in the span of 12 months.[48]

The following interventions are advisable for managing risk factors:

1. **Smoking**: Cessation counselling is provided to the patient and relatives.

2. **Obesity**: Dietary changes and physiotherapy can be recommended to the patient to reduce weight. Obstructive sleep apnoea should be ruled out.

3. **Anxiety or depression**: An asthmatic patient is susceptible to anxiety and depression.

4. **Food allergy**: The patient is advised to avoid suspected food edibles.

5. **Financial problems**: The patient is advised on the most cost-effective medicines.

6. **Continued allergen exposure**: The patient is advised SLIT therapy to house dust mite if sensitive,provided the FEV_1 is more than 70% of the predicted.

WRITTEN ASTHMA ACTION PLAN

In an asthma action plan, written instructions are given to a patient regarding treatment. Patients keep record of symptoms, medicines and their peak flow meter readings. Based on these, the patients are guided to change their medications.[1,2]

CONCLUSION

Asthma is a disease that can start at an early age and affects all age groups, from small children to the elderly. At every age group, asthma is characterized by its general features and the features that are unique to that age group. Management at every step is crucial, especially when we look at the magnitude of morbidity of asthma. The patient should become an active partner in asthma management. Both doctor related and patient related goals must be directed to achieve complete symptom control and allow the patient to lead a normal life. This can be achieved by taking proper steps to reduce asthma related deaths, activity limitation and exacerbations.

REFERENCES

1. National Asthma Education and Prevention Program: Expert panel report III: Guidelines for the diagnosis and management of asthma. Bethesda, MD: National Heart, Lung, and Blood Institute, 2007. (NIH publication no. 08-4051). www.nhlbi.nih. gov/guidelines/asthma/asthgdln.htm (Accessed on May 31, 2016).

2. Global Initiative for Asthma (GINA). Global Strategy for Asthma Management and Prevention. www. ginasthma.org (Accessed on March 27, 2020).

3. British Guideline on the Management of Asthma. https://www.brit-thoracic.org.uk/guidelines-and-quality-standards/asthma-guideline/ (Accessed on May 27, 2014).

4. McCoy K, Shade DM, Irvin CG, et al. Predicting episodes of poor asthma control in treated patients with asthma. J Allergy Clin Immunol 2006;118:1226–1233.

5. Patel M, Pilcher J, Reddel HK, et al. Metrics of salbutamol use as predictors of future adverse outcomes in asthma. Clin Exp Allergy 2013;43:1144–1151.

6. Ernst P, Spitzer WO, Suissa S, et al. Risk of fatal and near-fatal asthma in relation to inhaled corticosteroid use. JAMA 1992;268:3462–3464.

7. Melani AS, Bonavia M, Cilenti V, et al. Inhaler mishandling remains common in real life and is associated with reduced disease control. Respir Med 2011;105:930–938.

8. Denlinger LC, Phillips BR, Ramratnam S, et al. Inflammatory and comorbid features of patients with severe asthma and frequent exacerbations. Am J Respir Crit Care Med 2017;195:302–313.

9. Bousquet J, Khaltaev N, Cruz AA, et al. Allergic Rhinitis and its Impact on Asthma (ARIA) 2008 update (in collaboration with the World Health Organization, GA(2)LEN and AllerGen). Allergy 2008;63 Suppl 86:8–160.

10. Fitzpatrick S, Joks R, Silverberg JI. Obesity is associated with increased asthma severity and exacerbations, and increased serum immunoglobulin E in inner-city adults. Clin Exp Allergy 2012;42:747–759.

11. Murphy VE, Clifton VL, Gibson PG. Asthma exacerbations during pregnancy: incidence and association with adverse pregnancy outcomes. Thorax 2006;61:169–176.

12. Mazenq J, Dubus JC, Gaudart J, Charpin D, Viudes G, Noel G. City housing atmospheric pollutant impact on emergency visit for asthma: A classification and regression tree approach. Respir Med 2017;132:1–8.

13. Osborne ML, Pedula KL, O'Hollaren M et al. Assessing future need for acute care in adult asthmatics: the Profile of Asthma Risk Study: a prospective health maintenance organization-based study. Chest 2007;132:1151–1161.

14. Zeiger RS, Schatz M, Zhang F, et al. Elevated exhaled nitric oxide is a clinical indicator of future uncontrolled asthma in asthmatic patients on inhaled corticosteroids. J Allergy Clin Immunol 2011;128:412–414.

15. Lazarus SC, Boushey HA, Fahy JV, et al. Long-acting beta2- agonist monotherapy vs continued therapy

with inhaled corticosteroids in patients with persistent asthma: a randomized controlled trial. JAMA 2001;285:2583–2593.

16. LeMay KS, Armour CL, Reddel HK. Performance of a brief asthma control screening tool in community pharmacy: a cross-sectional and prospective longitudinal analysis. Prim Care Respir J 2014;23:79–84.

17. Juniper EF, Svensson K, Mork AC, Stahl E. Measurement properties and interpretation of three shortened versions of the asthma control questionnaire. Respir Med 2005;99:553–558.

18. Schatz M, Kosinski M, Yarlas AS, Hanlon J, Watson ME, Jhingran P. The minimally important difference of the Asthma Control Test. J Allergy Clin Immunol 2009;124:719–723.e1.

19. Chung KF, Wenzel SE, Brozek JL, et al. International ERS/ATS Guidelines on Definition, Evaluation and Treatment of Severe Asthma. Eur Respir J 2014;43:343–373.

20. Taylor YJ, Tapp H, Shade LE, Liu TL, Mowrer JL, Dulin MF. Impact of shared decision making on asthma quality of life and asthma control among children. J Asthma 2018;55:675–683.

21. Gibson PG, Powell H, Coughlan J, et al. Self-management education and regular practitioner review for adults with asthma. Cochrane Database Syst Rev 2003:CD001117.

22. Cabana MD, Slish KK, Evans D, et al. Impact of physician asthma care education on patient outcomes. Pediatrics 2006;117:2149–2157.

23. Osborne ML, Pedula KL, O'Hollaren M, et al. Assessing future need for acute care in adult asthmatics: the Profile of Asthma Risk Study: a prospective health maintenance organization-based study. Chest 2007;132:1151–1161.

24. Ulrik CS. Outcome of asthma: longitudinal changes in lung function. Eur Respir J 1999;13:904–918.

25. Rosi E, Stendardi L, Binazzi B, Scano G. Perception of airway obstruction and airway inflammation in asthma: a review. Lung 2006;184:251–258.

26. Boulet L-P, Vervloet D, Magar Y, Foster JM. Adherence: the goal to control asthma. Clin Chest Med 2012;33:405–417.

27. Petsky HL, Li A, Chang AB. Tailored interventions based on sputum eosinophils versus clinical symptoms for asthma in children and adults. Cochrane Database Syst Rev 2017;8:Cd005603.

28. Petsky HL, Kew KM, Chang AB. Exhaled nitric oxide levels to guide treatment for children with asthma. Cochrane Database Syst Rev 2016;11:Cd011439.

29. Petsky HL, Kew KM, Turner C, Chang AB. Exhaled nitric oxide levels to guide treatment for adults with asthma. Cochrane Database Syst Rev 2016;9:Cd011440.

30. Roche N, Reddel HK, Agusti A, et al. Integrating real-life studies in the global therapeutic research framework. Lancet Respir Med 2013;1:e29–e30.

31. Chung KF. New treatments for severe treatment-resistant asthma: targeting the right patient. Lancet Respir Med 2013;1:639–652.

32. Busse WW, Pedersen S, Pauwels RA, et al. The Inhaled Steroid Treatment As Regular Therapy in Early Asthma (START) study 5-year follow-up: effectiveness of early intervention with budesonide in mild persistent asthma. J Allergy Clin Immunol 2008;121:1167–1174.

33. O'Byrne PM, Pedersen S, Lamm CJ, Tan WC, Busse WW. Severe exacerbations and decline in lung function in asthma. Am J Respir Crit Care Med 2009;179:19–24.

34. Baur X, Sigsgaard T, Aasen TB, et al. Guidelines for the management of work-related asthma.[Erratum appears in Eur Respir J. 2012 Jun;39(6):1553]. Eur Respir J 2012;39:529–545.

35. Virchow JC, Prasse A, Naya I, Summerton L, Harris A. Zafirlukast improves asthma control in patients receiving high-dose inhaled corticosteroids. Am J Respir Crit Care Med 2000;162:578–585.

36. Hanania NA, Alpan O, Hamilos DL, et al. Omalizumab in severe allergic asthma inadequately controlled with standard therapy: a randomized trial. Ann Intern Med 2011 May 3; 154(9):573–582.

37. Abramson MJ, Puy RM, Weiner JM. Injection allergen immunotherapy for asthma. Cochrane Database Syst Rev 2010:CD001186.

38. Xu K, Deng Z, Li D, et al. Efficacy of add-on sublingual immunotherapy for adults with asthma: A meta-analysis and systematic review. Ann Allergy Asthma Immunol 2018;121:186–194.

39. Vasileiou E, Sheikh A, Butler C, et al. Effectiveness of Influenza Vaccines in Asthma: A Systematic Review and Meta-Analysis. Clin Infect Dis 2017;65:1388–1395.

40. Castro M, Rubin AS, Laviolette M, et al. Effectiveness and safety of bronchial thermoplasty in the treatment of severe asthma: a multicenter, randomized, double-blind, sham-controlled clinical trial. Am J Respir Crit Care Med 2010;181:116–124.

41. Cassim R, Russell MA, Lodge CJ, Lowe AJ, Koplin JJ, Dharmage SC. The role of circulating 25 hydroxyvitamin D in asthma: a systematic review. Allergy 2015;70:339–354.

42. Jolliffe DA, Greenberg L, Hooper RL, et al. Vitamin D supplementation to prevent asthma exacerbations: a systematic review and meta-analysis of individual participant data. Lancet Respir Med 2017;5:881–890.

43. Price DB, Buhl R, Chan A, et al. Fractional exhaled nitric oxide as a predictor of response to inhaled corticosteroids in patients with non-specific respiratory symptoms and insignificant bronchodilator

reversibility: a randomised controlled trial. Lancet Respir Med 2018;6:29–39.

44. Bateman ED, Bousquet J, Keech ML, Busse WW, Clark TJ, Pedersen SE. The correlation between asthma control and health status: the GOAL study. Eur Respir J 2007;29:56–62.

45. DiMango E, Rogers L, Reibman J, et al. Risk factors for asthma exacerbation and treatment failure in adults and adolescents with well-controlled asthma during continuation and step-down therapy. Annals of the American Thoracic Society 2018;15:955–961.

46. Usmani OS, Kemppinen A, Gardener E, et al. A randomized pragmatic trial of changing to and stepping down fluticasone/formoterol in asthma. J Allergy Clin Immunol Pract 2017;5:1378–87.e5.

47. Hagan JB, Samant SA, Volcheck GW, et al. The risk of asthma exacerbation after reducing inhaled corticosteroids: a systematic review and meta-analysis of randomized controlled trials. Allergy 2014;69:510–516.

48. Miller MK, Lee JH, Miller DP, Wenzel SE. Recent asthma exacerbations: a key predictor of future exacerbations. Respir Med 2007;101:481–489.

Index

Italicized and **bold** pages refer to figures and tables, respectively.

A

ABPA, *see* Allergic bronchopulmonary aspergillosis
ABPM, *see* Allergic bronchopulmonary mycosis
Absolute eosinophil counts, in AD diagnosis, 22
AC, *see* Allergic conjunctivitis
ACE inhibitors, 77
ACQ (Asthma Control Questionnaire), 227
ACT (Asthma Control Test), 227
Acute asthma, in pregnancy, 137; *see also* Asthma
Acute eosinophilic pneumonia (AEP), 181
Acute inflammatory response, in asthma, 99, *100*
Acute laryngeal angioedema, 39
Acute severe asthma, 154–159; *see also* Asthma
    biomarkers, 156
    clinical assessment, 156
    definition of, 154–155, **155**
    epidemiology, 155
    exacerbations
        genetics and, 155
        risk factors, 155, **155**
        triggers for, 155, **155**
    management, 156, *157–158*
        antibiotics, 156
        bronchodilators, 156
        corticosteroids, 156
        ECLS (extra corporeal life support), 159
        magnesium sulphate, 156
        mechanical ventilation, 158
        other therapies, 159
        oxygen therapy, 158–159
    overview, 154
    pathogenesis, 155–156
    pathophysiology, 156
Acute spontaneous urticaria (ASU), 26
Acute urticaria, 26
AD, *see* Atopic dermatitis
Add-on therapies, 254
Adherence 229; *see also* Non-adherence
Adipokines, 145
Adjunctive therapy, for anaphylaxis, 71
Adolescents; *see also* Asthma; Young adults
    AD in, 19–20
    asthma in
        biologics for, 236–241
        inhaler therapy, 218–223
        risk factors, 87–88
        transition of care, 130
        treatment recommendation, **117**
    corticosteroids role in allergic disorders, 211–216;
        see also Corticosteroid(s)
ADR, *see* Adverse drug reaction
Adrenaline, 208
Adrenergic urticaria, 27
Adverse drug reaction (ADR)/drug allergy, 53–60
    administration of potentially cross-reacting
        drugs, 59

    classification and mechanisms, 54–55, **55**
    clinical features, 56
    clinical significance, 54
    danger hypothesis, 56
    defined, 53
    diagnosis, 57
    differential diagnosis, 56, **57**
    drug provocation testing, 58
    drugs implicated, 56, **56**
    incidence, 53–54
    management, 58–59
    overview, 53
    pharmaco-vigilance, 59–60
    P–I concept, 56
    prevention of, 59
    prohapten-hapten concept, 55
    readministration of offending drug, 59
    risk factors, 53–54, **54**
    serological assays, 58
    skin testing, 57–58
    type A reactions, 54
    type B reactions, 54
AEP, *see* Acute eosinophilic pneumonia
Airway bronchial hyperresponsiveness, 102–103
Airway hyper-responsiveness (AHR), 144
Airway irritants, e-liquids, 109
AIT, *see* Allergen immunotherapy
Alarmins, 44
Allergen avoidance hypothesis, 43, 44
Allergen immunotherapy (AIT), 11, 42, 243–249
    accelerated schedules, 245–246
    adverse events, 248–249
    allergen preparations, 244–245
    in AR, 14–15, *15*
    contraindications for, 246
    diagnostic tests, 243–244
    effectiveness of VIT, 248
    food allergy, 246–247
    genetic vaccines, 249
    immunotherapy schedule, 247
    indications for, 243
    mucosal challenge test, 244
    overview, 243
    protocols, 248
    safety of, 246
    skin tests, 244
    subcutaneous immunotherapy, 245
    sublingual immunotherapy (SLIT), 246
    types of, 245
    venom immunotherapy, 247
    venom preparations, 247–248
    in vitro tests, 244
Allergen(s), 2, 3, 75
    in AD, 21
    allergy skin test, 78
    class I food allergens, 42
    class II food allergens, 42
    continued exposure, 257
    diagnostic tests for, 243–244
    indoor and outdoor, asthma and, 99

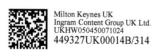

9 780367 646783